second edition

Compounding Sterile Preparations

E. Clyde Buchanan, M.S., FASHP

Senior Director
Pharmaceutical Services
Emory Healthcare
Atlanta, GA

Philip J. Schneider, M.S., FASHP

Clinical Professor and Director
Latiolais Leadership Program
Division of Pharmacy Practice and
  Administration
College of Pharmacy
The Ohio State University
Columbus, OH

American Society of Health-System Pharmacists®
Bethesda, Maryland

Any correspondence regarding this publication should be sent to the publisher, American Society of Health-System Pharmacists, 7272 Wisconsin Avenue, Bethesda, MD 20814, attn: Special Publishing. Produced in conjunction with the ASHP Publications Production Center.

Acquisitions Editor: Hal Pollard
Editorial Project Manager: Dana A. Battaglia
Senior Project Editor: Bill Fogle
Page Design: Carol Barrer
Cover Design: Armen Kojoyian

ISBN: 1-58528-105-0

To our wives, Jan Buchanan and Candy Schneider, for supporting us throughout the editing of this text.

Contents

Introduction

This is the second edition of a book that was titled *Principles of Sterile Product Preparation* and originally published in 1995, with a revised first edition in 2002. The circumstances surrounding the publication of this book were the public concern about the quality of pharmacy-prepared sterile products, some of which resulted in highly publicized harm to patients. This book and other products from ASHP were part of a concerted self-regulatory effort to improve standards of practice within pharmacy to avoid external regulation by the FDA and State Boards of Pharmacy. It would be nice to think that this effort was a success and that harm resulting from improperly compounded sterile preparations was less frequent. It would be nice to know that pharmacists were more often adhering to published guidelines for compounding sterile preparations. Sadly, this is not the case.

In addition to the same circumstances that prompted the publication of the first and revised first edition of this book, there is now the imperative of USP Chapter <797>, "Pharmaceutical Compounding—Sterile Preparations." Before this chapter was published, only guidelines existed for pharmacists. While these might have constituted a standard of practice, they did not have the force of regulation by State Boards of Pharmacy or accreditation standards from the Joint Commission on Accreditation of Healthcare Organizations (JCAHO®). It now seems clear that such force will be needed and now exists to provide for improving standards of practice. Thus, the revision *Compounding Sterile Preparations*, second edition, has been prepared. This revision includes the requirements from the USP Chapter <797> that will be used by the Food and Drug Administration, State Boards of Pharmacy, and the JCAHO in their oversight of organizations that compound sterile preparations.

This new edition has been reorganized into two sections: sterile preparation and quality management. The sterile preparation section contains information about actually compounding sterile preparations. Included in this section is a new chapter on the use of isolators as an alternative method for creating a suitable environment. The quality management section includes information about creating, monitoring, and managing the system of compounding sterile preparations. Included in this section are new chapters on dealing with latex allergies and outsourcing sterile compounding. Six new authors have written chapters in this revision.

The editors and authors hope that this revised textbook will be part of a recommitment among pharmacists to restore competency in performing one of the most important tasks within heath care—compounding sterile preparations. This book could be used as a textbook in pharmacy technician programs, by colleges of pharmacy as part of their pharmacy practice laboratory experiences, in training programs for pharmacy departments such as pharmacy practice residencies, and as a reference book by all pharmacists who compound sterile preparations. The public and regulatory and accreditation organizations are watching.

Philip J. Schneider, M.S., FASHP
Clinical Professor and Director
Latiolais Leadership Program
Division of Pharmacy Practice and
   Administration
College of Pharmacy
The Ohio State University
Columbus, OH
March 2, 2004

Contributors

Caryn M. Bing, R.Ph., M.S., FASHP
CB Healthcare Consulting
Las Vegas, NV

E. Clyde Buchanan, M.S., FASHP
Senior Director
Pharmaceutical Services
Emory Healthcare
Atlanta, GA

Stephen K. Hetey, M.S., R.Ph., FASHP
Pharmacy Manager and Clinical Assistant
Professor
Department of Pharmacy Practice
School of Pharmacy
Texas Tech University
Pharmacy Administration
Children's Medical Center of Dallas
Dallas, TX

Eric S. Kastango, R.Ph., M.B.A., FASHP
Principal
Clinical IQ, LLC
Florham Park, NJ

Patricia (Tish) Kuban, R.Ph., M.B.A.
Assistant Director
Sterile Products and Performance
Improvement
Department of Pharmaceutical Services
Emory Hospitals
Emory Healthcare
Atlanta, GA

Luci A. Power, MS, R.Ph.
Senior Pharmacist, Manager
IV Additive Service
Department of Pharmaceutical Services
University of California Medical Center
San Francisco, CA

Henry (Hank) Rahe, B.S.I.M., M.S.E.
Director of Technology
EnGuard Systems
Indianapolis, IN

Philip J. Schneider, M.S., F.A.S.H.P.
Clinical Professor and Director
Latiolais Leadership Program
Division of Pharmacy Practice and
Administration
College of Pharmacy
The Ohio State University
Columbus, OH

1 | Guidelines for Sterile Preparations

E. Clyde Buchanan

The Institute of Medicine recommended "have the central pharmacy supply high-risk intravenous medications" to reduce medical errors.[1] The compounding of sterile preparations is an integral part of any health-system setting. However, sterile compounding procedures vary widely across the country.[2-4] This lack of uniformity, combined with changing technology for sterile compounding and drug administration, has led to serious medication errors and, therefore, recommendations in a variety of professional practice guidelines. Professional organizations have focused on improving pharmacy sterile compounding practice for more than 30 years; still, few pharmacists are using proper garb, performing environmental sampling, end-product testing, or process validation, and the compounding of sterile preparations in uncontrolled environments outside pharmacies continues to be common.[5,6]

Adverse Drug Events

Over the past 25 years, pharmacists have been publicly cited many times for harming patients through a variety of errors in compounding sterile preparations.[7] Errors can be categorized as incorrect ingredients[8] (identity or purity of ingredients), incorrect strengths of ingredients (inaccurate measurements, instabilities or incompatibilities),[9] and contamination with pathogenic microorganisms, pyrogens or harmful ingredients.[10] The CDC cited one set of contaminated IV admixtures that resulted, in part from the pharmacy's failure to follow ASHP guidelines.[6] In five U.S. hospital pharmacies, Flynn et al. observed a 9% error rate in the compounding of IV admixtures.[11]

Other health professionals have also caused harm through poor aseptic technique. Anesthesia personnel in seven hospitals accidentally contaminated propofol, a lipid-based anesthetic, with a variety of pathogens leading to infectious complications in dozens of patients.[12] Dialysis personnel caused Serratia infections in at least 12 patients through multiple punctures of single-use vials and pooling of preservative-free epoetin alfa.[13] Pharmacists are obligated to train other personnel in handling sterile preparations even if pharmacists are not available to carry out aseptic manipulations themselves.

More Challenges Ahead

These adverse events are but a few examples of the dangers inherent in compounding sterile preparations. While many institutions have developed practices to prevent these dangers, new technologies and procedures are challenging pharmacists' abilities to compound, package, and label appropriately.[14-16]

New Technologies

New technologies, such as syringe pump infusion systems and patient-controlled analgesia (PCA) pumps, require pharmacists to repackage injectables into syringes, increasing the chance of errors.[17] Infusion pumps that allow a pharmacist to place multiple intermittent doses into a single IV bag also increase the risks of incorrect compounding, packaging, and labeling. Portable pumps and indwelling medication reservoirs permit longer infusion periods and higher compounding temperatures, possibly leading to mistakes in expiration dating.[18,19] Elastomeric infusion devices, which are simple to use but require special storage conditions, may lead to dosing errors.[20]

New Procedures

The use of high-risk routes of administration (e.g., intrathecal, intraocular) also increases the danger level. Additionally, the use of more toxic sterile preparations—highly concentrated injections of potassium chloride, dextrose, lidocaine, and doxorubicin—has led to fatal medication errors. The compounding of sterile drugs from nonsterile ingredients increases the level of risk. Common examples include concentrated morphine injection for epidural analgesia and reservoirs, alum for bladder irrigation,[21] and caffeine for neonatal respiratory distress.

Another technical, and possibly legal, issue for pharmacists is the use of automated compounders:

- How do such large devices affect laminar-airflow in an ISO Class 5 (Class 100) workbench?

- How does a pharmacist ensure that the right additives are hung on individual stations?[22]

●   How does a pharmacist ensure that the pump is measuring ingredients accurately?[23,24]

Other complexities arise because pharmacy compounded sterile preparations are now used in numerous settings, including patients' homes, physicians' offices, and long term care facilities. In these settings, pharmacists must ensure the efficacy and safety of any sterile preparation they compound or check.

FDA Authority and Actions

The technological and procedural issues described here have led to action by the Food and Drug Administration (FDA), which has the authority to regulate the quality of drug preparations compounded in pharmacies. Since 1990, the FDA has sent warning letters to retail pharmacies that may manufacture, distribute, and promote unapproved drugs for human use outside the bounds of licensed pharmacy practice. The FDA's position was stated in a 1980 compliance guide (see Appendix E). After recognizing some serious pharmacy errors in batch compounding, in 1990 the FDA formally reminded pharmacists that they are responsible for adhering to good manufacturing practices and safe packaging.[25]

Under its authority to regulate "new" drugs, the FDA allows physicians to prescribe "an unusual preparation that requires compounding by a pharmacist from drugs readily available for other uses and which is not generally regarded as safe and effective for the intended use"[26] (see Appendix E). However, processing and repackaging of approved drugs by pharmacists for resale to hospitals, other pharmacies, etc., are subject to premarket approval by the FDA as new drug preparations. The FDA's regulatory authority over extemporaneous and batch compounding is interpreted by its inspectors, who generally do not examine state-licensed pharmacies.

With strong support from pharmacy organizations, the U.S. Congress passed the Food and Drug Administration Modernization Act of 1997 (FDAMA).[27] Section 127 of this Act, which codified pharmacy compounding, states that pharmacy compounding must comply with an applicable United States Pharmacopeia–National Formulary (USP-NF) monograph, if one exists, and the USP-NF chapter on pharmacy compounding or the compounded substance must be a component of an FDA-approved drug product or, if neither of these apply to the ingredient being compounded, the substance must appear on a list of bulk drug substances developed by FDA and must be accompanied by a valid certificate of analysis and be manufactured in an FDA-registered establishment.

In February 2001, the Federal Ninth Circuit Court of Appeals declared pharmacy compounding provisions in the FDAMA entirely invalid.[28] This court agreed with the federal district court, which had found that the advertising restrictions contained in Section (c) of the law were unconstitutional because they abrogated the constitutional right to free speech. However, the court of appeals went further, stating that the advertising section could not be severed from the rest of the law because Congress would not have passed the law without the advertising prohibition. Although the Ninth Circuit covers only the western states, the FDA has suspended actions to complete regulations supporting FDAMA. The effect has been to leave pharmacy compounding primarily under state pharmacy laws but with no safe haven from federal inspections of compounding pharmacies. Recognizing the need for guidance for compounding pharmacists, the FDA revised its Compliance Policy Guide.[29] Although the FDA will continue to defer to state authorities regarding "less significant violations" related to pharmacy compounding, FDA will seriously consider enforcement action when it suspects a pharmacy of manufacturing and distributing unapproved new drugs in a manner that is clearly outside of traditional pharmacy practice and violates federal law. FDA identified nine factors that it will use to determine whether to initiate action against a pharmacy:

1.   Compounding of drugs in anticipation of receiving prescriptions, except in very limited quantities in relation to the amounts of drugs compounded after receiving valid prescriptions.

2.   Compounding drugs that were withdrawn or removed from the market for safety reasons.

3.   Compounding finished drugs from bulk active ingredients that are not components of FDA approved drugs without an FDA sanctioned investigational new drug application (IND) in accordance with 21 U.S.C. § 355(i) and 21 CFR 312.

4. Receiving, storing, or using drug substances without first obtaining written assurance from the supplier that each lot of the drug substance has been made in an FDA-registered facility.

5. Receiving, storing, or using drug components not guaranteed or otherwise determined to meet official compendia requirements.

6. Using commercial scale manufacturing or testing equipment for compounding drug products.

7. Compounding drugs for third parties who resell to individual patients or offering compounded drug products at wholesale to other state licensed persons or commercial entities for resale.

8. Compounding drug products that are commercially available in the marketplace or that are essentially copies of commercially available FDA-approved drug products. In certain circumstances, it may be appropriate for a pharmacist to compound a small quantity of a drug that is only slightly different than an FDA-approved drug that is commercially available. In these circumstances, FDA will consider whether there is documentation of the medical need for the particular variation of the compound for the particular patient.

9. Failing to operate in conformance with applicable state law regulating the practice of pharmacy.

The foregoing list of factors is not intended to be exhaustive. Other factors may be appropriate for consideration by FDA in a particular case.

NABP Actions and Guidelines

The National Association of Boards of Pharmacy (NABP) hold that prescription compounding is a pharmacist's responsibility and should be regulated by state boards of pharmacy.[30] To distinguish between compounding and manufacturing, NABP defined these terms in its Model State Pharmacy Practice Act[31]:

Compounding means the preparation, mixing, assembling, packaging, or labeling of a drug or device (1) as the result of a practitioner's prescription drug order or initiative based on the practitioner/patient/pharmacist relationship in the course of professional practice, or (2) for the purpose of, or as an incident to, research, teaching, or chemical analysis and not for sale or dispensing. Compounding also includes the preparation of drugs or devices in anticipation of prescription drug orders based on routine, regularly observed prescribing patterns.[32]

Manufacturing means the production, preparation, propagation, conversion, or processing of a drug or device, either directly or indirectly, by extraction from substances of natural origin or independently by means of chemical or biological synthesis, and includes any packaging or repackaging of the substance(s) or labeling or relabeling of its container, and the promotion and marketing of such drugs or devices. Manufacturing also includes the preparation and promotion of commercially available products from bulk compounds for resale by pharmacies, practitioners, or other persons.[32]

NABP published a model regulation, "Model Rules for Sterile Pharmaceuticals." This model regulation does not have the force of law and does not distinguish levels of sterile preparation risk to patients (see discussion of risk levels, below). They merely serve as a basis for individual state boards to develop rules and regulations.

ASHP Actions and Guidelines

ASHP has continually promoted appropriate pharmacy compounding in the institutional setting. In 1990, ASHP developed a multistep action plan to encourage and teach pharmacists to compound safe and effective sterile preparations.

Letter and Survey

The first step of this plan was to send a letter to pharmacy directors, assistant directors, and IV supervisors across the nation, urging them to review and revise their sterile compounding techniques.[33] In the second step, ASHP sent a survey to a representative sample of hospital pharmacy directors to assess the quality of sterile compounding procedures.[34] Some key findings were[1]:

● Nearly 96% of hospital pharmacies extemporaneously compounded sterile preparations; 61% also batch compounded such preparations.

- Almost all pharmacists (99.4%) who compounded sterile preparations used a laminar airflow workbench.

- About 75% of respondents used laminar-airflow workbenches in limited-access areas.

- About 50% of respondents said that their laminar airflow workbenches were certified every 6 months and that prefilters were changed monthly.

- Less than 33% of respondents reported sampling the environment in and around the hood for microbial contamination.

- About 33% of pharmacists used final filtration to sterilize some preparations compounded extemporaneously, and 16% of pharmacists filtered preparations in batch compounding.

Nearly half the survey respondents never tested the chemical purity, drug potency, sterility, or pyrogenicity of sterile preparations. Less than a third of the pharmacies tested their pharmacists or technicians, either by written exam or process validation, on aseptic technique. In other words, the majority of hospital pharmacists could not determine whether they were compounding safe and effective sterile preparations. ASHP concluded that certain quality-assurance procedures for sterile preparations needed significant improvement.

Conference

The third step in ASHP's plan was to invite key persons to participate in a conference[35] to list apparent problems with pharmacy compounded sterile preparations and to identify possible solutions. Attendees included representatives from the FDA, United States Pharmacopeial Convention, American Hospital Association (AHA), NABP, Intravenous Nurses Society, Association for Practitioners of Infection Control, American College of Apothecaries, Joint Commission on the Accreditation of Healthcare Organizations (JCAHO), AACP, Parenteral Drug Association, Pharmaceutical Manufacturers Association, American Biological Safety Association, Canadian Society of Hospital Pharmacists, American Nurses Association, and some members and staff of ASHP.

Conference participants listed 12 problems with pharmacy sterile compounding practices. These problems may be categorized into four groups:

1. A lack of appropriate policies and procedures.

2. A lack of personnel training and education materials.

3. A lack of consistent regulatory definitions, standards, and enforcement by professional and governing groups.

4. A lack of commercially available sterile preparations.

Twenty-six ideas were suggested for resolving the problems.

Educational Programs and Publications

ASHP began the fourth step of its plan with educational programs and publications to teach pharmacy personnel how to compound safe and effective sterile preparations. Several articles and editorials also have been published in the *American Journal of Health-System Pharmacy* (formerly the *American Journal of Hospital Pharmacy*) that explain the need for professional guidelines for compounding sterile preparations.[7, 36-39]

As a final step, ASHP developed a practice standard for the quality assurance of pharmacy compounded sterile preparations. First published in 1993 as a technical assistance bulletin, this standard was updated and republished in 2000 (Appendix A).[40] ASHP has also published a technical assistance bulletin on compounding ophthalmic preparations (Appendix B)[41] and guidelines on the safe use of automated compounding devices for compounding of parenteral nutrition admixtures (Appendix C).[42]

Risk Levels

The *ASHP Guidelines on Quality Assurance for Pharmacy-Prepared Sterile Preparations* designates three levels of risk to patients, increasing from the least (Risk Level 1) to the greatest (Risk Level 3) potential for harm. Risk levels are defined, and examples of sterile preparations in each level are given. Quality-assurance practices for patient safety and preparation effectiveness are also listed for each level. This categorization by risk levels allows pharmacists to match sterile compounding procedures to the preparations. When compounding a preparation under conditions that do not meet risk-level requirements, pharmacists are required to use their best judgment regarding the risk-to-benefit relationship for the patient.

Cleanrooms

A controversial part of these guidelines pertains to the suitable environment (or controlled area) for sterile compounding (see Chapter 17). While ASHP Risk Level 1 preparations require a separate, clean space of sufficient size, Risk Levels 2 and 3 require "cleanrooms." A cleanroom is a separate room that houses the laminar-airflow workbench; the room receives air filtered to a standard level of cleanliness (expressed in airborne particles per cubic foot). Airborne particles are the main vectors for microbes that contaminate preparations during processing. A properly maintained isolator also provides an acceptable environment (see Chapter 4).[43] An isolator provides an ISO Class 5 (Class 100) environment for sterile compounding; therefore, the isolator itself can be in a separate area of the pharmacy but need not actually be in a cleanroom.

The special environment requirement is controversial because of its cost-benefit ratio. The key to ensuring the best possible compounding environment is to ensure that airborne microbes do not enter the laminar-airflow workbench critical space. In 2002, Morris et al. found that only 6.3% of hospital pharmacies that compound Risk Level 3 preparations were compliant ASHP requirements for an ISO Class 7 (Class 10,000) cleanroom.[4] One study showed that simple changes in operating procedures can produce a clean environment without costly architectural changes.[44] Finally, a laminar-airflow workbench suited to the compounded preparations is the most important equipment, but it must be properly used and maintained to prevent contamination.

Garb

A discussion on garb (clothing, masks, gloves, and shoe covers) is also an integral part of the quality assurance guidelines (see Chapter 5). Operators should wear garb that sheds low levels of particulates, wash their hands frequently, and use proper hygiene. Sterile gloves are recommended in ASHP Risk Level 1 and are required in Risk Levels 2 and 3. In 2002, Morris et al. found that only 5.2% of hospital pharmacies that compound Risk Level 1 preparations were compliant ASHP garb requirements.[4]

Process Validation and Key Points

ASHP guidelines also describe the need for process validation to determine whether an operator, working under the most challenging conditions, can consistently produce a sterile preparation (see Chapter 20). Growth media are substituted for normal ingredients in the compounding process to validate the environment, equipment, supplies, and aseptic technique. Process validation (sometimes referred to as "media fills") is better than end-preparation sterility sampling, which can lead to accidental contamination, delayed results, and higher costs. ASHP guidelines stipulate process validation for individual operators in Risk Level 1, for each compounding process in Risk Level 2, and for each preparation in Risk Level 3.

Other key points in the ASHP guidelines include:

- Development and maintenance of up-to-date procedures.
- Training and competency testing of personnel.
- Storage and handling of ingredients, closures, containers, and supplies.
- Preparation stability (compatibility and physical and chemical stability) at the time of use.
- Beyond-use dating of compounded preparations.
- Labeling requirements.
- Final preparation inspection (sterility, nonpyrogenicity, drug potency, and stability).
- Documentation of all sterile compounding processes.
- Documentation of employee testing and validation, refrigerator temperatures, hood certification, batch control testing, and quarantine records.

USP Actions and Monographs

Well before pharmacy compounding errors came to public attention, USP decided that preparation of sterile IV preparations for home use involved special concerns (e.g., extended preparation storage and patient manipulations prior to use). Therefore, they established a Home Health Care Advisory Panel in 1989 to draft a monograph or guideline on compounding sterile preparations for home use. The first draft of this monograph was published in March 1992.[45] The official chapter appeared in the 1995 USP-NF[46] and was revised in the 2000 USP-NF.[47] This chapter, which was previously entitled "Sterile Drug Products for Home Use," was revised based on the FDA Advisory Committee on compounding recommendation from its July 2002 meeting, that the chapter be recognized as the national standard for compounded sterile preparation techniques and practices.

Comparison of ASHP Guidelines and USP Monograph

Like ASHP, USP defines three risk levels to patients, low-risk , medium risk and high-risk categories. However, USP risk levels are defined somewhat differently from the ASHP guidelines; therefore, some preparation types do not match ASHP's corresponding risk levels. Table 1-1 presents examples of which preparations fit into corresponding risk levels of the ASHP and USP documents. The ASHP and USP guidelines each have their advantages.

Features of ASHP Guidelines

1. Risk level sections and topics are organized and clear.

2. A single, extensive glossary defines terms.

3. Exhaustive references, 127 in number, cite original literature.

4. Laminar-airflow workbench recertification is specified for at least every 6 months, instead of every year.

5. Environmental cleaning standards and intervals are listed.

6. Calibration of automated compounder and pumps is specified. ASHP also published a separate guideline on the use of automated compounding devices for the compounding of parenteral nutrition admixtures (see Appendix C).

7. Provides list of recommended written policies and procedures for each of the 3 risk levels.

8. As an ASHP guideline, is a required level of pharmacy practice for pharmacies ASHP-accredited for residency and technician training.

9. As referenced in several state pharmacy regulations, is enforceable by pertinent state boards of pharmacy.

Features of USP Monograph

1. Covers "redispensing" of sterile preparations that have been rerouted from one patient who no longer needs the preparation to another patient who does need the preparation, in two sections: Storage and Beyond-Use Dating and Sterile Preparations for Institutional Use.

2. Extensively treats environmental control and monitoring.

3. Recommends an ISO Class 8 (Class 100,000) cleanroom environment for all risk levels.

4. Recommends nonshedding coats or coveralls for all risk level categories.

5. Recommends that each operator perform medial fills initially and annualy for low-risk operations plus gives a more thorough discussion of verification.

6. Provides a better discussion of sterilization by filtration and heat.

7. Provides a more thorough discussion on maintaining preparation quality and control after the sterile preparation leaves the pharmacy.

8. Covers responsibilities of off-site compounding pharmacies and corresponding receiving pharmacies.

9. Is enforceable by the U.S. Food and Drug Administration.[48]

10. Is enforceable by the Joint Commission on Health Care Organizations.[48]

11. USP allows longer storage periods after compounding but before administration of the sterile preparations (see Chapter 8).

12. Specifies responsibilities for pharmacies dispensing to patients in the home, including a patient monitoring and complaint system.

A.S.P.E.N. Guidelines for Parenteral Nutrition

Recognizing the importance of safe practices associated with these preparations, the National Advisory Group on Standards and Practice Guidelines for Parenteral Nutrition was

Table 1-1

Examples of Sterile Products by Risk-Level Category

ASHP Guidelines USP 797 Monograph	USP 797 Monograph
Risk Level 1	*Low-Risk Category*
Single-patient admixture	● Single transfers of sterile dosage forms from ampuls, bottles, bags, and vials using sterile syringes with sterile needles, other administration devices, and other sterile containers. The contents of ampuls require sterile filtration to remove any glass particles.
Single-patient ophthalmic, preserved	
Single-patient syringes without preservatives used within 28 hours	
Batch-prefilled syringes with preservatives	● Manually measuring and mixing no more than three manufactured products to compound drug admixtures and nutritional solutions.
Total parenteral nutrient (TPN) solution made by gravity transfer of carbohydrates and amino acids into an empty container with the addition of sterile additives with a syringe and needle	*Medium Risk Category*
	● Compounding of total parenteral nutrition fluids using manual or automated devices during which there are multiple injections, detachments, and attachments of nutrient source products to the device or machine to deliver all nutritional components to a final sterile container.
Risk Level 2	
Injections for use in portable pump or reservoir over multiple days	● Filling of reservoirs of injection and infusion devices with multiple sterile drug products and evacuation of air from those reservoirs before the filled device is dispensed.
Batch-reconstituted antibiotics without preservatives	
Batch-prefilled syringes without preservatives	● Filling of reservoirs of injection and infusion devices with volumes of sterile drug solutions that will be administered over several days at ambient temperatures between 25° and 40°.
TPN solutions mixed with an automatic compounding device	
	● Transfer of volumes from multiple ampuls or vials into a single final sterile container or product.
Risk Level 3	*High Risk Category*
Alum bladder irrigation	● Dissolving nonsterile bulk drug and nutrient powders to make solutions, which will be terminally sterilized.
Morphine injection made from powder or tablets	● Sterile ingredients, components, devices, and mixtures are exposed to air quality inferior to ISO Class 5 of opened or partially used packages of manufactured sterile products that lack antimicrobial preservatives.
TPN solutions made from dry amino acids	
TPN solutions sterilized by final filtration	● Measuring and mixing sterile ingredients in nonsterile devices before sterilization is performed.
Autoclaved IV solutions	● Assuming, without appropriate evidence or direct determination, that packages of bulk ingredients contain at least 95% by weight of their active chemical moiety and have not been comtaminated or adulterated between uses.

formed, consisting of five pharmacists who were members of the American Society for Parenteral and Enteral Nutrition (A.S.P.E.N.). Their report, "Safe practices for parenteral nutrition formulations," was published in 1998.[49] This document is currently being revised and it is expected that the revision will be published in 2004.[50]

The A.S.P.E.N. guidelines are organized into six sections, each of which includes evidence to support the need for a practice guideline, specific practice guidelines based on a consensus of the National Advisory Group, a summary of areas requiring further study, and a list of references. The six sections include:

- Introduction
- Labeling parenteral nutrition formulations
- Standard nutrient ranges and sample parenteral nutrition formulations
- Extemporaneous compounding of parenteral nutrition formulations
- Stability and compatibility of parenteral nutrition formulations
- In-line filtration of parenteral nutrient admixtures

Compliance with these guidelines was assessed by O'Neal et al.[51] They found compliance ranging from 15.4% to 86.9%, suggesting a need to improve practices in the preparation of parenteral nutrition formulations. Areas of high compliance included use of filters, verification of stability and compatibility by a pharmacist or computer, evaluating aseptic technique of staff, clarification of doses out of range, and use of standard order forms. Areas of low compliance included use of dosing weight on the label, including daily ingredient amounts on the label, having pharmacist-to-pharmacist communication during patient transfer, end-preparation sterility testing, and use of 2-in-1 formulations in neonatal and infant patients.

Miscellaneous Governmental Agencies

NIOSH and OSHA

The Occupational Safety and Health Act of 1970 created both The National Institute for Occupational Safety and Health (NIOSH) and the Occupational Safety and Health Administration (OSHA). OSHA is in the U.S. Department of Labor and is responsible for developing and enforcing workplace safety and health regulations. NIOSH (a part of Centers for Disease Control and Prevention, CDC) is an agency established to help assure safe and healthful working conditions for workers by providing research, information, education, and training in the field of occupational safety and health. NIOSH is finalizing a communication—which it calls an alert—to help hospitals and other health care institutions to reduce occupational exposures from hazardous drugs to health care workers[52] (see Chapter 4). OSHA is updating is own standards on work place exposures and safety procedures for hazardous drugs.[53]

ISO

International Organization for Standardization (ISO) is a nongovernmental organization, i.e., its members are not delegations of national governments. ISO occupies a position between the public and private sectors. Some member institutes are part of the governmental structure of their countries, or are mandated by their government. Other members have their roots in the private sector, having been set up by national partnerships of industry associations. ISO is in the process of publishing a series of standards for cleanrooms and associated controlled environments. The U.S. federal government now uses the terminology set forth by the ISO in place of its former standard (Federal Standard 209e) (see Chapter 17). Table 1-2 summarizes the new ISO monographs.

Summary

Pharmacists who are responsible for compounding sterile preparations face many issues unknown 10–15 years ago. With current publicity, governmental scrutiny, and technological changes, pharmacists are greatly challenged to meet this responsibility. To compound sterile preparations appropriately, pharmacists must understand the guidelines of NABP, ASHP, USP, and A.S.P.E.N. Each guideline has a unique perspective and offers information not covered in the others. However, professional judgment is required in applying these guidelines to individual practice settings.

Table 1-2.

ISO Standards for Cleanrooms and Associated Environments

ISO 14644-1 Cleanrooms and associated controlled environments—Part 1: Classification of airborne particulates. May 1999.

ISO 14644-2 Cleanrooms and associated controlled environments—Part 2: Specifications for testing monitoring to prove continued compliance with ISO 14644-1 after July 2000.

ISO 14644-4 Cleanrooms and associated controlled environments—Part 3: Metrology and test methods (in press).

ISO 14644-4 Cleanrooms and associated controlled environments—Part 4: Design, construction, and start-up.

ISO 14644-4 Cleanrooms and associated controlled environments—Part 5: Operations 2000- (contamination risk assessment, training procedures, mechanical equipment operation and maintenance, and safety and proper documentation to prove that appropriate procedures are in place and being followed). (In press.)

ISO 14644-4 Cleanrooms and associated controlled environments—Part 6: Terms and definitions (in press).

ISO 14644-4 Cleanrooms and associated controlled environments—Part 7: Enhanced clean devices mini-environments, isolators, glove boxes, and clean workbenches). (In press.)

References

1. Kohn LT, Corrigan JM, and Donaldson MS, editors. *To Err Is Human: Building a Safer Health System.* Washington, DC: National Academy Press; 1999. p. 167.

2. Santell JP, Kamalich RF. National survey of quality assurance activities for pharmacy-prepared sterile preparations in hospitals and home infusion facilities–1995. *Am J Health-Syst Pharm.* 1996; 53:2591–605.

3. Ringold DJ, Santell JP, Schneider PJ. ASHP national survey of pharmacy practice in acute care settings: dispensing and administration–1999. *Am J Health-Syst Pharm.* 2000; 57:1759–75.

4. Morris AM, Schneider PJ, Pedersen CA, Mirtallo JM. National survey of quality assurance activities for pharmacy-compounded sterile preparations. *Am J Health-Syst Pharm.* 2003; 60:2567–76.

5. Myers CE. Needed: serious attention to sterile products. *Am J Hosp Pharm.* 1996; 53:2582.

6. Selenic D. Dodson DR, Jensen B et al. Enterobacter cloacae bloodstream infections in pediatric patients traced to a hospital pharmacy. *Am J Health-Syst Pharm.* 2003; 60:1440–6.

7. ASHP gears up multistep action plan regarding sterile drug products. *Am J Hosp Pharm.* 1991; 48:386–9.

8. Pierce LR, Gaines A, Varricchio R, et al. Hemolysis and renal failure associated with use of sterile water for injection to dilute 25% human albumin solution. *Am J Health-Syst Pharm.* 1998; 55:1057, 1062, 1070.

9. Food and Drug Administration. Safety alert: hazards of precipitation associated with parenteral nutrition. *Am J Hosp Pharm.* 1994; 51:1427–8.

10. Gebhart F. Fatal meningitis linked to compounding by California pharmacy. *Drug Topics.* 2001 (Jul 2); 145:32,35.

11. Flynn EA, Pearson RE, Barker KN. Observational study of accuracy in compounding i.v. admixtures at five hospitals. *Am J Health-Syst Pharm.* 1997:904–12.

12. Bennet SH, McNeil MM, Bland LA, et al. Postoperative infections traced to contamination of an intravenous anesthetic, propofol. *N Engl J Med.* 1995 (Jul 20); 333 (3):147–54.

13. Grohskopf LA, Roth VR, Reikin DR, et al. Serratia liquefaciens bloodstream infections from contamination of epoetin alfa at a hemodialysis center. *N Engl J Med.* 2001(May 17); 344:1491–97.

14. Kwan JW. High-technology i.v. infusion devices. *Am J Hosp Pharm.* 1991; 48 (Suppl 1):S36–51.

15. Kwan JW, Anderson RW. Pharmacists' knowledge of infusion devices. *Am J Hosp Pharm.* 1991; 48 (Suppl 1):S52–3.

16. Johnson R, Coles BJ, Tribble DA. Accuracy of three automated compounding systems determined by end-product laboratory testing and comparison with manual preparation. *Am J Health-Syst Pharm.* 1998; 55:1503–7.

17. Mulye NV, Turco SJ, Speaker TJ. Stability of ganciclovir sodium in an infusion-pump syringe. *Am J Hosp Pharm.* 1994; 51:1348–9.

18. Stiles ML, Tu Y-H, Allen LV Jr. Stability of morphine sulfate in portable pump reservoirs during storage and simulated administration. *Am J Hosp Pharm.* 1989; 46:1404–7.

19. Duafala ME, Kleinberg ML, Nacov C, et al. Stability of morphine sulfate in infusion devices and containers for intravenous administration. *Am J Hosp Pharm.* 1990; 47:143–6.

20. Kaye T. Prolonged infusion times with disposable elastomeric infusion devices. *Am J Hosp Pharm.* 1994; 51:533–4.

21. Levchuk JW. Rapid preparation of alum bladder irrigation. *Hosp Pharm.* 1991; 26:577. Letter.

22. Davis NM. Unprecedented procedural safeguards needed with the use of automated i.v. compounders. *Hosp Pharm.* 1992; 27:488. Editorial.

23. Brushwood DB. Hospital liable for defect in cardioplegia solution. *Am J Hosp Pharm.* 1992; 49:1174–6.

24. Murphy C. Ensuring accuracy in the use of automatic compounders. *Am J Hosp Pharm.* 1993; 50:60. Letter.

25. Bloom MZ. Compounding in today's practice. *Am Pharm.* 1991; NS31 (Oct):31–7.

26. Office of Enforcement, Division of Compliance Policy. Regulatory action regarding approved new drugs and antibiotic drug products subjected to additional processing or other manipulations. FDA Guide 7132c.06. Washington, DC: Food and Drug Administration; Jan 18, 1991: Chap 32c.

27. Food and Drug Modernization Act of 1997, Pub. L No. 105-115 Stat.2296.

28. Harteker LR. Federal court strikes down compounding regulations. *Am J Health-Syst Pharm.* 2001; 58:638, 640, 643.

29. Anon. Compliance policy guidance for FDA staff and industry, Chapter 4, Subchapter 460 Section 460.200 *Pharmacy Compounding.* May 2002.

30. Delegates approve 20 resolutions at annual meeting, resolution No. 89-1-93. *NABP Newsl.* 1993; 22:57.

31. Good compounding practices applicable to state licensed pharmacies. Part I. *Natl Pharm Compliance News.* 1993; May:2–3.

32. Anon. Model State Pharmacy Practice Act and Model Rules of the National Association of Boards of Pharmacy, Fall 1999.

33. ASHP urges review of sterile drug product procedures. *ASHP Newsl.* 1991; 24 (Jan):1.

34. Next step in sterile product action plan: a survey of hospital pharmacists. *ASHP Newsl.* 1991; 24 (Feb): 1.

35. ASHP invitational conference on quality assurance for pharmacy-prepared sterile products. *Am J Hosp Pharm.* 1991; 48:2391–7.

36. Zellmer WA. Upgrading quality assurance for pharmacy-prepared sterile products. *Am J Hosp Pharm.* 1991; 48:2387–8. Editorial.

37. Tormo VJ. Perspective on sterile compounding practices and the draft guidelines. *Am J Hosp Pharm.* 1992; 49:946–7.

38. Trissel LA. Compounding our problems. *Am J Hosp Pharm.* 1994; 51:1534. Editorial.

39. Hasegawa GR. Caring about stability and compatibility. *Am J Hosp Pharm.* 1994; 51:1533–4. Editorial.

40. ASHP Council on Professional Affairs. ASHP guidelines on quality assurance for pharmacy-prepared sterile products. *Am J Health-Syst Pharm.* 2000; 57:1150–69.

41. ASHP Council on Professional Affairs. ASHP technical assistance bulletin on pharmacy-prepared ophthalmic products. *Am J Hosp Pharm.* 1993; 50:1462–3.

42. ASHP Council on Professional Affairs. ASHP guidelines on the safe use of automated compounding devices for the preparation of parenteral nutrition admixtures. *Am J Health-Syst Pharm.* 2000; 57:1343–8.

43. Pilong A, Moore M. Conversion to isolators in a sterile preparation area. *Am J Health-Syst Pharm.* 1999; 56:1978–80.

44. Lau D, Shane R, Yen J. Quality assurance for sterile products: simple changes can help. *Am J Hosp Pharm.* 1994; 51: 1353. Letter.

45. Dispensing practices for sterile drug products intended for home use. *Pharmacopeial Forum.* 1992; 18:3052–75.

46. Sterile drug products for home use. In: United States pharmacopeia, 23rd rev./ national formulary, 18th ed. Rockville, MD: United States Pharmacopeial Convention; 1994:1963–75.

47. Sterile drug products for home use. In: United States pharmacopeia, 24th rev./ national formulary, 19th ed. Rockville, MD: United States Pharmacopeial Convention; 2000; 2130–43.

48. Thompson CA., USP publishes enforceable chapter on sterile compounding. *Am J Health-Syst Pharm.* 2003; 60:1814, 1817, 1818, 1822.

49. Safe practices for parenteral nutrition formulations. *J Parenter Enteral Nutr.* 1998; 22:49–66.

50. USP Center for the Advancement of Patient Safety (CAPS). *CAPSLink* [on-line newsletter]. 2004 (Feb).

51. O'Neal BC, Schneider PJ, Pedersen CA, Mirtallo JM. Compliance with safe practices for preparing parenteral nutrition formulations. *Am J Health-Syst Pharm.* 2002;59:264–9.

52. Gebhart F. NIOSH finalizing chemotherapy alert for healthcare workers. *Drug Topics Health-System Ed.* 2003 (Feb 17); HSE14.

53. Controlling occupational exposure to hazardous drugs. In: OSHA Technical Manual (OSHA Instruction CPL 2-2.20B CH-4). Washington: Directorate of Technical Support, Occupational Safety and Health Administration.1995:Chap 21. (Accessed 03/12/2004.)

2 | Sterile Preparation Formulation

E. Clyde Buchanan

The objective of formulating and compounding sterile preparations is to provide a dosage form of a labeled drug, in the stated potency, that is safe to use if administered properly.[1] This chapter explains the federal regulations, professional standards, and operating procedures that should be followed during formulation and compounding. The components, containers, and closures also are described, as well as the physiologic and physical norms of preparing formulations for parenteral and ophthalmic use. However, this chapter does not cover stability and incompatibility of drugs (see Chapter 8), sterilization methods (see Chapter 13), labeling (see Chapter 9), documentation (see Chapters 10 and 14), and end preparation evaluation (see Chapter 21).

Federal Regulations

When formulating and compounding sterile preparations, pharmacists must follow both state laws and Food and Drug Administration (FDA) regulations. State pharmacy practice acts and board of pharmacy regulations cover these activities. The FDA also regulates formulation and compounding under adulteration, misbranding, and new drug provisions of the Federal Food, Drug and Cosmetic Act (see Appendix F).[2]

Adulteration and Misbranding

Section 501(a)(2)(B) of the Act states that a drug is adulterated if "the methods used in, or the facilities or controls used for its manufacture, processing, packing, or holding do not conform to current good manufacturing practice"[3] (see Appendix F).

Pharmacists who compound sterile preparations must meet purported norms (i.e., what is implied on the label is actually true). Purported norms include identity and strength of ingredients, quality, and purity (i.e., absence of pyrogens, particulates, microbes, and other contaminants). Failure to ensure purported norms renders the preparation adulterated and misbranded.

New Drug Regulations

FDA Guide 7132.06 states that "a physician may prescribe an unusual preparation that requires compounding by a pharmacist from drugs readily available for other uses and which is not generally regarded as safe and effective for the intended use." If the pharmacy merely fills each prescription as received, clearance under the "new drug" provisions is not required.[3]

Compounding investigational drugs for an investigator's use also does not require new drug registration but falls under current good manufacturing practice. If the preparation has been or will be shipped in interstate commerce for clinical trials, however, the investigator must file a new drug application. Moreover, if a pharmacist compounds finished drugs from bulk active ingredients that are not obtained from an FDA-approved facility or are not compliant with compendial standards (i.e., U.S. Pharmacopoeia/National Formulary), these finished preparations must be covered by a new drug application.[3]

If a pharmacist changes the strength, dosage form, or components of a commercially available preparation in a compounded prescription, good compounding procedures should be used.[4] Pharmacists are responsible for compounding and dispensing finished preparations in accordance with a prescription or a prescriber's order or intent and to dispense those preparations in compliance with established Boards of Pharmacy and other regulatory agencies. Such requirements vary from state to state.

Professional Standards

Formulating, compounding, and sterilizing a pharmaceutical from nonsterile ingredients or in nonsterile containers is the most difficult and risky procedure in sterile drug preparation. Under Risk Level 3 section on aseptic technique and product preparation, ASHP says that nonsterile components must meet USP standards for identity, purity and endotoxin levels, as verified by a pharmacist.[5] Batch master worksheets should include comparisons of actual with anticipated yields, sterilization methods, and quarantine specifications. Presterilized containers should be used if feasible. Final containers must be sterile and capable of maintaining product integrity through the beyond-use date. Sterilization method is to be based on properties of the preparation.

USP says that nonsterile active ingredients and added substances, or excipients, for compounded sterile preparations should preferably be official USP and NF articles.[6] When nonofficial ingredients are used, they must be accompanied by certificates of analysis from their suppliers to aid compounding personnel in judging the identify, quality and purity in relation to the intended use in a particular compounded sterile preparation. Bulk, or unformulated, drug substances and added substances, or excipients, must be stored in tightly closed containers under temperature, humidity, and lighting conditions that are either indicated by official monographs or approved by suppliers; also the date of receipt in the compounding facility must be clearly and indelibly marked on each package of ingredient. After receipt by the compounding facility, packages of ingredients that lack a supplier's expiration date cannot be used after one year, unless either appropriate inspection or testing indicates that the ingredient has retained its purity and quality for use in compounded sterile preparations. Careful consideration and evaluation of nonsterile ingredient sources is especially warranted when the compounded sterile preparation will be administered into the vascular, central nervous system, and eyes. Upon receipt of each lot of the bulk drug substance or excipient, the individual compounding the preparation performs a visual inspection of the lot for evidence of deterioration, other types of unacceptable quality and mislabeling.

Written Procedures

Any individual who formulates and compounds sterile preparations should develop and comply with the following written procedures (see also Chapters 10, 14, and 22):

Pharmacies must have a specifically designated and adequate area (space) for the orderly placement of equipment and materials to be used in compounding. Compounding of sterile preparations should be in a separate and distinct area from nonsterile compounding.[4]

Ingredients must meet requirements of USP/NF monographs. When compendial monographs are not available another high-quality source may be acceptable, e.g., certified analytical reagent, certified by American Chemical Society or Food Chemicals Codex grade.[7]

The pharmacist ensures that the sterile components under his supervision meet acceptable criteria of stability and sterility by[8]:

- Dispensing the oldest stock first and observing expiration dates.

- Storing components under the environmental conditions stated in the individual monographs and/or in the labeling.

- Observing components for evidence of instability. Although chemical degradation ordinarily cannot be detected by the pharmacist, some physical changes not necessarily related to chemical potency, such as change in color and odor, or formation of a precipitate, or clouding of solution, may alert the pharmacist to the possibility of a stability problem. If a component has undergone a physical change not explained in the labeling, such a preparation is never to be dispensed.

- Observing components for evidence of lack of sterility. The presence of microbial contamination in sterile components usually cannot be detected visually, but haze, color change, cloudiness, surface film, particulate or flocculent matter, or gas formation is sufficient reason to suspect possible contamination. Evidence that the integrity of the seal has been violated should make the component suspect of microbial contamination.

- Properly handling and labeling preparations that are repackaged, diluted, or mixed with other products.

- Dispensing in the proper container with the proper closure.

- Sterile compounding equipment must be appropriate in design, size, and composition so that surfaces contacting components are not reactive, additive, or absorptive. These surfaces should not alter the required safety, identity, strength, quality, and purity of the components.[4] Moreover, prescription balances and volume-measurement devices should meet United States Pharmacopeial Convention (USP) specifications.[9]

- Dispensing pharmacists must inspect and approve or reject all formulas, calculations, substances, containers, closures, and in-process materials.

Pharmacists who compound batches of parenteral preparations must follow a master formula sheet to reproduce preparations that meet all purported norms.

Components

Components are any ingredients used in compounding, whether or not they appear in the final preparation (i.e., intermediate ingredients). Whenever available, commercially sterile components should be used. Commercial ingredients should be made in an FDA-approved facility and meet official compendial requirements.[10] If these requirements cannot be met, pharmacists should determine if alternative substances should be procured.[4]

Vehicles

Vehicles for most liquid sterile preparations have no therapeutic activity or toxicity. Rather, they serve as solvents or mediums for the administration of therapeutically active ingredients. For parenteral preparations, the most common vehicle is water. Vehicles must meet USP requirements for the pyrogen or bacterial endotoxin tests.[11,12] Several vehicles that are official in the compendia are discussed here.[1]

Water for Injection

Water for injection is purified by distillation or reverse osmosis and is free of pyrogens. Sterile water for injection USP is sterilized and packaged in single-dose containers not exceeding 1000 ml. Bacteriostatic water for injection is sterilized and contains one or more bacteriostatic agents in a container no larger than 30 ml.

Sterile water for inhalation is sterilized and packaged in single-dose containers that are labeled with the full name. As implied, this component cannot be used to prepare parenterals. Sterile water for irrigation is sterilized and packaged in single-dose containers with no added substances. Although this component may be packaged in containers larger than 1000 ml, it is not intended for parenteral use.

Aqueous Isotonic Vehicles

Aqueous isotonic vehicles are often used in sterile preparations. A common vehicle is sodium chloride injection, a 0.9% solution (also known as normal saline) that is sterilized and packaged in single-dose containers no larger than 1000 ml. Bacteriostatic sodium chloride injection is a 0.9% sodium chloride injection that contains one or more bacteriostatic agents in a container no larger than 30 ml. Sodium chloride irrigation also is a 0.9% solution. However, it has no preservatives and may be packaged in a container larger than 1000 ml.

Other isotonic vehicles include Ringer's injection, dextrose injection 5%, and lactated Ringer's injection. None of these components is available in containers larger than 1000 ml.

Water-Miscible Solvents

Several water-miscible solvents are used as a portion of the vehicle in sterile preparations (i.e., as cosolvents). These solvents (e.g., ethyl alcohol, liquid polyethylene glycol, and propylene glycol) dissolve drugs with low water solubility. Preparations compounded with these components are usually administered intramuscularly.[13] Examples of drugs in cosolvent formulations include some barbiturates, antihistamines, and cardiac glycosides. When the solvent has toxic properties or produces toxic decomposition preparations (e.g., polyethylene glycol 300), the formulation requires extra caution (e.g., limiting cosolvent concentrations).[1]

Nonaqueous Vehicles

Nonaqueous vehicles, such as fixed oils, can be used to formulate parenteral preparations. USP specifies that fixed oils must be vegetable (metabolizable) in origin and odorless (or nearly so) and also have no rancid odor or taste.[14] Examples include peanut, cottonseed, corn, and sesame oils. Some vitamins and hormones can only be solubilized in these oils. Moreover, oil-based parenterals can only be given intramuscularly. However, two emulsified oils (i.e., soybean and safflower) are marketed for their caloric contribution in IV nutrition support.

Solutes

Solute chemicals dissolved in vehicles should be USP grade or better since their contaminants (especially metals) can:

- Alter solubility and compatibility of other solutes.
- Cause catalytic chemical reactions.
- Cause toxicity to patients.

Many chemicals used in sterile preparation formulations are available in a pharmaceutical grade that meets compendial standards. The safest solutes already exist in a finished pharmaceutical preparation, free from microbial and pyrogenic contaminants (e.g., commercially available electrolyte additives). Solutes may be active ingredients, i.e., drugs that exert a therapeutic effect, or added substances.

Added substances can increase stability or usefulness if they are harmless in their administered amounts and do not interfere with therapeutic efficacy or responses to assays and tests.[18] Examples include antimicrobial preservatives, pH buffers, antioxidants, chelating agents, tonicity agents, solubilizers and emulsifiers. Although added substances may prevent a reaction or negative result, they can induce others. Therefore, a pharmacist must consider the total formulation of active ingredients and added substances. Moreover, no coloring agent should be added to a sterile preparation solely to color it.

Antimicrobial Preservatives

Antimicrobial preservatives may be added up to a concentration that is considered bacteriostatic or fungistatic. Some preservatives, however, have innate toxicity within these concentrations (e.g., phenylmercuric nitrate 0.01%, benzalkonium chloride 0.01%, and phenol 0.5%). Because of their toxicity, these preservatives are used mostly in ophthalmics and seldom in injectables.

Benzyl alcohol (usually 0.9%) and the parabens (methyl 0.18% combined with propyl 0.02%) are commonly used in injectables. In oleaginous preparations, no antimicrobial is highly effective. However, hexylresorcinol 0.5% and phenylmercuric benzoate 0.1% are reported to be moderately bacteriocidal.[13]

An antimicrobial agent may be effective in one formula of ingredients but not in another. For example, large molecule components such as polysorbate 80, polyvinylpyrrolidone, and polyethylene glycol form complexes that inactivate the parabens. To select a preservative, an appropriate reference[16] should be consulted and its effectiveness should be verified. USP provides a test for the efficacy of antimicrobial preservatives.[17]

pH buffers

Buffering agents stabilize an aqueous solution of a chemical against degradation. Buffer systems are formulated at the lowest concentration needed for stability so that the body's physiologic pH is not disturbed. Acid salts such as citrates, acetates, and phosphates are commonly used as buffers.[13] For an in-depth review of parenteral buffering systems, pharmacists should consult reference 18.

Antioxidants

Antioxidants help to prevent oxidation of the component drug. The most common antioxidants are the sodium and potassium salts of metasulfite and sulfite ions.[19] However, the choice of salt depends on the pH of the system to be stabilized. Metabisulfite is used for low pH values, bisulfite for intermediate pH values, and sulfite for high pH ranges. The administration of large amounts (500 mg/L) of sodium bisulfite in peritoneal dialysis fluids causes toxicity with large volumes (10–40 L/day).[1]

Other antioxidants include acetone metabisulfite, ascorbic acid, thioglycerol, and cysteine hydrochloride.

Chelating Agents

Chelating agents enhance the effectiveness of antioxidants. They form complexes with trace amounts of heavy metals, thereby eliminating the catalytic activity of metals during oxidation. The most commonly used chelating agent is edetate disodium.

Tonicity Agents

Some injectable preparation monographs require that the osmolar concentration appear on the preparation's label. Ideally, parenteral preparations are formulated to be isotonic by use of an isotonic vehicle (e.g., normal saline). When the desired concentration of the active ingredient is hypertonic, the drug must be administered by slowing the rate of injection or by infusion into a large vein (e.g., administration of TPN into subclavian vein).[1]

Solubilizers

Pharmacists must know the solubility characteristics of new drug substances (especially in aqueous systems), since they must possess some aqueous solubility to elicit a therapeutic response. To maintain some drugs in solution, pharmacists may have to include either a miscible cosolvent or a chemical solubilizer. Polyethylene glycols 300 and 400, propylene glycol, glycerin, and ethyl alcohol frequently are used. However, toxic levels of these solvents must be avoided as well as amounts that make the preparation too viscous for parenteral use.

Emulsifiers

Some drugs are minimally soluble in water. Emulsifiers are used to suspend tiny oil globules in water to create an emulsion that contains a uniform concentration of the active drug throughout the volume of the liquid. Emulsions may serve as a caloric source in parenteral nutrition. One example is a soybean oil and water emulsion manufactured with egg yolk phospholipids 1.2% and glycerol 1.7% as emulsifiers.* An example of an active drug is propofol that is dissolved in soybean oil which is emulsified at a concentration of 100 mg/ml in water with glycerol (22.5 mg/ml) and egg lecithin (12 mg/ml) as emulsifiers.†

Containers

Containers are defined as "that which holds the article and is or may be in direct contact with the article. The closure is part of the container."[21] All containers for sterile preparations must be sterile, free of both particulate matter and pyrogens. These containers should not interact physically or chemically with formulations to alter their required strength, quality, or purity. Containers also must permit inspection of their contents.[14]

Container volumes are set by USP. Each container of an injection is filled with liquid, slightly in excess of the labeled size or volume that is to be withdrawn. USP provides a guide showing recommended excess volumes for both mobile and viscous liquids.[14]

Single or Multiple Dose

Sterile, single-dose containers are intended for parenteral, inhalation, irrigation, otic, and ophthalmic administration. Examples are prefilled syringes, cartridges, ampuls, and vials (when labeled as single-use).

Multiple-dose containers permit withdrawal of successive portions of their contents without changing the strength, quality, or purity of the remaining portion. Sterile, multiple-dose

containers may be used for preserved parenterals, ophthalmics, and otics.[22]

Glass

Glass is the most popular material for sterile preparation containers. USP classifies glass as Type I (borosilicate glass), Type II (soda-lime-treated glass), Type III (soda-lime glass), or NP (soda-lime glass unsuitable for parenteral containers).[23] Different glass types vary in their resistance to attack by water and chemicals. For pharmaceutical containers, glass must meet the USP test for chemical resistance.[25] Because most pharmacists do not have the time or facilities to perform glass chemical interaction studies, they should use only Type I glass to minimize sterile preparation incompatibilities.[24]

Plastic

Plastic polymers can be used as sterile preparation containers but present three problems:

1. Permeation of vapors and other molecules in either direction through the container.

2. Leaching of constituents from the plastic into the preparation.

3. Sorption of drug molecules onto the plastic.

Plastics must meet USP specifications for biological reactivity and physicochemicals.[21, 25] Most plastic containers do not permit ready inspection of their contents because they are unclear. Most plastics also melt under heat sterilization.[13]

Closures

Rubber closures must be rendered sterile, free from pyrogens and surface particles. To meet these specifications, multiple washings and autoclavings are required. Closures are made of natural, neoprene, or butyl rubber. In addition, rubber contains[26]:

- Sulfur as a vulcanizing agent.
- Guanidines or sulfide compounds as accelerators.
- Zinc oxide or stearic acid as an activator.
- Carbon, kaolin, or barium sulfate as a filler.
- Dibutyl phthalate or stearic acid as a plasticizer.

---

*Intralipid manufactured by Fresenius Kabi Clayton, L.P. Clayton, NC 27520 USA.

†Diprivan 1%, manufactured by AstraZeneca S.p.A. Caponago, Italy.

● Aromatic amines as antioxidants.

Thus, the rubber sealing of a vial or the plug in a syringe is a complex material that can interact with the ingredients of a formula. Rubber closures also are subject to coring. Therefore, pharmacists should consult compendial or literature standards when selecting a rubber closure for sterile preparations.

Parenteral Formulations

Parenteral preparations are classified into six general categories[13]:

1. Solutions ready for injection.
2. Dry, soluble preparations ready to be combined with a solvent before use.
3. Suspensions ready for injection.
4. Dry, insoluble preparations ready to be combined with a vehicle before use.
5. Emulsions.
6. Liquid concentrates ready for dilution prior to administration.

Most compounded sterile parenteral preparations are aqueous solutions (first category). Other categories usually require the equipment and expertise of a licensed pharmaceutical manufacturer. In addition to using the appropriate vehicle, solvent, and container, the pharmacist must ensure that the final aqueous solution maintains the appropriate physiologic and physical norms.

Physiologic Norms

When injectable solutions are formulated, every effort should be made to mimic the body's normal serum values for pH and tonicity and to create a pyrogen-free preparation.

pH

Normal human serum pH, a logarithmic measure of the hydronium ion concentration in solution, is 7.4. Drugs that are acids or bases or their salts sometimes must be buffered to a pH near normal (e.g., 3–8) to prevent pain or tissue damage. As mentioned previously, acid salts are commonly used as buffers. Stranz and Kastango have provided a good review of pH considerations in parenteral products.[27]

Tonicity

Any chemical dissolved in water exerts a certain osmotic pressure (i.e., a solute concentration related to the number of dissolved particles—un-ionized molecules, ions, macromolecules, and aggregates per unit volume).[28] Blood has an osmotic pressure corresponding to sodium chloride 0.9%; thus, its common name is normal saline. Normal saline is said to be "isosmotic" with blood and other physiologic fluids.

In the medical setting, the term "isotonic" is used synonymously with isosmotic. A solution is isotonic with a living cell if no net gain or loss of water is experienced by the cell and no other change is present when the cell contacts that solution. Very hypotonic IV preparations can cause hemolysis of red blood cells. Very hypertonic injections can damage tissue and cause pain on injection or crenation of red blood cells. Parenteral solutions usually exert an osmotic pressure of 150–900 mOsm/kg compared to a physiologic norm of 282–288 mOsm/kg for blood. The greater the volume of solution to be injected, the closer the parenteral preparation should be to isotonicity.

Pyrogenicity

Pyrogens are contaminants that are unacceptable in final compounded sterile preparations. Pyrogens are fever-producing endotoxins from bacterial metabolism. As large proteins, pyrogens are not removed by normal sterilization procedures and can exist for years in aqueous solution or dried form.

The sources of pyrogens in sterile preparations are:

● Aqueous vehicles.
● Equipment.
● Containers and closures.
● Chemicals used as solutes.
● Human touch.

If sterile water for injection is the vehicle, the risk of pyrogens in water is eliminated. Equipment, containers, and closures can be decontaminated by dry heat or by washing or soaking with acids or bases. Bulk supplies of chemicals may be specified as pyrogen free, although they usually are not. Therefore, sterile preparations made from bulk chemicals must undergo a USP test.[11] Touch contamination is most easily prevented with proper aseptic technique. The maximum limit of endotoxin in a drug product labeled for intrathecal use is set at 0.2 USP endotoxin units/Kg/hr. Thus, to prepare intrathecal dosage forms, the compounding pharmacist must be much more critical during the procedural protocol than during that for intravenously administered preparations.[29] Various methods can be used to test for endotoxins in nonsterile components.[30]

Physical Norms

Particulates

Parenteral solutions must be free of particulate matter—mobile, undissolved solids not intended for sterile preparations. Examples include lint, cellulose and cotton fibers, glass, rubber, metals, plastics, undissolved chemicals, rust, diatoms, and dandruff. To determine levels of particulates, USP sets limits and provides tests.[31] Sources of particulate matter are:

- Vehicles and solutes.
- Environment.
- Equipment.
- Containers and closures.
- Personnel.

However, a careful choice of components, containers, and closures can minimize particulate contamination. Moreover, filtration can remove particles and bacteria from sterile preparations.[32] Lipid emulsions and irrigating solutions are exempt from USP's particulate matter limits.

Stability

Stability of parenteral preparations must be assured so that patients receive the intended dose. Hydrolytic and oxidative drug degradation are the most common forms of instability but rarely show as cloudiness, precipitates, or color changes. The rate of hydrolysis may be affected by storage temperature or pH of the solution. Oxidation is affected by temperature, pH, exposure to light, oxygen concentration of the solution, impurities (e.g., heavy metals), and concentration of the oxidizable drug. Other types of degradation (e.g., racemization, polymerization, isomerization, and deamination) also can occur in solution.

Because numerous factors affect the stability of drug molecules, pharmacists who compound parenterals from bulk chemicals should use a short beyond-use date or know from the literature that longer stability exists. Antioxidant and/or chelation additive systems should be reserved for formulas that are verified in the literature as stable for a given period. The choice of packaging also is important for parenteral drug stability. ASHP publishes the following guides that include information about sterile preparation stability:

- Bing CM. *Extended Stability for Parenteral Drugs, 2nd ed.* Bethesda, MD. American Society of Health-System Pharmacists; 2003.
- Trissel LA. *Handbook on Injectable Drugs, 12th ed.* Bethesda, MD. American Society of Health-System Pharmacists; 2003.

Impurities

Effective July 26, 2004, the FDA requires that large volume parenterals used in total parenteral nutrition therapy (TPN) limit the aluminum content to 25 micrograms per liter.[33] Aluminum may reach toxic levels with prolonged parenteral administration if kidney function is impaired. Premature neonates are particularly at risk because their kidneys are immature, and they require large amounts of calcium and phosphate solutions, which contain aluminum.[33] The FDA requires that small volume parenterals used to compound TPN show on the product container the maximum concentration of aluminum at expiry or state that the product contains no more than 25 micrograms per liter of aluminum. Renally-impaired patients who receive parenteral aluminum at greater than 4 to 5 micrograms per kilogram per day accumulate aluminum at levels associated with central nervous system and bone toxicity.[33] In formulating TPN, pharmacists should measure and/or calculate the soluble aluminum load that a patient will receive and notify the patient's physician if the FDA limit will be exceeded. The physician is responsible for making a clinical decision as to patient risk for aluminum exposure versus the risk of a reduced or different treatment.

Heavy metals (like lead and mercury) are also to be minimized in sterile preparations. Heavy metals can be toxic and can catalyze the degradation of active ingredients and preservatives. Introduction of these impurities is most likely when nonsterile, raw materials are used in compounding. This is why the pedigree of a chemical source is necessary either by meeting USP/NF standards or by written manufacturer certification of analysis and purity.

Of particular concern for formulators of TPN is the relative concentrations of calcium salts and phosphate salts. If either is too high, an insoluble calcium phosphate precipitate results and has led to deaths.[34] While some pharmacists rely on a "magic sum" of calcium and phosphorus to prevent calcium phosphate precipitates, this practice is unsafe because many variables affect the likelihood of precipitation, e.g., type of calcium salt (chloride or gluconate), amount of magnesium, amount of proteins (as amino acids). The best guide is to use a computer program to calculate how much calcium and phosphate can safely be added.[35]

Parenteral Formulas

APhA has published a collection of 168 formulas, some of which are parenteral, organized by therapeutic category, including analgesics, antiemetics, anti-infective agents, and anti-inflammatory agents.[36] The *International Journal of Pharmaceutical Compounding*[37] maintains a website (www.ijpc.com) that lists formulas for many parenteral products, including some products that have been discontinued by pharmaceutical manufacturers. The *IJPC* website lists compact discs for sale that contain articles and formulations from back issues of the journal, including sterile product compounding, stability and compatibility studies. The *IJPC* sterile compounding CD contains 30 articles and 60 formulas on parenteral preparations.

Ophthalmic Formulations

Ophthalmic preparations share many of the same properties as parenteral preparations but present additional concerns. For example, ophthalmic formulations may use different added substances (e.g., buffers, antimicrobial preservatives, tonicity-adjusting chemicals, and thickening agents). Furthermore, ophthalmic preparations include solutions (eye drops or washes), suspensions, and ointments. Since pharmacists rarely compound sterile suspensions or ointments, this discussion is limited to solutions.

Physiologic Norms

Buffers and pH

Lacrimal fluid has a pH of approximately 7.4 and limited buffering capacity. Ophthalmic solutions of weak bases (e.g., alkaloids), for which therapeutic efficacy depends on the bioavailability of the alkaloid base, are buffered to acidity but as near pH 7.4 as possible while keeping the alkaloid in solution after instillation.[38] The buffer system (e.g., phosphate or acetate) should maintain pH within the drug's solubility range for the duration of expiration dating.[39] A moderately acidic solution does not cause discomfort on instillation unless the buffer system overcomes the buffer capacity of lacrimal fluid. Nonisotonic ophthalmic solutions below pH 6.6 or above pH 9.0 have been associated with irritation, reflex tears, and blinking.[40]

Tonicity

Lacrimal fluid has an osmotic pressure or tonicity similar to aqueous sodium chloride 0.9% solution. Eye tissue can tolerate tonicities of 0.5%–1.8% without much discomfort.[38] However, the tonicity of eyewashes is more important than drops because a larger volume of solution contacts the eye. The tonicity of intraocular solutions also should be as close as possible to physiologic.

When formulating ophthalmic solutions, pharmacists should adjust the tonicity to approximate lacrimal fluid by adding a substance such as sodium chloride. Several methods can be used to calculate the amount of sodium chloride needed. The following example uses the colligative property, freezing-point depression. Lacrimal fluid lowers the freezing point of water by 0.52° C. To make a boric acid 1% solution isotonic, sodium chloride crystals are added. Boric acid lowers the freezing point by 0.29° C; therefore, sodium chloride must be added to lower the freezing point further by 0.23° C. To use a proportion:

$$\frac{0.52°\ C}{0.9\%} = \frac{0.23°\ C}{X}$$

Therefore, $X = 0.4\%$. Thus, sodium chloride crystals are added to a boric acid 1% solution to make it a sodium chloride 0.4% solution.[41]

Another easy method of calculation is to add the sodium chloride equivalent. Appendix A of Remington's Chapter 18 gives the sodium chloride equivalents, freezing-point depressions, and hemolytic effects of 375 medicinal chemicals.[28] Remington's Chapter 18, Appendix B, lists volumes of water to add to 300 mg of 82 drugs to make an isotonic solution.

Viscosity

Viscosity is important in ophthalmic preparations. Viscosity sometimes is increased to extend contact between the solution and eye. Moreover, water-dispersible polymers (e.g., methylcellulose, hydroxyethylcellulose, hydroxypropylcellulose, and polyvinyl alcohol) are used as thickening agents. A good review of viscosity agents, including their maximum concentrations may be found in the *International Journal of Pharmaceutical Compounding*.[42] Although USP discusses use of cellulose derivatives, precautions are necessary. Cellulose derivative solutions cannot be filtered. When autoclaved, the derivative precipitates from solution because of decreased water solubility at high temperatures but redissolves at room temperature.[41]

When a heat-labile drug is formulated with a cellulose derivative, all components must be sterilized separately and then recombined aseptically. The drug in solution is sterilized by filtration, and the cellulose derivative is sterilized by autoclaving.[41] Viscosity of 25–50 centipoises improves contact time with the eye, whereas higher viscosity offers no contact advantage but usually leaves a residue on eyelid margins.[38]

Sterility

To ensure sterility of ophthalmic solutions, pharmacists must prepare them in single-dose containers or use antimicrobial preservatives in multiple-dose containers. The microbe that causes great concern is *Pseudomonas aeruginosa*; however, no preservative is 100% effective against all strains of it.

The most common preservative is benzalkonium chloride (0.004%–0.02%), but high concentrations of it irritate the eye. This preservative is incompatible with large anions (e.g., soaps) as well as with nitrates and salicylates. Other preservatives include phenylmercuric acetate and nitrate (0.001%–0.01%), phenyl-ethanol (0.5%), parabens (0.1%), and chlorobutanol (0.5%). Since chlorobutanol is stable only near pH 5–6, it is used only with solutions in this range.

Remington's Chapter 43 discusses different ophthalmic preservatives.[38] The properties of various ophthalmic preservatives have been discussed.[43] Some ophthalmologists prefer nonpreserved solutions because of allergic reactions to common preservatives. This is particularly true for ophthalmic solutions injected during cataract surgery.[44]

Physical Norms

Required physical characteristics of ophthalmics include clarity, stability, and compatibility. Ophthalmics are made clear or particle free by filtration; therefore, nonshedding filters, containers, and closures must be used.

Stability depends on the chemical nature of the drug, preparation pH, preparation method (especially temperature), solution additives, and packaging. If oxidation is a problem, sodium bisulfite (up to 0.3%), ascorbic acid, or acetylcysteine can be added. Surfactants are used in low concentrations to achieve solution or suspension of active ingredients. APhA has published a handbook that contains some ophthalmic formulas along with their stability information.[45]

Ophthalmic Formulas

The *International Journal of Pharmaceutical Compounding* published an issue containing formulas for fifteen ophthalmic preparations:[46]

- Acetylcysteine 15% ophthalmic solution
- Amphotericin B 2 mg/ml ophthalmic solution
- Ascorbic acid 10% ophthalmic solution
- Calcium gluconate 1% ophthalmic irrigation solution
- Cyclosporin 2% ophthalmic solution
- Dexamethasone sodium phosphate 0.05% ophthalmic ointment
- Fluconazole 0.2% ophthalmic solution
- Fortified gentamicin ophthalmic solution
- Glucose 40% ophthalmic ointment
- Idoxuridine 0.5% ophthalmic ointment
- Idoxuridine 0.1% ophthalmic solution
- Lissamine Green 0.5% ophthalmic solution
- Ophthalmic lubricant
- Rose Bengal 1% ophthalmic solution

● Vancomycin 25 mg/ml ophthalmic solution

These formulas are accompanied by the method of preparation, packaging, labeling, stability, discussion, and references.

ASHP has published extemporaneous formulations from The Children's Hospital of Philadelphia[47] for ophthalmics, including:

● Bacitracin ophthalmic solution 10,000 units/ml

● Cefazolin ophthalmic solution 33 mg/ml

● Cidofovir intravitreous solution 0.2 mg/ml

● Gentamicin ophthalmic solution 13.6 mg/ml (fortified)

● LET (lidocaine 4%/epinephrine 0.1%/tetracaine 0.5%) gel

● Tobramycin ophthalmic solution 13.6 mg/ml (fortified)

● Tobramycin ophthalmic solution 15mg/ml

● Vancomycin ophthalmic solution 31 mg/ml

Summary

In many cases, no commercial preparation is available for a final sterile preparation. Legally, pharmacists may compound these preparations under the regulations of the Food, Drug and Cosmetic Act. However, various sterile components (e.g., vehicles, buffers, and solubilizers) are required. It is the pharmacist's responsibility to ensure that they meet the appropriate compendial requirements.

When formulating either parenteral or ophthalmic preparations, a pharmacist should use components so that the final sterile preparation achieves both physiologic and physical norms.

References

1. Turco SJ. Composition. In: Turco SJ, ed. *Sterile Dosage Forms, Their Preparation and Clinical Application*, 4th ed. Philadelphia, PA: Lea & Febiger; 1994:1127.

2. Office of Enforcement, Division of Compliance Policy. Manufacture, distribution, and promotion of adulterated, misbranded, or unapproved new drugs for human use by state-licensed pharmacies. FDA Guide 7132.16. Washington, DC: Food and Drug Administration; Mar 16, 1992:Chap 32.

3. Food and Drug Administration. Chap 32, Division of Field Regulatory Guidance. Hospital pharmacies status as drug manufacturer. FDA Guide 7132.06. Washington, DC: Oct 1, 1980.

4. National Association of Boards of Pharmacy. *Appendix C. Good compounding practices applicable to state licensed pharmacies. Model State Pharmacy Act and Model Rules of the National Association of Boards of Pharmacy.* http://nabp.org; accessed September 9, 2003.

5. American Society of Health-System Pharmacists. ASHP Guidelines on quality assurance for pharmacy-prepared sterile products. *Am J Health-Syst Pharm.* 2000; 57:1150-69.

6. United States Pharmacopeial Convention. Chapter 797 Pharmaceutical compounding–sterile preparations. *United States Pharmacopeia, 27th rev./National Formulary.* 2004. On-line version www.uspnf.com. Accessed 4/01/04.

7. Anon. Standard operating procedure: Certificates of analysis of materials used for pharmaceutical compounding. *Internat J Pharma Compound.* 2001 (Mar/Apr); 5:147.

8. United States Pharmacopeial Convention. Chapter 1191 Stability considerations in dispensing practice. In: *United States Pharmacopeia, 27th rev./National Formulary 22nd* http://uspnf.com; accessed August 1, 2003.

9. United States Pharmacopeial Convention. Chapter 1176 Prescription balances and volumetric apparatus. In: *United States Pharmacopeia, 27th rev./National Formulary 22nd* http://uspnf.com; accessed August 1, 2003.

10. Food and Drug Administration. Chap. 4 Subchap. 460.200 Pharmacy compounding. http://fda.gov/ora/compliance_ref/cpg/default.htm. accessed September 12, 2003.

11. United States Pharmacopeial Convention. Chapter 151 Pyrogen test. In: *United States Pharmacopeia, 27th rev./National Formulary 22nd* http://uspnf.com; accessed August 1, 2003.

12. United States Pharmacopeial Convention. Chapter 85 Bacterial endotoxins test. In: *United States Pharmacopeia, 27th rev./National Formulary 22nd* http://

uspnf.com; accessed August 1, 2003.

13. Avis KE, Levchuk JW. Chapter 41. Parenteral preparations. In: Gennaro AR, ed. *Remington: The Science and Practice of Pharmacy*, 20th ed. Baltimore, MD: Lippincott Williams & Wilkins; 2000. p. 780–806.

14. United States Pharmacopeial Convention. Chapter 1 Injections. In: *United States Pharmacopeia, 27th rev./National Formulary 22nd* http://uspnf.com; accessed August 1, 2003.

15. Ando HY, Radebaugh GW. Chap 38. Preformulation. In: Gennaro AR, ed. *Remington: The Science and Practice of Pharmacy*, 20th ed. Baltimore, MD: Lippincott Williams & Wilkins; 2000. p. 700–20.

16. Akers MJ. Considerations in selecting antimicrobial preservative agents for parenteral product development. *Pharm Technol*. 1984; 8:36.

17. United States Pharmacopeial Convention. Chapter 51 Antimicrobial effectiveness testing. In: *United States Pharmacopeia, 27th rev./National Formulary 22nd* http://uspnf.com; accessed August 1, 2003.

18. Wang YJ, Kowal RR. Review of excipients and pHs for parenteral products used in the United States. *J Parenter Drug Assoc*. 1980; 34:452–62.

19. Akers MJ. Preformulation screening of antioxidant efficacy in parenteral products. *J Parenter Drug Assoc*. 1979; 33:346–56.

20. United States Pharmacopeial Convention. Chapter 785 Osmolarity. In: *United States Pharmacopeia, 27th rev./National Formulary 22nd* http://uspnf.com; accessed August 1, 2003.

21. United States Pharmacopeial Convention. General notices and requirements. In: *United States Pharmacopeia, 27th rev./National Formulary 22nd* http://uspnf.com; accessed August 1, 2003.

22. Turco SJ. Characteristics. In: Turco SJ, ed. *Sterile Dosage Forms, Their Preparation and Clinical Application, 4th ed.* Philadelphia, PA: Lea & Febiger; 1994:28–38.

23. United States Pharmacopeial Convention. Chapter 661 Containers. In: *United States Pharmacopeia, 27th rev./National Formulary 22nd* http://uspnf.com; accessed August 1, 2003.

24. Turco SJ. Extemporaneous preparation. In: Turco SJ, ed. *Sterile Dosage Forms, Their Preparation and Clinical Application, 4th ed.* Philadelphia, PA: Lea & Febiger; 1994:57–78.

25. United States Pharmacopeial Convention. Chapter 87 Biological reactivity tests, in-vitro. In: *United States Pharmacopeia, 27th rev./National Formulary 22nd* http://uspnf.com; accessed August 1, 2003.

26. Turco SJ. Large-scale preparation. In: Turco SJ, ed. *Sterile Dosage Forms, Their Preparation and Clinical Application, 4th ed.* Philadelphia, PA: Lea & Febiger; 1994:39–56.

27. Stranz M, Kastango ES. A review of pH and osmolarity. *Internat J Pharma Compound*. 2002 (May/Jun) 6:216–20.

28. Reich I, Poon CY, Sugita ET. Chap. 18. Tonicity, osmoticity, osmolality and osmolarity. In: Gennaro AR, ed. *Remington: The Science and Practice of Pharmacy*, 20th ed. Baltimore, MD: Lippincott Williams & Wilkins; 2000. p. 246–62.

29. Jones M. Bacterial endotoxins and pyrogens. *Internat. J. Pharma. Compound*. 2001 (Jul/Aug); 5:259–63.

30. Joiner TJ, Kraus PF and Kupiec TC. Comparison of endotoxin testing methods for pharmaceutical products. *Internat J Pharma Compound*. 2002 (Nov/Dec); 6:408-9.

31. United States Pharmacopeial Convention. Chapter 788 Particulate matter in injections. In: *United States Pharmacopeia, 27th rev./National Formulary 22nd* http://uspnf.com; accessed August 1, 2003.

32. McKinnon BT, Avis KE. Membrane filtration of pharmaceutical solutions. *Am J Hosp Pharm*. 1993; 50:1921–36.

33. Food and Drug Administration. Aluminum in large and small volume parenterals used in total parenteral nutrition: Delay of effective date. *Fed Reg*. 2003 (Jun 3); 68:32979–81.

34. Food and Drug Administration. Safety alert: hazards of precipitation associated with parenteral nutrition. *Am J Hosp Pharm*. 1994; 51:1427–8.

35. Trissel LA. *Trissel's Ca/P Check*. Bethesda, MD: American Society of Health-System Pharmacists; 2003.

36. Allen LV. *Allen's Compounded Formulations: The Complete U.S. Pharmacist Collection.* Washington, DC: American Pharmacists Association; 2003.

37. *International J. Pharmaceutical Com-*

pounding. (www.ijpc.com); website accessed, September 18, 2003.

38. Hecht G. Chap. 43. Ophthalmic preparations. In: Gennaro AR, ed. In: Gennaro AR, ed. *Remington: The Science and Practice of Pharmacy,* 20th ed. Baltimore, MD: Lippincott Williams & Wilkins; 2000. p. 821–835.

39. Leiter CW. Buffer solutions for ophthalmic preparations. *Internat J Pharma Compound.* 1998 (May/Jun) 2:190–191.

40. Mobley C. Anatomical and physiological considerations for pharmacy compounding. *Drug Topics.* 2003 (June 2); 147:64–72.

41. Turco SJ. Ophthalmic preparations. In: Turco SJ, ed. *Sterile Dosage Forms, Their Preparation and Clinical Application, 4th ed.* Philadelphia, PA: Lea & Febiger; 1994: 344–54.

42. Anon. Compounding ophthalmic preparations. *Internat J Pharma Compound.* 1998 (May/June) 2:184–8.

43. Anon. Preservation, sterilization and sterility testing of ophthalmic preparations. *Internat J Pharma Compound.* 1998 (May/June) 2:192–5.

44. Anderson NJ, Edelhauser HF. Ophthalmic solutions in cataract surgery. *Internat J Pharma Compound.* 1998 (May/June) 2:196–202.

45. Trissel LA. *Trissel's Stability of Compounded Formulations, 2nd Ed.* Washington, DC American Pharmacists Association; 2000.

46. Anon. Formulations. *Internat J Pharma Compound.* 1998 (May/Jun) 2:221–236.

47. Jew RK, Mullen RJ and Soo-Hoo W. *Extemporaneous Formulations.* Bethesda, MD: American Society of Health-System Pharmacists; 2003. pp. 75–82.

3 | Equipment for Compounding Sterile Preparations

Philip J. Schneider

Although most sterile preparations are compounded using aseptic technique, some are made under nonsterile conditions and then are terminally sterilized. Both methods require the critical area to be as sterile as possible. Supplies also should be stored in a clean environment (the controlled area). Both the critical and controlled areas must be maintained appropriately (see Chapter 21), and a major determinant in their maintenance is the equipment used in them.

The most common piece of equipment used in sterile compounding areas is a laminar-airflow hood. Automated compounding devices, refrigerators, freezers, computer terminals, shelving, chairs and tables, carts, lockers, and miscellaneous items also influence the cleanliness of critical and controlled areas.

To ensure meeting environmental standards, as much of this equipment as possible should be separated from the critical area. Other than the laminar-airflow hood, most equipment should be stored in the controlled area or the pharmacy itself.

Clean Air Environments

In the critical area, air should meet ISO 5 (Class 100) conditions. ISO 5 (Class 100) cleanrooms can be constructed to meet this requirement (see Chapter 6). Offsite modular cleanrooms also can be purchased, but their cost may limit usage to settings where large quantities of sterile preparations (e.g., home care companies) or high-risk products are compounded. Two other options for maintaining a ISO 5 (Class 100) environment are laminar-airflow hoods and barrier isolators (see Chapters 4 and 17).

Laminar-Airflow Hoods

A laminar-airflow hood with either horizontal or vertical airflow is a cost-effective, efficient way to provide the ISO 5 (Class 100) environment required for pharmacy use (see Chapter 18). A laminar-airflow hood includes a high-efficiency particulate air (HEPA) filter to retain airborne particles and microorganisms, and its use decreases the chance of contamination of compounded preparations.[1] According to a recent survey, most pharmacies compounding sterile preparations had a laminar-airflow hood.[2]

Horizontal Laminar-Airflow Hoods

Horizontal airflow hoods are used to compound most sterile preparations because they do not require expensive venting to outside air and can be easily moved to different locations. These hoods produce air of a specified quality that flows horizontally over work areas (see Figure 3-1).

Horizontal hoods are available in various widths (26 inches to 8 feet) and with different electrical requirements (120 or 220 volts). Work surfaces are of either high-density laminated composition board or stainless steel. Some models are for use on counter tops and others are stand-alone floor units.

Vertical Laminar-Airflow Hoods

Since horizontal laminar-airflow hoods blow air toward the operator, vertical laminar-airflow hoods are preferred when working with hazardous substances (see Figure 3-2). Vertical flow hoods are part of a family of equipment called biohazard cabinets or biological safety cabinets. Three types of biohazard cabinets are available:

1. Class I cabinets have a HEPA filter on their exhaust outlet but not for inward airflow. They protect personnel and the environment but do not prevent contamination of compounded preparations. This class of hoods has no application in compounding sterile preparations.

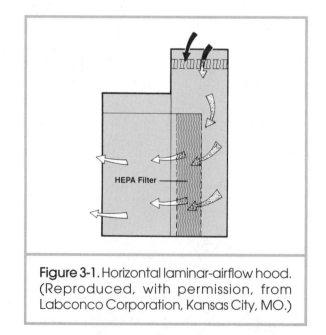

Figure 3-1. Horizontal laminar-airflow hood. (Reproduced, with permission, from Labconco Corporation, Kansas City, MO.)

2. Class II cabinets have HEPA-filtered inward air for protection of compounded preparations and HEPA-filtered exhaust air to protect personnel. They are suitable for compounding sterile preparations.

3. Class III cabinets are totally enclosed, vented, and gastight units. Operations are conducted through attached rubber gloves, and the cabinet is maintained under negative pressure. These cabinets have limited applications in the preparation of sterile products and are intended for the handling of extremely hazardous substances or virulent microorganisms. They include, but are not limited to barrier isolators (Chapter 4).

Types of Class II cabinets. Class II cabinets are classified according to how their exhaust air is vented.

A Class II, Type A cabinet

- Maintains a minimum calculated average inflow air velocity of 75 ft/min through the work area access opening.

- Has HEPA-filtered air from a common plenum (some air is exhausted from the cabinet and some is supplied to the work area).

- May have air exhausted back into the controlled area.

- May have positive-pressure-contaminated ducts and plenums.

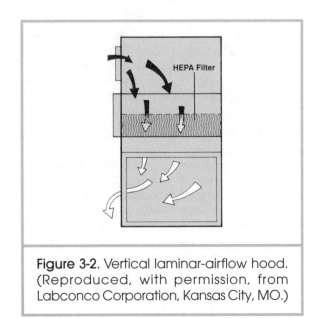

Figure 3-2. Vertical laminar-airflow hood. (Reproduced, with permission, from Labconco Corporation, Kansas City, MO.)

A Class II, Type B cabinet exhausts some or all air outside the controlled area. These cabinets are further classified as II B1, II B2, or II B3 (or A/B3) cabinets.

A II B1 cabinet

- Maintains an average air velocity of 100 ft/min.

- Has HEPA-filtered downflow air composed largely of uncontaminated, recirculated inflow air.

- Exhausts *most* contaminated air to the atmosphere through a dedicated duct and HEPA filter.

- Has all contaminated ducts and plenums under negative pressure.

A II B2 cabinet, sometimes called a total exhaust cabinet, differs from a II B1 cabinet in that it

- Has *all* downflow air drawn through a HEPA filter from the controlled area or outside, not recirculated from the cabinet.

- Exhausts *all* air to the atmosphere after HEPA filtration, not to recirculation in the cabinet or controlled area.

A II B3 cabinet, sometimes referred to as a convertible cabinet

- Has HEPA-filtered air that is a portion of the mixed downflow and inflow air from a common exhaust plenum.

- Exhausts all air to the atmosphere after HEPA filtration.

- Can be converted from a Type B to a Type A cabinet if desired.

The airflow characteristics of different types of biohazard cabinets are shown in Figure 3-3.

Cabinet safety. The safest biohazard cabinet for compounding sterile preparations (e.g., chemotherapy) is a II B2 unit. It is recommended for programs where a limited number of staff handle or compound extensive amounts of preparations using hazardous materials. These cabinets require expensive venting and cannot be easily installed. A less expensive alternative, the Class II, Type A cabinet, does not need to be vented to the outside atmosphere if the controlled area is large and the quantity of compounded preparations prepared is low.

Class	II	II	II	II	II	II
Type	A	A/B3	A	A/B3	B3	B2
Sash opening (inches)	10	8	10	8	8	8
Inflow (fpm)*	80	105	80	105	105	105
Downflow (fpm)*	80	80	80	80	80	60–65
% Recirculation	70	70	70	70	70	0
Exhausts to	room	room	outside	outside	outside	outside
Exhaust duct connection**	none	none	canopy	canopy	hard duct	hard duct

*Inflow and downflow velocities are shown at nominal fpm.
**Varies according to local codes.

Figure 3-3. Airflow characteristics of Class II vertical laminar-airflow hoods. (Reproduced, with permission, from Labconco Corporation, Kansas City, MO.)

Hood Selection

Vertical laminar-airflow hoods are the preferred choice. These cabinets prevent cumulative exposure to potentially toxic medications, especially if the staff routinely compound hazardous preparations for a long time.

When sterile preparations are compounded, aerosols can form and be blown toward the operator using a horizontal hood. Long-term exposure to cytotoxic agents as well as other drugs, especially antibiotics, is a great concern. Vertical airflow hoods, however, minimize such exposure.

The disadvantage of vertical airflow versus horizontal airflow hoods are expense and ease of use. Class II, Type B hoods are more expensive than horizontal hoods and can be very costly to install due to venting requirements. Hoods that vent air to the room (Class II, Type A) are less expensive but are still more costly than horizontal airflow hoods. Furthermore, vertical airflow hoods generally are more restrictive and may slow workflow.

When selecting a laminar-airflow hood, several questions should be addressed.

- *Is a horizontal or vertical airflow hood (biohazard cabinet) needed?* If hazardous materials are being used to compound preparations routinely, a vertical airflow hood should be used.

- *If a biohazard cabinet is required, does it need to be ventilated to the atmosphere?* If large quantities of hazardous materials are being used to compound preparations regularly and the controlled area is small, operators may be exposed to high amounts of aerosols. In this case, the vertical cabinet should be vented to the outside atmosphere.

- *What are the counter length, depth, and height limitations in cabinet selection?* These dimensions depend on the size and layout of the controlled area, workload, and number of staff working in the controlled area. Hood manufacturers readily supply cabinet dimensions on request.

- *What are the electrical requirements?* Manufacturers offer various hoods requiring either 120 or 220 volts. Institutional policies or procedures relating to equipment voltage and the facility's capacity must be determined.

- *Should a counter top or stand-alone unit be purchased?* This decision should be based on the space available and the work area required. Generally, smaller hoods can be placed on counter tops, but they require enough ceiling clearance to provide intake air. Door openings also must be considered when a hood is to be put in an existing cleanroom.

Compounding Devices

Many tools have been developed to assist personnel in compounding sterile preparations. Compounding devices, syringe systems, automatic systems based on peristaltic pump principles, and robotics are frequently used for batch compounding, nutrition solutions, and cardioplegia preparations. Before these devices are employed, however, three questions should be answered:

1. Do standardized formulations lend themselves to an automated system?

2. Does the workload justify the use of the device to improve efficiency?

3. Are appropriate quality-assurance controls in place to monitor the products compounded with these devices?

Syringe-Based Devices

The Cornwall syringe, an example of a manual device, uses a two-way valve. This valve is attached to a diluting fluid and to the syringe, and spring mechanism refills the barrel after each use. This device is used for mass reconstitution of powdered drugs in vials or to add a set quantity of one ingredient to other preparations (e.g., electrolyte addition to nutrition formulas).

Electronically powered versions of this device also have been introduced (e.g., FasPak).

Peristaltic Pump Devices

The automated compounding device, based on peristaltic pump principles similar to infusion pumps, is a recent technological development for compounding sterile preparations. It is useful for complex multicomponent sterile preparations (e.g., nutrition formulations and cardioplegia solutions).

Automated compounding devices are available for both large volume (e.g., sterile water, dextrose, and amino acids) and small volume (e.g., electrolytes and micronutrients) components. Some devices have computer operating systems that perform calculations, record doses, maintain manufacturing records, and run the device itself.

For pharmacies compounding large numbers of complicated preparations, these devices can improve both efficiency and accuracy. Since they involve a high capital cost, monthly lease payments, or the purchase of expensive infusion sets, their application to small operations is limited. An organization that purchases numerous products from a company that sells an automated compounding device may be able to obtain one on a contractual basis based on preparation usage.

The accuracy of the final preparations compounded with these devices has been questioned. Patients have received preparations containing inaccurate quantities of ordered ingredients.[3-5] In most reported cases, pediatric patients received nutrition formulas containing the wrong concentration of dextrose. The accuracy of these formulations can be verified using weight or refractometry measurements,[6,7] as discussed in Chapter 21.

Robotic Devices

The next generation of automation will be robotic devices that actually compound the final sterile preparation. While these devices are not yet widely available to pharmacists, they potentially can automate the entire process, minimizing human error and breaks in technique. These devices probably will be expensive (hundreds of thousands of dollars), however, limiting application to the largest programs or regional pharmacies.

Other Equipment

In addition to the cleanroom itself, many important equipment decisions have to be made concerning the compounding of sterile preparations. The relationship of equipment from refrigerators to computers and special precautions for their operation must be considered.

Refrigerators

Many drugs and compounded sterile preparations require refrigeration to maintain stability. The *United States Pharmacopeia/National Formulary (USP/NF)* defines a refrigerator as "a cold place in which the temperature is maintained thermostatically between 2 and 8 degrees centigrade (36 to 46 degrees Fahrenheit)." The *USP/NF* also defines storage conditions:

- Cold temperatures not exceeding 8°C (46°F).

- Cool temperatures between 8 and 15°C (46 and 59°F).

The *USP/NF* also states that articles requiring storage in a cool place (e.g., insulin) can be refrigerated unless otherwise indicated.[8]

Ordinary consumer refrigerators are often used for sterile preparations programs. Although these refrigerators are adequate, a quality-assurance program must ensure that appropriate temperatures are maintained. At the very least, a thermometer in the refrigerator should be checked (and documented) daily.

Commercial refrigerators often are more durable and have valuable features for pharmacy applications. One desirable feature is an alarm that sounds if the temperature varies from control limits (due to power failure or equipment malfunction). Since this alarm should be monitored 24 hr/day, it should be wired to a security office. Staff responsible for monitoring temperatures or temperature alarms should be familiar with the effects of temperature changes on stored products.

Refrigerator location

Refrigerator placement can cause pharmacy design problems. The refrigerator ventilation motor can create air movement in a controlled or critical area. If a refrigerator must be in the controlled area, it should be as far as possible from the laminar-airflow hood.

Storage refrigerators should not be in any ISO 5 (Class 100) cleanroom. To supply refrigeration to a ISO 5 (Class 100) cleanroom, refrigerators with two-sided, pass-through doors should be used. These refrigerators, with doors on both sides, permit access to sterile preparations by both operators in the controlled area and personnel outside it. If the facility is properly designed, this arrangement eliminates unnecessary entry of personnel to the controlled area to retrieve sterile preparations.

Refrigerator size

Since refrigerators come in many sizes, proper selection depends on the volume of drugs and final preparations to be stored. Having several small units instead of one large unit may be desirable because they

- Provide both a safeguard and a backup if one unit fails.
- Permit segregation of drugs and final preparations for safety purposes (e.g., some pharmacists prefer to store chemotherapy or investigational preparations separately).

The simplest method to determine the refrigerator size needed is to add (1) the space required for the maximum inventory of drug supplies and final preparations on the busiest day of the week and (2) additional capacity for future growth. Then possible storage areas must be identified so the decision can be made between one large and several small refrigerators. Furthermore, if the facility is already built, the maximum size refrigerator that can be moved through the door and ceiling limitations must be considered. Power requirements also should be checked against institutional policies before any unit is purchased.

Freezers

Some sterile preparations must be kept frozen to extend their stability and shelf life. According to the *USP/NF*, a freezer is "a cold place in which the temperature is maintained thermostatically between $-20°$ and $-10°$ C ($-4°$ and $14°$ F)."[8] The same quality-control issues (e.g., monitoring temperatures) that apply to refrigerators also apply to freezers, as do concerns for location, size, and selection.

Computer Terminals and Software

To maintain records and generate labels, most sterile preparations programs now use computers. In large institutions, these programs are part of the pharmacy computer system. Small pharmacies, however, may use commercially available software written specifically for compounding sterile preparations.

Computer equipment has fans to cool units and paper to print reports and labels. Both features are undesirable in the cleanroom fans disrupt airflow and printers generate particulates. Therefore, computer equipment must be located as far as possible from the critical area and never in it. (Automated compounding devices are not considered computer equipment.) Space, noise, cable installation, hardware needs, and workflow should all be considered when locating computer equipment.

Shelving

Storage of supplies should be minimized in the controlled area, and no cardboard should be kept on any shelving. Shelving for plastic bags and glass containers in the controlled area should be easy to clean and provide minimal horizontal surface for particulates to settle. Stainless steel wire shelving units are ideal.

Chairs and Tables

Stainless steel furniture should be standard for the cleanroom because it can be easily cleaned and does not generate particles. For comfort, chairs may be covered with a cleanable vinyl but not porous fabric. Chairs and tables should have wheels so that they can be easily moved to clean and disinfect the flooring.

Carts

Components and final preparations should be moved in and out of critical and controlled areas on large, heavy duty, stainless steel carts. These carts should have 6-inch swivel wheels and brakes. Their shelving should be made of heavy wire (mesh) to prevent the collection of dust and dirt on horizontal surfaces. Cardboard boxes should not be used.

Drugs and supplies should be unpacked from cardboard shipping containers outside the controlled area and then placed on these carts. Once in the controlled area, supplies and drugs can be further opened for patient-specific or batch compounding. These materials can be taken into the critical area on smaller stainless steel carts with smooth surfaces. As an alternative, supplies can be placed on trays or bins and then into the laminar-airflow hood.

Carts for delivery out of the controlled area (to patient areas) should be selected on the basis of size and quantity of the sterile preparations involved. Large quantities of large size sterile preparations should be transported on heavy duty, stainless steel wire carts, similar to those used for supplies in the controlled area.

Locker Facilities

Since personnel compounding sterile preparations should wear special garb (gowns, gloves, masks, etc.), they need a place to change their clothing before entering the cleanroom. This area, with individual lockable storage containers and necessary garb, should be as close to the controlled area as possible. A sink (with floor controls) and soap dispensers for hand washing also should be in this locker area.

Miscellaneous Equipment

Other items that may be useful for compounding sterile preparations are

- A digital readout microwave oven.
- A warming cabinet to store drugs prone to crystallization (e.g., mannitol).
- A balance (i.e., scale) for measuring compounding powders.

Special Equipment for Cytotoxic and Hazardous Drugs

Special equipment is required when cytotoxic and hazardous drugs are compounded.[9] Shelves, carts, counters, and trays must be designed to prevent breakage. Bin shelves must have barriers at the front or other features that keep drug containers from falling to the floor. Appropriate protective apparel (e.g., disposable gloves and long sleeve gowns) must be readily available.

Other supplies such as disposable plastic-backed absorbent liners, gauze pads, cytotoxic waste disposal bags and warning labels, and plastic containers for used needles, ampuls, etc., should be conveniently located. Syringes and IV sets should have Luer-lok fittings.

Spill kits for cleaning up cytotoxic drugs also should be readily accessible. Each kit should include sealable plastic waste disposal bags (appropriately labeled), disposable dust and mist respirators, splash goggles, absorbent sheets or powders, two or more pairs of disposable gloves, and a small scoop for collecting glass fragments.

Cytotoxic drugs should be compounded in a Class II containment cabinet. Whether or not this hood must be vented to the outside atmosphere, however, is still being debated. If a Class II cabinet is unavailable, the drugs should be prepared in a quiet workspace, away from heating and cooling vents and other personnel.

Summary

The maintenance of sterility depends more on technique than any other single factor. Therefore, having the appropriate equipment should not give personnel a false sense of security there is no substitute for good aseptic technique. Nevertheless, appropriate equipment can further minimize contamination of sterile preparations by providing a contaminant-free environment.

The laminar-airflow hood is the most important piece of equipment used to compound sterile preparations; it establishes the critical area for compounding ingredients. Other items (e.g., refrigerators, freezers, and shelving) also must ensure the proper environment for the storage of ingredients and final preparations.

All equipment should be selected on the basis of preventing inadvertent introduction of microbes and particulates into controlled and critical areas.

References

1. Brier KL, Latiolais CJ, Schneider PJ, et al. Effect of laminar air flow and clean room dress on contamination rates of intravenous admixtures. *Am J Hosp Pharm.* 1981; 38:1144–7.
2. Morris AM, PJ Schneider, CA Pedersen, et al. National survey of quality assurance activities for pharmacy-compounded sterile preparations. *Am J Health-Syst Pharm.* 2003; 60(24):2567–76.
3. Brushwood DB. Hospital liable for defect in cardioplegia solution. *Am J Hosp Pharm.* 1992; 49:1174–6.
4. Silverberg JM. Automix error neonatal TPN. *Formul Inf Exch Bull Board.* 1991; Mar 20.
5. Faulty cardioplegia solution leads to $492,000 verdict. *Hosp Pharm Rep.* 1990; 4 (Aug):1.
6. Murphy C. Ensuring accuracy in the use of automated compounders. *Am J Hosp Pharm.* 1993; 50:60. Letter.
7. Silverberg JB, Webb B, Pawlak R. Specific gravity-based determination of dextrose content of total parenteral nutrient solutions for neonates. *Am J Hosp Pharm.* 1993; 50:2090–1.
8. General notices and requirements. In: USP 26 AND NF 21. Rockville, MD: United States Pharmacopeial Convention; 2003:9.
9. American Society of Hospital Pharmacists. ASHP technical assistance bulletin on handling cytotoxic and hazardous drugs. *Am J Hosp Pharm.* 1990; 47:1033–49.

4 | Isolators

Henry Rahe

Isolators are one of the two means of satisfying USP 797 requirements for proper facilities for compounding sterile preparations.[1] Isolators are an alternative to an ISO class 8 (Class 100,000) cleanroom with a ISO class 5 (Class 100) for compounding sterile preparations. Isolation technology has its roots in the following three industries: the nuclear industry, electronics, and health care.

The nuclear industry first developed the technology as a means for safe handling of radioactive materials without exposing personnel, in order to reduce the potential of radiation poisoning. The isolators shielded the radioactive source with lead that would not allow the rays to penetrate. The isolator's function was personnel protection with no concern for the internal isolator cleanliness.

The electronic industry adopted isolation technology to provide a clean environment in which to manufacture, transport, and store microchips. The motivation for use of isolators was productivity through increased yields as any chip on which an airborne particle landed becomes scrap.

The health care industry has adopted isolation technology in several areas. Pharmaceutical companies have utilized the technology for two applications which at times overlap. The first application is for aseptic manipulation of sterile preparations during manufacturing and testing. Isolators provide an environment which reduces the potential for contamination of the preparations by airborne particles during processing operations. The second application is to prevent personnel from coming in contact with hazardous drugs which may be inhaled or absorbed through skin or mucous membranes. Hospital pharmacy is another area in which the health care industry has adopted isolation technology. The initial use of isolators in hospital pharmacy was in the United Kingdom where over 400 isolators are currently in use for both preparation and personnel protection.[2]

Isolation technology for health care applications has developed at a rapid rate since its debut in the 1980s. The progress of this technology is reflected in the health care literature's evolution of recommendations and guidelines. For example, in the 1994 publication *Isolators for Pharmaceutical Applications*,[3] it is recommended that isolators in a hospital pharmacy be located in a separate room, which was a reaction to the misuse and bad design of an isolator. The particular design had a feature that allowed the front wall to be opened. When the wall was opened for cleaning, personnel were exposed to the toxic chemical being used in the isolator. Rather than addressing the design problem that allowed the isolator front to be opened, the authors recommended placing the isolator in a separate room. The Food and Drug Administration published draft pharmaceutical industry guidelines for sterile preparations produced by aseptic processing in 2003.[4] These guidelines identify the use of properly designed isolators as having significant advantages over the more traditional processing methods which employ cleanrooms.

Recommendations in USP Chapter 797 *Pharmaceutical Compounding—Sterile Preparations* also confirm that the use of properly designed isolators offer advantages over cleanrooms.[1] Advantages of the isolators over cleanrooms include flexibility of installation, less initial cost, and lower operating cost (see Chapter 17). The most important advantage, however, is improved sterility assurance from separating personnel from the critical zone for compounding preparations.

Sterility Assurance of Sterile Preparations

Maintaining sterility assurance of parenteral preparations during manipulation is critical to the safety of patients. Pharmaceutical manufacturers seek to achieve a quality assurance level of less than one preparation in one million having potential contamination. This level of sterility can only be achieved by terminal sterilization of the preparation after filling the container. The majority of commercial parenteral products are manufactured using aseptic processing without terminal sterilization due to the inability of many ingredients to withstand the high temperature or other stress of the sterilization process. Sterility assurance levels of preparations produced by aseptic processing are considered to have sterility assurance levels of ten to the minus third or fourth as compared to the ten to minus seven for terminally sterilized preparations. The FDA has acknowledged improved sterility assurance in preparations processed in isolators[4] which reinforces the use of isolation technology in handling sterile preparations by aseptic processing. After the vial or ampoule has been manufactured, the base level of sterility assurance is established and can only be reduced by further manipulation in the health care setting.

Two things are critical to maintaining an aseptic environment in the pharmacy: (1) air quality that is created by HEPA air filtration and (2) sanitization of surfaces to kill microorganisms. An effective sanitization procedure that includes rotation of sanitizing agents, methods of applying sanitizers, and adequate dwell time after application.

Definition of an Isolator

The term isolator has been adopted to describe a controlled environment that is defined by fixed walls, floor and ceiling. Transfers of materials in and out of the environment as well as the interaction technologies are separated by barriers such as gloves, sleeves, and airlocks that prevent the internal environment from being exposed to the surrounding environment's conditions of air quality. An isolator can be defined by the following four elements:

1. The physical structure or the materials that make up the walls, floor, and ceiling;

2. The air-handling system which is made up of the blower and filters;

3. The personnel interaction system which can be glove ports, half suits, or robotics;

4. The material transfer system, that can be airlocks, bag rings, or rapid transfer ports (RTP)

Certain attributes support the specific use of isolators and help to provide additional protection for aseptic processing. For example, positive pressure is required for processing sterile preparations. Additional attributes include the monitoring systems that indicate the isolator is operating within the control parameters, ergonomics that impact personnel fatigue that could lead to errors, and efficiency that impacts both capital and operating costs.

A number of terms that describe similar systems are found in the literature. These include isolators, glove boxes, controlled environments, and class III biological safety cabinets (BSC). Neither terminology nor definition for this class of equipment has been standardized. When comparing equipment called by other terms, it is important to compare both the basic elements and the attributes for the specific application to those described in the isolator definition.

Pharmacy Applications of Isolators

Isolators are used for three primary applications in the pharmacy. The preparation of IV admixtures, total parenteral nutrition (TPN) solutions, and hazardous drugs (Figure 4-1). Each application places different requirements on the configuration of the isolator.

Types of Isolators

Isolators can be defined by either their intended use or physical structure of the shell of the isolator. Intended use usually dictates the pressurization scheme used for secondary protection of preparation or personnel. Positive pressure for sterility or negative pressure for containment are the intended use categories. In the case of hazardous drugs, both containment and the need for sterility exist; so choices must be made regarding pressurization as to whether to provide secondary protection of preparation or personnel during the preparation of hazardous drugs.

The materials of construction of the physical structure are another means of differentiating of isolators. Choices for construction materials fall into two categories: either soft shell (flexible plastic) or hard shell, which could include a variety of materials from rigid plastic to different grades of stainless steel.

This chapter will discuss the use of pressurization as an attribute within the framework of isolators defined by the materials of construction of the physical structure.

Elements of an Isolator

The four elements of an isolator define both its physical appearance and functionality. The functionality of the isolator is dependant on the attributes selected to be incorporated into the equipment.

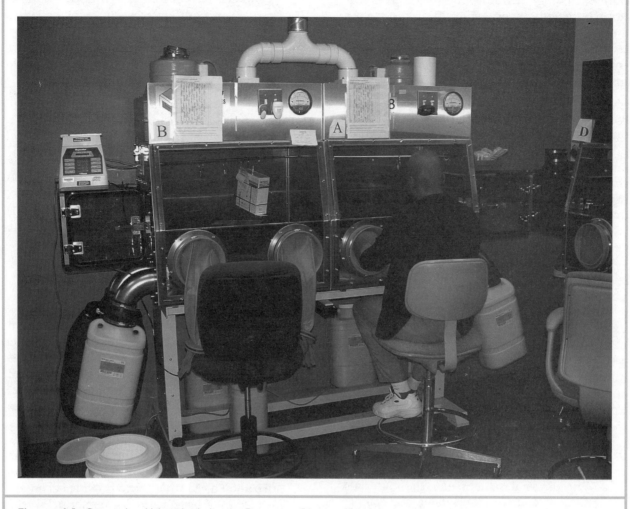

Figure 4-1. Operator Using Isolator to Prepare Chemotherapy

Physical Structure

Flexible isolators are not recommended for pharmacy applications. Rigid isolators are made of rigid plastic, anodized aluminum, 304 stainless steel, or 316L stainless steel. Stainless steel is the recommended material of construction with the author's strong preference for 316L grade. Stainless steel is manufactured in different grades with the number designation usually an indication of higher quality. The "L" indicates higher levels chrome or nickel. The importance of the higher level is that they tend not to leach iron causing corrosions and pitting of the stainless steel. The viewing areas can be fabricated from either glass or engineered plastic.

Air-Handling System

The air-handling system includes HEPA fil-tration both into and out of the isolator with a powered blower to move the air. The two alternative airflows are unidirectional (at one time called laminar) and turbulent flow. Both are acceptable for isolators.[5] However, the volume of airflow within an isolator should be much less than that used for horizontal and vertical directional airflow workbenches and Class II biological safety cabinets.

The laminar air flow workbenches and class II BSC cabinets typically have air movement in the range of 600 to 800 cubic feet per minute and attempt to achieve velocities of 90 feet per minute to meet the requirements of standards such as Federal Standard 209e.

Because isolators totally closed do not require these large volumes or velocities of air, air deflections and eddies are much more likely with higher velocities and volumes of air flow and will create areas that can have little or no airflow. This lack of airflow will create areas within the isolator that can have high particulate counts, increasing the probability of contamination.

Personnel Interaction System

Interaction with the interior of the isolator to perform manipulations of objects inside can be accomplished in any of three ways: (1) through glove ports, (2) half units, or (3) robotics. Each method has advantages and disadvantages.

Glove ports are openings in the isolator wall that have attached sleeves and gloves to allow the user to perform manipulations inside the isolator. This method of interaction has the advantage of ease of use, flexibility of location, and lower cost of replacement materials. Disadvantages include limited range of motion and inability to lift heavy objects. The typical range of motion is 22–24 inches in arc from the centerline of the two glove ports.

Half suits incorporate the upper half of the user's torso. This technology is typically used if expanded reaches or lifting of heave objects is required inside the isolator. The disadvantage of the half suit is that it is typically built into the floor of the isolator and the person entering the half suite must bend and crawl into the suit. Additional issues arise with multiperson use of the same half suit.

Robotics requires exact repetitive motions, extensive training and programming. This alternative is most likely not practical for compounding sterile preparations in the typical pharmacy.

Material Transfer Systems

Material transfer systems include the use of air locks, bag rings or RTPs. The selection of specific technology depends on the particular application requirements for maintaining the internal environment and containment of materials that may exist in the environment.

Air locks act as a buffer or anteroom to the isolator. Therefore the air lock must be independent of each area with a gas tight seal between both the outside and internal environments. Air lock transition zones offer the most flexibility because they can be built to any size required to allow the efficient movement between the external and internal environments. Airlocks also offer the advantage of being rectangular in shape.

Bag rings can be used to transfer materials into and out of the controlled environment of an isolator through a plastic tubular material. This technology is commonly used for containment applications and has several drawbacks for sterile applications. Disadvantages are the inability to sanitize the internal section of the tubing and difficulty in handling materials being introduced or removed because of the circular configuration of the tubing.

RTPs originated in the nuclear industry for transferring radioactive materials. This system offers a closed connection between the receiving vessel and the isolator. The system has been used in some pharmaceutical applications but is expensive to install, slow to operate and expensive to maintain.

Attributes of Isolators

Attributes of isolators are not necessary for functionality but add value in terms of effectiveness of use, safety, and ease of use. Examples of items that are attributes are materials of construction, monitoring systems for pressure differential, pressurization of the isolator, external venting, efficiency of use, ergonomics, and cleanability.

Monitoring Systems for Pressure Differential

Monitoring the pressure differential between the internal pressure of the isolator and the outside environment assures the air-handling system is operating properly. A continuous pressure differential indicates that the isolator has no leaks in any sealed area such as doors, gloves, or disposal systems. The typical monitor is a pressure differential gauge that measures the level of pressure difference between the internal environment of the isolator and the outside room in which the isolator is located. Any leak will cause the pressure to be equalized between the two environments and will alert personnel that the isolator requires attention to correct the problem.

Pressurization

The internal environment of an isolator can be pressurized to be either positive or negative to the surrounding environment. The pressurization acts as a secondary means of protection if there is a breach in the integrity of the isolator.

Positive pressure protects the internal environment from any foreign materials entering the environment if a breach occurs by pushing airflow through the breach toward the outside environment. Negative pressure causes air to be pulled into the isolator.

Isolators used for sterile preparations are recommended to operate with positive pressure.[4] Isolators used for containment of hazardous drugs are recommended to be operated at negative pressure.[1] This creates a dilemma for the preparation of sterile hazardous drugs such as chemotherapy drugs.

Gas-tight construction of the isolator with properly designed airlocks along with proper procedures for glove and sleeve change limits the potential for exposure of the internal environment to the external environment. Either approach will work and it will be up to the regulatory bodies (FDA and OSHA) to select a preferred approach.

The FDA argument is to protect the internal environment of the isolator from outside environment by positive pressure to the outside and an airlock system that would maintain positive pressure. The personnel safety argument is to protect the worker from any potential exposure by using a negative pressure internal environment. To support the negative pressure argument a number of isolators are today operating with negative pressure and maintaining an ISO class 5 environment.

External Venting

The use of external venting is a means of removing the air that passes through the isolator if the air is potentially contaminated with hazardous drugs such as chemotherapy agents. An alternative to venting is a recirculating system that keeps the air internal to the isolator. The recirculating system offers advantages in isolator placement within a facility and operating cost of isolator. Key to the use of recirculating air-handling systems is having a gas-tight environment including the isolator, ductwork and blower. External vented isolators tend to be the units that are moving large volumes of air.

Efficiency in Use of Isolators

Efficiency of isolator use includes functional issues such as the placement of airlocks, the movement of materials into and out of the isolator, placement of hanger bars, removal of

trash and sharps waste, and proper policies and procedures that support the correct use of the isolator.

Ergonomics

Ergonomic design of isolators is critical to effective use of the technology. Design issues, such as the proper height are important to both visibility of the internal environment and personnel fatigue that can occur if the person does not have the proper viewing angle and working height. Background lighting can also cause eye strain and the isolator should be positioned so that overhead lights do not directly reflect off the viewing area.

Ability to Clean

The user's ability to clean the internal surfaces of the isolator is important. Surfaces should be smooth with coved junctures of walls, ceiling and floor to facilitate cleaning. The critical surface is the floor where aseptic manipulations take place and this area should be free of obstructions such as air vent returns. Cleaning of all internal surfaces is critical. Attention should be paid to HEPA filter areas and air vent returns which, if difficult to clean and sanitize, may be a major contributor to contamination that leads to a breach of the aseptic within the isolator. The materials of construction of the isolator should be smooth with all welds ground smooth and polished.

Recommendations for both cleaning and sanitizing the internal environment should come from the manufacturer of the isolator and be consistent with recommended practices and regulatory guidance.

Maintenance of Isolators

Isolator maintenance is critical to the controlled environment necessary for sterile compounding. The sealing sections of the isolator such as the door seals, gloves, and sleeves should be checked daily. A visual inspection should occur at the start of the day and be verified by a comparison of the pressure differential indicated on the gauge to the recommended setting.

A routine schedule should be set for changing gloves and sleeves based on usage level and time. Some isolators use a two-piece glove sleeve system while others use a single glove sleeve. Both systems should be changed based on usage. For high use, the gloves on the two-piece system should be changed at least weekly and the sleeves every 6 months. History of condition should be the most important thing in determination of frequency of change, and if wear becomes apparent the change schedule should be modified.

Hazardous drugs can possibly leach through the glove material. The frequency of glove change for isolators used for this application should be based on usage and thickness of gloves. Gloves should be at least two times the thickness of current disposable gloves used in biological safety cabinets (i.e., 4 microns).

HEPA filters should be checked based on state board of pharmacy requirements. If the HEPA filter requires changing, contact the isolator manufacturer for recommendations as to proper replacement filter and procedures for removal and reinstallation.

Consult the manufacturers' manuals for additional recommendations for type and frequency of maintenance.

Recommended Use Procedures for Isolators

Some manufacturers provide policies and procedures for use of their isolator. Important considerations for use are preparation of materials for entry into the isolator, recommended practices for cleaning and sanitizing, and utilization of any special features includes on the isolator.

Passage of syringes and other support materials into and out of the isolator is critical to the safe and efficient use of the unit. Consult the manufacturer as to recommendations for material handling.

Cleaning is the removal of material form soiled surfaces and requires polices and procedures for frequency and method. The frequency should be based on usage. A designated time should be set to clean the isolator. Cleaning involves wetting of all surfaces with water and a mild detergent. For hard to clean areas a more aggressive preparation may be required. Cleaning is not sanitizing but simply the removal of soil from surfaces so cleaning must be followed with sanitization.

Sanitization is the use of an agent that will kill microorganisms. It is important to select a sanitizing agent capable of destroying a broad range of organisms and rotating it with another agent to prevent organisms from developing resistances to the sanitizing agent. Application of sanitizing agents has been debated in the literature in terms of spray method or wiping. The spray method offers a more uniform application. Length of contact of sanitizing agents is critical to effectiveness. Consult with the supplier of the sanitizing agent as to recommended duration and range of organisms the agent is effective against. Some organisms can live in sanitizing agents such as alcohol. It is good practice to sterile filter sanitizing agents before use.

Manufacturers' Technical Support

Purchasing isolators to be compliant with regulatory facility[6] requirements is a major decision affecting not only capital cost but also operation of the pharmacy sterile compounding area. When evaluating this decision, the technical support provided by the manufacturer of the isolator should be a major factor in the decision process. Technical support in terms of installation, personnel training, documentation and after-purchase service are all factors that should be carefully weighed in the selection process. Bargains in capital equipment such as isolators may turn into long-term problems if these quality issues are not considered initially.

Cost Considerations

Evaluation of cost and feasibility of implementation should be considered in the selection of which alternative best meets regulatory requirements for the individual pharmacy location. The primary evaluation of selecting a cleanroom or isolator alternative should include the total cost, i.e., capital cost, of purchase of equipment, renovation cost and cost to operate the new facility (see Chapter 17).

Operating cost considerations include the cost of disposables such as gowns, gloves, and other disposables required based on technology selection. Additional costs to consider are the costs of operation of the technology including cost of energy and energy back-up systems.

Table 4-1.

Isolator Attributes and Preferred Configurations

Attribute	Preferred Configuration
Physical structure	Rigid structure
Air handling system	HEPA filtration in and out
Personnel interaction system	Glove ports
Material transfer system	Air locks
Materials of construction	316L stainless steel
Monitoring system	Pressure differential gauge

Summary

Isolators are compliant with USP <797> facility requirements and offer a flexible alternative to cleanrooms. Isolator attributes and the authors preferred configurations appear in Table 4-1. Establishing the proper pharmacy configuration to meet the functional needs for capacity to prepare IV admixtures, large-volume parenteral nutritionals, and hazardous drugs is important in determining the number of isolators required to meet needs and capacity requirements of each facility.

References

1. United States Pharmacopeial Convention. Chapter <797> Pharmaceutical Compounding—Sterile Preparations United *States Pharmacopeia 27th Ed./ National Formulary 22nd Rev. First Supplement.* On-line www.uspnf.com. Effective January 1, 2004.

2. Lee GM, Midcalf B, eds. *Isolators for Pharmaceutical Applications.* Printed in the United Kingdom. 1994 Document Number ISBN 0 11 701829 5. pp. 9–10.

3. Lee GM, Midcalf B, eds. *Isolators for Pharmaceutical Applications.* Printed in the United Kingdom. 1994 Document Number ISBN 0 11 701829 5. p. 1.

4. U. S. Department of Health and Human Services. Food and Drug Administration. *Guidance for Industry. Sterile Drug Preparations Produced by Aseptic Processing – Current Good Manufacturing Practices.* August 2003. http://www.fda.gov/cber/gdlns/steraseptic.pdf Accessed November 2003.

5. ASHP. Guidelines on Quality Assurance of Pharmacy-Prepared Sterile Products. *Am J Health-Syst Pharm.* 2000; 57:1150–69.

6. Lee GM, Midcalf B, Editors. *Isolators for Pharmaceutical Applications.* Printed in the United Kingdom. 1994 Document Number ISBN 0 11 701829 5. p. 6.

5 | Personnel Behavior and Garb

E. Clyde Buchanan*

*The author acknowledges Barbara T. McKinnon, who authored this chapter in the previous edition.

By itself, strict adherence to aseptic technique cannot prevent microbial contamination during the compounding of sterile preparations. Personnel behavior and proper garb use are also critical factors and are covered in this chapter. This chapter does not cover the use of personnel protective equipment or garb for handling hazardous drugs (see Chapter 7) or for use with isolators (see Chapter 4); or large compounding equipment (see Chapters 3 and 17); or personnel education about garb (see Chapters 15 and 16).

Personnel Preparation

Proper preparation for performing assigned responsibilities includes personal dress and grooming. Prior to entering the controlled area (i.e., cleanroom or buffer room), personnel should remove outer laboratory jackets and cover both their head and facial hair. Cosmetics that are likely to flake, such as powder and mascara, should also be removed. Similarly, hair spray, perfume, and other scented cosmetics should not be used. Furthermore, finger and wrist jewelry should be minimized or eliminated.[1]

Health Status

Employees involved in compounding should be free of infectious diseases that can be transmitted through contaminated preparations. Especially harmful to the compounding environment are individuals with respiratory ailments accompanied by fluid discharge, sneezing, or excessive perspiration. Similarly, conditions that cause shedding of skin particles, such as rashes and sunburn, increase the risk of contamination. During the period when severely affected, the employee should be excluded from compounding sterile preparations until the condition is remedied, especially for high-risk sterile preparations.[2]

Hand Washing

For nearly 200 years, cleansing hands with an antiseptic agent has been recommended to prevent transmitting contagious diseases to patients.[3] Before compounding, personnel should scrub hands and arms to the elbows with an appropriate cleanser. Although the United States Pharmacopeial Convention[2] (USP) recommends the use of plain soap and

water, the American Society of Health-System Pharmacists[1] (ASHP) and the Centers for Disease Control and Prevention[4] (CDC) suggest an antimicrobial skin cleanser. The CDC Guidelines for Hand Hygiene in Health-Care Settings make the following points that are relevant to compounding sterile preparations:

- Surfaces under fingernails harbor higher concentrations of bacteria than other parts of the hand, even after hand cleansing.

- Artificial nails are more likely to harbor gram-negative pathogens that natural nails, both before and after hand washing.

- Bacteria are transferred to various types of surfaces in much larger numbers from wet hands than from hands that are thoroughly dried.

- Frequent use of hand-hygiene products, particularly soaps and other detergents, is a primary cause of chronic dermatitis among health care workers. Other antiseptic agents cause irritant contact dermatitis (in order of decreasing frequency) including iodophores, chlorhexidine, chloroxylenol, triclosan, isopropyl and ethyl alcohols.

- When hands are visibly dirty, wash hands first with either a non-antimicrobial soap or an antimicrobial soap. If hands are not visibly soiled, use an alcohol-based hand rub for routinely decontaminating hands.

- The effectiveness of gloves in substantially reducing contamination of health care workers hands has been confirmed in several clinical studies. However, wearing gloves does not provide complete protection against hand contamination.

- Gloves should not be reused.

Antimicrobial Cleansing Products

Plain soaps have minimal, if any, antimicrobial activity. Six antimicrobial ingredients are currently are available as hand-washing products[4]:

- *Isopropyl and ethyl alcohol hand rinses, gels, or foams.* Alcohol solutions containing 60%–95% alcohol are the most effective against gram-positive and gram-negative bacteria, various fungi and viruses. Alcohols have poor activity against bacterial spores, protozoan oocysts and non-lipophilic viruses (e.g., hepatitis A). Alcohols have no appreciable residual activity on the skin. Alcohols reduce bacterial counts on hands more than washing hands with cleansers containing povidone-iodine, chlorhexidine, or triclosan. The addition of skin-conditioning agents (e.g., glycerin) to alcohol rinses, gels, or foams results in less skin irritation than soaps and detergents. Moisturizing alcohol hand gels are gaining acceptance as hand cleansing agents of choice in hospitals.[5]

- *Chlorhexidine gluconate* is a cationic bisguanide that is an effective disinfectant but is slower acting than alcohol. Chlorhexidine 2%–4% has good activity against gram-positive bacteria but has somewhat less activity against gram-negative bacteria and fungi, and minimal activity versus tuberculosis bacilli and bacterial spores. Chlorhexidine inactivates enveloped viruses like herpes simplex type 1 and HIV type 1 but is ineffective versus human coronavirus and non-enveloped viruses (e.g., Coxsackie, adenovirus, and polio).[6] Several applications may be required to reduce skin flora significantly. Chlorhexidine has some residual antimicrobial activity. On contact with the eye, chlorhexidine products with greater than 1% concentration cause conjunctivitis and possibly severe corneal damage.

- *Chloroxylenol (also known as PCMX)* is a halogen-substituted phenolic compound. It has good activity against gram-positive bacteria and fair activity against gram-negative bacteria and mycobacteria. Chloroxylenol inactivates enveloped viruses like herpes simplex type 1 and HIV type 1 but is ineffective versus human coronavirus and non-enveloped viruses (e.g., Coxsackie, adenovirus, and polio).[6] Chloroxylenol has less residual activity than chlorhexidine.

- *Iodophors* are iodine combined with polymers like povidone or with poloxamers. They are bacteriocidal against gram-positive, gram-negative and certain spore-forming bacteria and are active against mycobacteria, viruses and fungi. They are not usually sporicidal. There is some residual activity from 1 to 6 hours after hand cleansing. The iodophors cause more skin irritation than the alcohols or other effective skin-cleansing agents.

- *Quaternary ammonium compounds* are composed of a nitrogen atom linked to four alkyl groups (e.g., benzethonium chloride). They are primarily bacteriostatic and fungistatic, are more active against gram-positive than gram-negative bacteria, and are weakly active versus mycobacteria, fungi, and non-lipophilic viruses. Therefore, these compounds are seldom used in hand cleansing.

- *Triclosan* is a trichloro-diphenyl ether that is less effective than the other agents but is mild and may produce some sustained residual activity. The FDA has not found triclosan products to be safe and effective for use as an antiseptic hand wash.

Hexachlorophene was widely used in the 1960s and 1970s but is no longer recommended because of its limited antibacterial coverage and potential toxicity.[4]

When a hand-washing product is chosen to prepare hands for sterile compounding, safety, efficacy, cost, comfort, and the concentration of the active ingredient are the most important considerations. Generally, an institution's infection control committee will select the hand cleansing antiseptic agent for use throughout the institution.

Duration, Frequency, and Preparation

First prepare hands prior to hand washing. Since most microbes come from beneath the fingernails, nails should be trimmed short and scrubbed carefully. Rings should not be worn because they increase bacterial counts on the hands,[7] interfere with washing, and may tear gloves. Other factors that discourage effective hand washing, such as artificial nails and nail polish, also should be avoided.[4] The duration, frequency, and technique of hand washing are all important factors. The CDC makes the following recommendations on hand-hygiene technique[4]:

- When washing hands with soap and water, wet hands first with water, apply an amount of product recommended by the manufacturer to hands, and rub hands together vigorously for at least 15 seconds, covering all surfaces of hands and fingers. Rinse hands with water and dry thoroughly with a disposable towel. Use towel to turn off the faucet. Avoid using hot water because repeated exposure to hot water may increase risk of dermatitis.

- When decontaminating hands with an alcohol-based hand rub, apply product to palm of one hand and rub hands together, covering all surfaces of hands and fingers, until hands are dry. Follow the manufacturer's recommendations regarding the volume of product to use.

- Multiple-use cloth towels of the hanging or roll type are not recommended for use in health-care settings.

- Hand washing is sometimes incorrectly omitted when gloves are worn, the assumption being that they provide enough hand protection. In fact, microorganisms multiply rapidly inside warm moist gloves and then can leak through them. The CDC has stated that gloving does not replace hand washing and that hand washing is imperative after gloves are removed.[8]

Gloves and Gloving

Humans are probably the greatest source of particulate contamination in cleanrooms (Table 5-1). The purpose of cleanroom garb is to contain particles generated from human bodies. Gloves are available in powdered, nonpowdered, sterile, and nonsterile versions. Gloves can be made from latex, neoprene, nitrile, nylon, polyester, polyethylene, polyurethane, or vinyl.[9] Nitrile is a soft, elastic material known for greater puncture and abrasion resistance than latex or vinyl disposable gloves. Vinyl is less expensive. Latex disposable gloves are easily cleaned, cost-effective but are allergenic.

Controversy exists as to whether operators should use sterile gloves during sterile com-

Table 5-1.

Human Particle Generation Rate (Greater than 0.3 Microns per Minute)

Motionless/sitting/standing	100,000
Head, arm, neck, leg motion	500,000
All of above with foot motion	1,000,000
Standing to sitting position and vice-versa	2,500,000
Walking at 2.0 miles per hour	5,000,000
Walking at 3.5 miles per hour	7,500,000
Walking at 5 miles per hourt	10,000,000

Adapted from: Eudy J. Human contamination. *Am Assoc Contain Control.* 2003 (Apr); 6:7–11.

pounding. A primary disadvantage of these gloves is that wearers may believe that the gloves remain sterile during operations when they do not. They contain bacteria-laden particles that may be shed, even from properly scrubbed hands.[2] Actually, the gloves are not sterile once they contact the air outside the laminar-airflow workbench, supplies, work counters, and other surfaces that are clean but not sterile. During extended compounding work, personnel should intermittently resanititize their gloves with 70% isopropyl alcohol.[2]

The ASHP[1] and USP[2] recommend glove use for all risk levels (Table 5-2). When gloves are used, their selection should be based on the type of compounding to be performed as well as on the material's durability, reliability, comfort, allergenicity, and protection from bacteria or hazardous drug penetration. Although gloves made of different materials have comparable barrier properties when removed from the box, their effectiveness as barriers can be compromised by rigorous hand and finger movements. In one study, latex and nitrile gloves held up better than vinyl gloves.[10]

Glove Recommendations

Sterile Versus Nonsterile Gloves

Sterile gloves are recommended for ASHP Risk Levels 2 and 3 compounding activities.[1] Nonsterile gloves, wiped with a disinfectant, may be acceptable for Risk Level 1 compounding or to protect hands during cleaning activities and while handling nonsterile supplies or equipment. During sterile compounding, all gloves should be rinsed thoroughly with a disinfectant (e.g., sterile 70% isopropyl alcohol) and changed if punctured, torn, or contaminated.[1]

Sterile gloves are available packaged in individual pairs or in bulk and in hand-specific or ambidextrous styles. Hand-specific gloves fit more comfortably for long periods, but ambidextrous gloves are cheaper. Individually packaged glove pairs provide better assurance of sterility but at the cost of increased particulates when the paper packaging is opened. Some gloves come in polyethylene bags to minimize particulate shedding.

Powdered Versus Nonpowdered Gloves

Powdered gloves increase the particulate level of filtered air within laminar-airflow work-

Table 5-2.

ASHP Recommendations for Aseptic Compounding Garb

Activity	Clean, Low-particulate Clothing	Gown or Coat with Elastic Cuffs	Hair Cover	Mask	Gloves	Double Gloves	Shoe Covers	Coverall	Approved Resiprator	Goggles
Risk Level 1	X	X	X	X						
Risk Level 2	X	X	X	X	X		X			
Risk Level 3	X		X	X	X		X	X		
Chemotherapy compounding	X	X*				X				X
Chemotherapy spill handling		X†			X		X	X†	X	X

*Disposable.
†Either gown or coverall is acceptable.

benches or other high-efficiency particulate air (HEPA) filtered work stations. A powder residue also can be deposited on supplies, products, and hands. Therefore, powdered gloves are to be avoided.

Latex Versus Non-Latex Gloves†

The CDC makes these statements about latex glove hypersensitivity[11]:

- Since the introduction of universal precautions, the use of latex gloves has become commonplace in health care settings. The increased use of latex gloves has been accompanied by increasing reports of allergic reactions to natural rubber among health care personnel.

- In studies of health care personnel, the reported prevalence of IgE-mediated allergy to latex varies from 2.9% to 17%.

- Allergic reactions may vary from local to systemic, including anaphylactic shock and death.

- Local and systemic reactions to latex may result from direct skin contact or from exposure to airborne latex allergens adsorbed to glove powder.

- Occupational asthma from latex is becoming increasingly recognized. Asthmatic responses to latex may occur early (less than 8 hours) or late (more than 8 hours) after

exposure. Because latex proteins can be aerosolized when powdered gloves are donned or removed, systemic symptoms caused by latex aeroallergens may not be alleviated by simply avoiding latex products, particularly if coworkers of the affected worker continue to use powdered latex gloves.

Some health care authorities recommend using only non-powdered, non-latex gloves.[12] Gloves suitable for a variety of aseptic compounding uses are available from several manufacturers. Good sources for finding aseptic compounding gloves are through your institution's infection control officer, your group purchasing organization, or at the buyers page of *Clean Rooms* (http://cleanrooms.365media.com/cleanrooms/search.asp).

Protective Gloves

See Chapter 7 for a discussion of personal protective equipment including gloves, gowns, and eye and face protection during the handling of hazardous drugs.

Garments

When garments are selected, the preparations to be prepared, type of compounding facility, and cost must be considered. To be most efficient, garments should be appropriate for the

---

†See also Chapter 19.

majority of preparations compounded, with only minor revisions (exception: donning of double gloves for handling hazardous drugs). The effectiveness of garments in preventing human-borne contamination in the environment depends upon garment construction and fabric barrier properties. Garment construction refers to seam containment and closures at the neck, ankles and wrists. Fabrics must provide a barrier for very small particles (e.g., viruses at 0.005 to 1 micron and bacteria 0.3 to 10 microns), must not shed fabric particles and must dissipate electrostatic charges (i.e., reduce static cling). Garments made of nonwoven fabrics are not particularly durable and are usually limited to a single use but they do provide better protection for workers from the material they are handling.[13] Tyvek by DuPont is a commonly-used nonwoven garment material.

Coats

Laboratory coats made of a low-particulate material (e.g., polyester) are adequate for compounding low-risk (Risk Level 1) preparations (lab coats worn elsewhere in the facility are not acceptable for compounding areas). Because of particulate shedding, sleeves should be fitted with elastic cuffs, not ribbed knit fabric.

Sleeve covers are an alternative to lab coats for compounding in a vertical laminar-airflow workbench or biological safety cabinet (BSC). To minimize particulate contamination from clothing, sleeve covers often are worn with clean uniforms ("scrubs").

Gowns and Coveralls

Gowns and coveralls should be made of a low-particulate material that protects against bacterial passage and drug permeability. The tighter the fabric weave, the more particles are contained. However, the tighter the weave, the harder it usually is for the garment to breathe, making the wearer feel warmer.[14]

Newer washable, reusable gowning materials, such as multifilament high-density polyester taffeta, provide comparable bacterial filtration to Tyvek, with improved appearance. The fabric is breathable and so allows the evaporation of perspiration, enhancing worker comfort. These garments can be laundered, withstanding high temperatures and chlorine, and are steam autoclave, ethylene oxide, and gamma radiation compatible for sterilization.

Shoe Covers

Shoe covers should be put on before the feet touch the floor on the "clean" side of a bench or line of demarcation. Most pharmacists use slip-on shoe covers; for high-risk compounding, however, some pharmacists prefer ankle-high booties for complete coverage between pant cuffs and shoes.

Masks

Masks should be donned just prior to work at a horizontal laminar-airflow workbench because normal talking, sneezing, or coughing generates air velocities that exceed the velocity of air from the workbench. Masks are optional in a vertical flow laminar-airflow workbench or BSC where a solid transparent shield establishes a physical barrier between the operator's face and workspace.[2] A tightly fitting surgical mask provides some barrier protection against bacteria, but its protective properties are reduced when wet. Masks should be changed each time personnel leave the compounding area and whenever their integrity is compromised.

Coats, gowns, masks, and shoe covers suitable for a variety of aseptic compounding uses are available from several manufacturers. Good sources for finding aseptic compounding garb are through your institution's infection control officer, your group purchasing organization, or at the buyers page of *CleanRooms* (http://cleanrooms.365media.com/cleanrooms/search.asp).

Gowning

Garb and Garment Selection

Recommendations for aseptic compounding garb are found in Table 5-2. Selection of appropriate garments is based on the risk level (see Chapter 1) of the preparations to be compounded[1] as well as the cleanliness level required in the compounding area.

Risk Level 1 Garb

Low-risk preparations are often compounded in an ISO Class 5 (Class 100) laminar-airflow workbench in a limited-access area. (Note that USP requires an ISO 8 (Class 100,000) cleanroom for low risk level sterile compounding.)

Clean clothing, low in particulates, should be worn. Clothing that produces lint, such as fuzzy sweaters, should be avoided. Some practitioners choose to wear uniforms (e.g., scrub suits), because typical clothing may carry a substantial particulate load after contact with environmental pollutants, cigarette smoke, pets, etc.

For compounding activities, a clean gown or closed coat with elastic sleeve cuffs is recommended.[1] Masks and hair coverings, including beard covers if necessary, should be worn. Hands and arms should be scrubbed to the elbows with an appropriate antimicrobial skin cleanser.[1] Workers in the anteroom or other limited-access area, who are not actually compounding sterile preparations, may wear clean low-particulate clothing and hair covers.

Risk Level 2 Garb

For Risk Level 2 compounding, all requirements for Risk Level 1 should be met. Gloves, gowns or closed coats, hair covers, and masks should be worn. Shoe covers also are recommended to help maintain cleanliness of controlled areas.[1]

Risk Level 3 Garb

For Risk Level 3 compounding, full cleanroom garb is necessary. Attire should consist of a low-shedding coverall, head cover, face mask, and shoe covers as well as sterile gloves. If personnel leave the controlled or support area during compounding, they should regown with clean garments before re-entering.

Gowning Techniques

Proper gowning techniques protect the compounding environment and allow the correct garments to perform optimally. Gowning normally takes place in an anteroom equipped for hand washing and storage of both personal clothes and cleanroom garments. To enter the gowning area, employees should walk over an adhesive mat; this mat removes loose particles from shoes. Outer personal garments are then stored, and scrubs or other uniforms are donned. Jewelry and makeup should be removed, and hands should be washed thoroughly before cleanroom garments are worn.

Gowning Order

Prior to entering the buffer (or clean) room, operators should remove outer lab jackets or similar garments, make-up, and jewelry and should thoroughly scrub hands and arms to the elbow.[2] Then, dry their hands and arms with a lint-free towel.

USP Low- and Medium-Risk Compounding[2]

Ideally, gowning should be performed from the head down before the compounding area is entered.

1. Hair should be covered with a bouffant head cover to confine particles released from hair and to keep hair from protruding into the compounding area.

2. A mask (and beard cover if needed) must be worn.

3. Shoe covers should be donned to capture particles on shoes.

4. The gown or closed coat should then be donned.

5. Gloves should be put on last.

Should the operator need to leave the cleanroom, the coat may be carefully removed at the entrance and hung inside-out for donning on re-entry, but only during the same shift. Hair covers, masks, shoe covers, and gloves should be discarded and new ones donned prior to re-entry.[2]

USP High-Risk Compounding

Typically, the order of gowning for high-risk compounding, assuming shoe covers and a hair cover are in place before the compounding area is entered, would be

1. Hood

2. Face mask

3. Coverall

4. Over-boots or a second pair of shoe covers

5. Gloves

A hood minimizes shedding of particles from the head, particularly if open reservoir mixing is planned. To wear a detachable face mask, the nose piece should be bent first to ensure a snug facial fit and then the strings should be tied on the outside of the hair cover.

Goggles then can be added for eye protection.

For high-risk operations, it is critical to minimize the risk of contamination on gowns or coveralls and other garb to be work in the cleanroom. Fresh clean garb should be donned upon each entry in to the cleanroom to avoid liberating contaminants from previously worn garb. Alternatively, garb that has been worn may be removed with the intention of regarding for re-entry into the cleanroom and stored during the interim under proper control and protection in the anteroom. Garb worn or taken outside the anteroom cannot be worn in the cleanroom.[2]

Preventing Contamination

Cleanroom garments should never touch or drag on the floor as they could carry dirt and particles into the cleanroom. The garment's outside surface should be kept as clean as possible. When coveralls are donned, the hems should be turned up several inches to prevent pant legs from touching the floor. If sterile garments are used for high-risk compounding, personnel should don gloves before handling these garments to protect them from contamination by body secretions and skin flakes.

When donning shoe covers or over-boots for high-risk compounding, some practitioners use a bench between clean and nonclean areas. With both feet on the nonclean side of the bench, a shoe cover is carefully placed on one foot and this leg then is transferred to the clean side. The process is repeated for the other foot.

Finally, cleanroom gloves should be donned. For the first glove, only the upper cuff area should be touched, and as little as possible. Only sterile areas of the second glove should be touched by sterile areas of the previously gloved hand. For maximum reduction of particulate shedding, the second glove should be placed over the sleeve.

Garment Fit and Integrity

Cleanroom garments must fit properly to prevent their billowing as well as the shedding of particles through openings. Garment cuffs should form a snug seal. To check this seal, a noncontaminating pencil-sized object can be slid between the wrist and the cuff with the arm hanging straight down. A properly fitting garment will hold the object. Similarly, if the collar is too large, particles will be emitted. The collar should be snug but not uncomfortable.

The use of rewashable garments has been prompted by environmental concerns. Although scrubs and uniforms can be washed by normal laundry procedures, they should be separated from other contaminated laundry (e.g., patients' linens). Low-particulate coats or coveralls made of tightly woven polyester, may be laundered but only by a special cleanroom laundry service to avoid introduction of particulates. Normally, hair covers, masks, shoe covers, and gloves are disposed after a single use.

Reusable cleanroom garments should be inspected regularly, and any damage should be promptly repaired. Particles may leak through garment holes or from weak and broken garment fibers. Regular inspection and repair will extend a garment's life and help protect sterile preparations from particulates.[15]

Summary

The prevention of contamination in the compounding of sterile preparations requires more than proper aseptic technique. Personnel must ensure appropriate grooming, hand washing, and attire. The use of gloves, gowns, hair covers, masks, and shoe covers is critical in preventing microbial contamination. Both the garments and the gowning technique should be selected based on the risk level of the prepared preparations.

References

1. American Society of Health-System Pharmacists. ASHP Guidelines on quality assurance for pharmacy-prepared sterile products. *Am J Health-Syst Pharm.* 2000; 57:1150–69.
2. United States Pharmacopeial Convention Chapter 797 Pharmaceutical Compounding—Sterile Preparations. *United States Pharmacopeia 27th Ed/ National Formulary 22nd rev., First Supplement.* Official Date, January 1, 2004. On-line version www.uspnf.com. Accessed 04/01/04.
3. Labarraque, A.G. Instructions and observations regarding the use of the chlorides of soda and lime. Porter J. ed. [French]

New Haven, CT: Baldwin and Treadway, 1829.

4. Centers for Disease Control and Prevention. Guidelines for hand hygiene in health-care settings. *Morbidity and Mortality Weekly Report (MMWR)*. 2002; 51 (October 25):1–45.

5. Jones, RD, Jampani J, Mulberry G, Rizer RL. Moisturizing alcohol hand gels for surgical hand preparation. *AORN Journal*. 2000 (Mar);71:584–93.

6. Wood A, Payne D. The action of three antiseptics/disinfectants against enveloped and non-enveloped viruses. *J Hosp Infect*. 1998; 38:283–95.

7. Salisbury DM, Hutfilz P, Treen LM, et al. The effect of rings on microbial load of healthcare workers' hands. *Am J Infect Control*. 1997 (Feb); 25:24–7.

8. Update: universal precautions for prevention of transmission of human immunodeficiency virus, hepatitis B virus, and other bloodborne pathogens in health-care settings. *MMWR*. 1988; 37 (Jun 24): 377–82, 387–8.

9. DeSorbo MA. Getting a handle on gloves. *Cleanrooms* 2002. (Jun) 16:34–6.

10. Rego A, Roley L. In-use barrier integrity of gloves: latex and nitrile superior to vinyl. *Am J Infect Control*. 1999; 27:405–10.

11. Bolyard EA, Tablan OC, Williams WW, et al. Guideline for infection control in health care personnel, 1998. *Am J Infect Control*. 1998; 26:289–354.

12. Keller KM and Altman GB. Practice powder-free and latex safe. *Nurse Practitioner: Am J Primary Health Care*. 2003 (Aug); 28:55–7.

13. Anderson C. One suit fits all. *Cleanrooms*. 2000 (Dec) 14:15–7.

14. Soules WJ. Considerations in garment selection. *Cleanrooms*. 1993; 7:32–8.

15. Goldwater M. The "best-dressed" follow stringent gowning procedures. *Cleanrooms*. 1994; 8:22–3.

6 | Aseptic Technique

Philip J. Schneider

Compounding sterile preparations requires the use of aseptic technique to maintain sterility. Although the term aseptic technique describes sterile techniques used in other areas (e.g., surgery and various medical procedures), this chapter only addresses aseptic technique used in the pharmacy.

While the importance of sterility was first recognized in the late 1800s, the concept of aseptic technique was not described until years later.[1,2] The need to sterilize solutions and equipment became accepted in the 1920s and 1930s.[3-5] Moreover, the development of sterile and pyrogen-free products and their applications continues today.

In the late 1960s, improperly manufactured and compounded IV solutions caused a rash of complications in patients.[6-11] Following these incidents, the National Coordinating Committee on Large Volume Parenterals (NCCLVP) published recommendations for techniques to compounding sterile preparations for pharmacists and other health professionals.[12-18]

A training manual for IV admixture personnel, largely intended for pharmacy technicians who prepare sterile products, was first published in 1972. This manual was revised in 1990.[19]

The American Society of Health-System Pharmacists (ASHP) published a videotape and study guide on aseptic technique.[20] This combination product was the first comprehensive guide to aseptic technique with practical application to many pharmacy settings. ASHP and the United States Pharmacopeial Convention (USP) publish guidelines regarding aseptic technique and further established practice standards for compounding sterile preparations (see Appendixes A and F).[21,22] ASHP's *Manual for Pharmacy Technicians, third edition* also includes a chapter on technician training as it relates to aseptic technique and compounding sterile preparations and ASHP's *Competency Assessment for Health-System Pharmacies, third edition* provides competency tests on the use of aseptic techniques.[23]

Proper Aseptic Technique

Aseptic technique describes the methods used to manipulate sterile products so that they remain sterile. Technique is a separate element in the compounding of sterile preparations, independent from equipment and the environment. Proper technique does not eliminate the need for good equipment and a proper environment. Conversely, good equipment and an ideal environment do not change the need for a good technique.

Equipment and Environment

In this chapter, the laminar airflow workbench (LAFW) is considered critical equipment for good aseptic technique. Issues related to handling and compounding of cytotoxic agents and using a biological safety cabinet are not addressed here, but are covered in Chapter 7. This chapter generally refers to techniques used in a horizontal, not a vertical LAFW. Although these workbenches are similar, the source and direction of the airflow differ. Vertical LAFWs are addressed in Chapter 7.

The critical principle in the use of LAFWs is that nothing should interrupt the airflow between the high-efficiency particulate air (HEPA) filter and the sterile object. This aseptic compounding space is referred to as the "critical area," and any foreign object can increase wind turbulence within this area. Contaminants from the foreign object may be blown or carried onto the sterile injection port, needle, or syringe. Large materials placed within the LAFW also can disturb the patterned flow of air from the HEPA filter. This "zone of turbulence" created behind an object could extend outside the workbench, pulling or allowing contaminated room air into the aseptic environment (Figure 6-1).

When laminar airflow is accessible to all sides of an object, the zone of turbulence extends approximately three times the diameter of that object. When airflow is not accessible on all sides (e.g., adjacent to a vertical wall), a zone of turbulence may extend six times the diameter of an object. For these reasons, objects should be at least 6 inches from the sides and front edge of the workbench, without blocking air vents and without obstructing airflow. Hands also should not block airflow.

The following are general principles for proper operation of LAFWs:

1. All aseptic manipulations should be performed at least 6 inches within the LAFW. This distance prevents reflected contamination from the worker's body and "backwash" contamination from turbulent air patterns developing at the LAFW–room air interface.

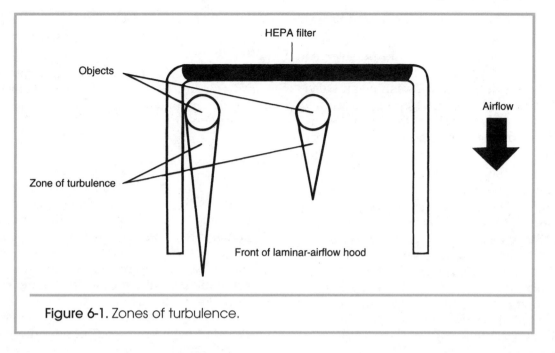

HEPA filter

Objects

Airflow

Zone of turbulence

Front of laminar-airflow hood

Figure 6-1. Zones of turbulence.

2. A LAFW should operate continuously. If the LAFW is turned off, it should not be used for a specified time when reactivated, depending on the manufacturer's recommendations (e.g., 30 minutes). This downtime allows all room air to be purged from the critical area.

3. Before use, all interior working surfaces of the LAFW should be cleaned with 70% isopropyl alcohol or another disinfecting agent and a clean, lint-free nonshedding cloth. Cleaning should be performed from back to front, so that contaminants are moved away from the HEPA filter. Throughout the compounding period, the LAFW should be cleaned often. Some materials are not soluble in alcohol and may initially require water for removal. To avoid damage, Plexiglas sides should be cleaned with warm, soapy water rather than alcohol.

4. Nothing should touch the HEPA filter, including cleaning solution, aspirate from syringes, and glass from ampuls. Ampuls should not be broken directly toward the filter.

5. A LAFW should be positioned away from excess traffic, doors, air vents, fans, and air currents capable of introducing contaminants.

6. Hand and wrist jewelry should not be worn; jewelry may introduce bacteria or particles.

7. Actions such as talking and coughing should be directed away from the critical

area, and any unnecessary motion should be avoided to minimize airflow turbulence.

8. Only objects that are essential to compounding sterile preparations should be placed in the LAFW, no paper, pens, labels, or trays.

9. LAFWs should be tested and certified by qualified personnel every 6 months, whenever the LAFW is moved, and if filter damage is suspected. Tests can certify airflow velocity and HEPA filter integrity.

10. Food and drink should not be permitted within the aseptic preparation area (controlled or critical areas).

Although the LAFW provides a sterile environment, strict aseptic technique must be used to ensure the sterility of the final preparation. The two most critical aspects of aseptic technique are proper hand washing and use and manipulation of syringes, needles, vials, and ampuls.

Hand Washing

Touch is the most common means of contaminating a pharmacy-compounded sterile preparation. Since the fingers harbor bacterial contaminants, hands should be washed properly (see Chapter 5). Before aseptic manipulations are performed, the hands, nails, wrists, and forearms should be scrubbed vigorously for at least 10 to 15 seconds (longer if visibly soiled) with a brush, warm water, and bactericidal soap.[24]

Hand-washing agents should be selected based on their ability to kill microorganisms on the hands at the time of washing and also to provide a residual effect. Isopropyl and ethyl alcohol hand rinses, gels, or foams, or a solution of 4% chlorhexidine gluconate are the best agents for reducing resident flora and transient microorganisms (see Chapter 5).

Results vary with isopropyl alcohol products for initial reduction of microorganisms, but these products clearly have little residual effect. Since most alcohol products are solutions, gels, or foams, they serve as hand disinfectants rather than hand-washing agents. Therefore, hand washing with soap before application of these agents sometimes is recommended. However, this additional step might lower compliance with procedures.

Povidone-iodine products have a slightly lower initial reduction in microorganisms and less residual effect compared to chlorhexidine, but they are acceptable. These products may cause more irritation and allergic reactions than other agents. Triclosan products and hexachlorophene provide poor initial reduction in microorganisms but have a good residual effect. Use of hexachlorophene over large surfaces of the body has been associated with absorption and related toxicity.

Hands should be washed frequently, especially when the compounding area is reentered, to reduce contamination. USP chapter <797> states that personnel should don sterile gloves as the last step in the gowning process.[22] However, gloves are only sterile as long as the wearer does not touch a surface that is not sterile.

In addition to hand washing, aseptic preparation requires the correct use and handling of sterile equipment and supplies, including syringes and needles.

Syringes

Syringes are made of either glass or plastic. Glass syringes are used when medication is to be stored for an extended period and when drug stability requires glass. Disposable plastic syringes cost less and are used when the contact time is short, minimizing the potential for incompatibility with the plastic. Glass syringes made for reuse have virtually been replaced by disposables. Disposables cost less, eliminate the risk of transmitting blood-borne pathogens, and do not break.

Syringes are composed of a barrel and plunger (Figure 6-2). The plunger, which fits inside the barrel, has a flat disk or lip at one end and a rubber piston at the other. The top collar of the barrel prevents the syringe from slipping during manipulation, while the tip is where the needle attaches. Most syringes have a locking mechanism (e.g., Luer Lok) at the tip, which secures the needle within a threaded ring. Manipulations of hazardous drugs requires syringes with this locking mechanism.

Syringes are available in many sizes, with volumes ranging from 0.5 to 60 ml. Graduation marks represent different increments, depending on the size of the syringe. If the sy-

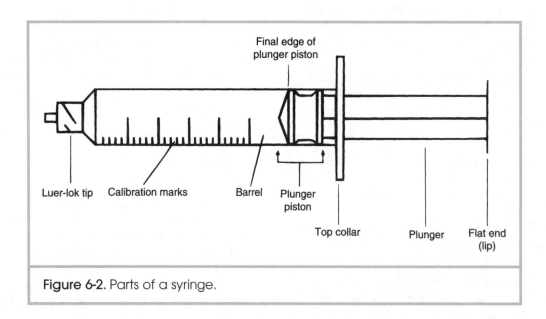

Figure 6-2. Parts of a syringe.

ringe capacity is large, the intervals between graduation lines usually are large. For example, each line on 10-ml syringes represents 0.2 ml; on a 30-ml syringe, each line represents 1 ml.

To maximize accuracy, the smallest syringe that can hold a desired amount of solution should be used. Syringes are accurate to one half of the smallest increment marking on the barrel. For example, a 10-ml syringe with 0.2-ml markings is accurate to 0.1 ml and can be used to measure a volume of 3.1 ml accurately. A 30-ml syringe with 1-ml markings is accurate to 0.5 ml and should not be used to measure a volume of 3.1 ml.

When measuring fluid in a syringe, the user should line up the final edge of the plunger piston to the desired graduation mark on the barrel (Figure 6-3). To maintain sterility, two parts of a syringe cannot be touched: the tip or the plunger.

Syringes are sent from the manufacturer already assembled and individually packaged in paper over-wraps or plastic covers. The sterility of the contents is guaranteed as long as the outer package remains intact. Therefore, these packages should be inspected for holes or tears and discarded if damaged. The syringe package should be opened in the laminar-airflow workbench to maintain sterility. To minimize contamination, however, the discarded packaging should not be laid on any surface within the workbench.

Most syringes also are packaged with a protector over the tip. This protector should be left in place until attaching the needle. When needles are attached to Luer-Lok-type syringes, a quarter turn should secure them.

Needles

Like syringes, needles are commercially available in many sizes. Needle sizes are described by two numbers, gauge and length. The gauge of the needle corresponds to the diameter of its bore. The smallest needles have a gauge of 27, and the largest needles have a gauge of 13. The length of a needle shaft usually ranges from $\frac{3}{8}$ to 3 inches.

The components of a simple needle are the shaft and the hub (Figure 6-4). The hub attaches the needle to the syringe and often is color-coded for a specific gauge size. The tip of the needle shaft is slanted to form a point; this slant is called the bevel, and the point is the bevel tip. The opposite end of the slant is the bevel heel.

Needles are sent from the manufacturer individually packaged in paper and plastic over-wraps. Sterility is guaranteed as long as the package remains intact. Therefore, damaged packages should be discarded. The hub of the needle should not be touched when removing the over-wrap.

A needle shaft usually is metal and is lubricated with a sterile silicone coating for smooth, easy access into rubber closures. Therefore, needles should never be swabbed with alcohol or touched. They should be handled by their

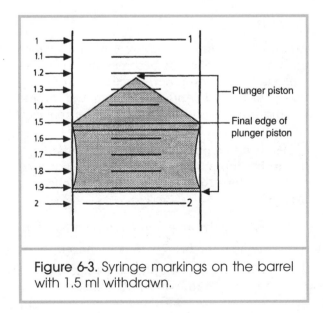

Figure 6-3. Syringe markings on the barrel with 1.5 ml withdrawn.

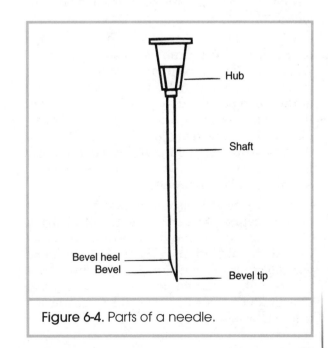

Figure 6-4. Parts of a needle.

protective covers only, and these covers should be left in place until the needles or syringes are used. Used needles should not be recapped, but rather discarded into a sharps container while still attached to the syringe.

Vials

Injectable medications usually are supplied in vials or ampuls, each requiring different techniques for withdrawal of the medication. A vial is a plastic or glass container with a rubber closure secured to its top by a metal ring. Multidose vials contain preservatives that allow their contents to be used after the rubber stopper is punctured. This stopper usually is protected by a flip-top cap or metal cover, but most caps do not guarantee sterility of the rubber closure. Therefore, all vials should be swabbed with 70% isopropyl alcohol before needle entry and left to dry. The correct technique is several firm strokes in the same direction over the rubber closure, using a clean, unused portion of a swab on each pass. The swabbing is effective in two ways:

● The alcohol acts as a disinfecting agent.

● The physical act of swabbing in one direction removes particles from the vial diaphragm.

Bottles or trays of isopropyl alcohol should not be used. Because alcohol may harbor resistant spores, repeated use of a nonsterile tray or bottle could promote this problem. Individually packaged swabs are sterile from the manufacturer.

When vials are pierced with needles, cores or fragments of the rubber closure can form. To prevent this problem, the needle should be inserted so that the rubber closure is penetrated at the same point with both the tip and heel of the bevel. This noncoring technique is accomplished by first piercing the rubber closure with the bevel tip and then applying lateral (away from the bevel) and downward pressure to insert the needle (Figure 6-5).

Vials are closed-system containers, since air or fluid cannot pass freely in or out of them. Therefore, the volume of fluid to be removed from a vial should be replaced with an equal volume of air to avoid creating a vacuum. But this technique should not be used with drugs that produce gas when they are reconstituted (e.g., ceftazidime).

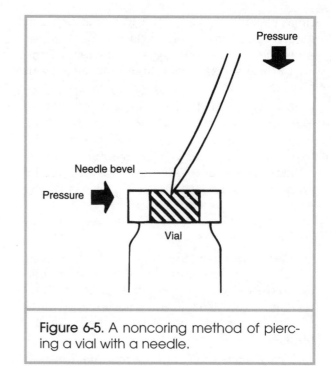

Figure 6-5. A noncoring method of piercing a vial with a needle.

If the drug within a vial is in a powdered form it must be reconstituted first. The desired volume of the diluent (e.g., sterile water for injection) is injected into the vial. As the diluent is added, an equal volume of air must be removed to prevent a positive pressure from developing inside the vial. This procedure may be accomplished by allowing air to flow into the syringe before removing the needle from the vial. Although most drugs dissolve rapidly when shaken, personnel must be sure that a drug is completely dissolved before proceeding.

Ampuls

Ampuls are composed entirely of glass. Once an ampul is broken, it becomes an open-system, single-use container. Since air or fluid may now pass freely in and out of them, the volume of fluid removed does not have to be replaced with air.

Before an ampul is opened, any solution visible in the top portion (head) should be moved to the bottom (body) by one of the following methods:

● Swirling the ampul in an upright position.

● Tapping the head with one's finger.

● Inverting the ampul and then quickly swinging it into an upright position.

To open an ampul properly, its neck should be cleansed with an alcohol swab and the swab should be left in place. This swab can prevent accidental cuts to the fingers as well as spraying of glass particles and aerosolized drug. The head of the ampul should be held between the thumb and index finger of one hand, and the body should be held with the thumb and index finger of the other hand. Pressure should be exerted on both thumbs, pushing away from oneself in a quick motion to "snap" the ampul open at the neck. Ampuls should not be opened toward the HEPA filter of the laminar airflow workbench (LAFW) or toward other sterile products within the workbench. Extreme pressure may result in crushing the head between the thumb and index finger. Therefore, if the ampul does not open easily, it should be rotated so that pressure on the neck is at a different angle.

To withdraw medication from an ampul, it should be tilted and the bevel of the needle placed in the corner space (or shoulder) near the opening. Surface tension should keep the solution from spilling out of the tilted ampul. The syringe plunger is then pulled back to withdraw the solution.

The use of a filter needle (e.g., a needle with a 5-µm filter in the hub) eliminates glass or paint chips that may have fallen into a solution from being drawn up into the syringe. Sometimes, a medication (e.g., a suspension) may need to be withdrawn from an ampul with a regular needle; a filter needle should then be used to push the drug out of the syringe. In all cases, the same filter needle should not be used for both withdrawing and injecting, since it will nullify the filtering effort.

Compounding a Sterile Preparation

Sterile preparations may be compounded in various final containers, including flexible plastic bags, glass bottles, semirigid plastic containers, and syringes, or as the drug vial itself. Flexible plastic bags made of polyvinyl chloride (PVC) or polyolefin are easy to store compared to glass bottles, less likely to break, and do not need to be vented.

PVC bags are available in several sizes and solution types. These bags are supplied in plastic over-wraps, which limit fluid loss. Once this over-wrap is removed, the remaining solution should be used as soon as possible. The injection port of a PVC bag, covered by a protective rubber tip, should be positioned toward the HEPA filter when an IV admixture is prepared. This positioning minimizes air turbulence in the critical area.

Before compounding, all materials should be assembled. Vials, ampuls, and IV solution containers should be inspected for cloudiness, particulate matter, cracks or punctures, expiration dates, and any indications of defects. Only necessary materials should be placed within the LAFW.

Next, all injection surfaces should be disinfected. Drug fluid should be withdrawn from its container in the amount needed, using the syringe size just larger than the volume to be injected. To obtain an accurate measurement, air bubbles should be removed by the following method:

1. Pulling back slightly on the plunger to remove any fluid trapped in the needle.
2. Tapping the syringe.
3. Depressing the plunger.

The instillation of drug into a PVC bag requires insertion of a needle into the alcohol-swabbed injection port and injection of the appropriate volume of fluid. The injection port has two diaphragms that must be pierced (Figure 6-6):

- Outside latex tip.
- Plastic diaphragm about $\frac{3}{8}$ inch inside the injection port.

To ensure fluid transfer into the IV bag, a needle longer than $\frac{3}{8}$ inch should be used.

Adding medication to a glass infusion container begins with removal of the protective cap from the IV bottle. A drug additive then is injected through the alcohol-swabbed rubber stopper or latex diaphragm. Needles should be inserted through rubber stoppers using the non-coring technique previously described for vials. Following admixture, a protective seal is placed over the stopper of a glass container before it is removed from the laminar-airflow workbench.

If the final sterile preparation is in a syringe, the needle used in compounding should be removed and discarded. The syringe should then be capped with a sterile tip. A small volume of air or overfill may be left in the syringe

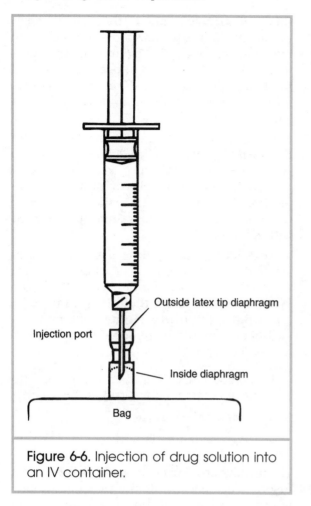

Figure 6-6. Injection of drug solution into an IV container.

for priming the needle or tubing before administering the dose. The syringe should be placed in a plastic bag or other container for transport, which minimizes the potential for plunger depression and/or leakage.

Syringes and needles used in the compounding of a sterile preparation should be discarded according to institutional policy. Syringes and needles (uncapped to prevent accidental needlestick) should be placed into a puncture-resistant, sealable container for proper disposal (usually incineration).

Once the sterile preparation is compounded, it should be properly labeled and inspected for cores and particulates. All drug and IV solution containers should be checked by a pharmacist to verify that the technician added the proper amount of the correct drug to the correct IV solution and the correct label affixed to the compounded preparation. Aseptic technique is slightly different for compounding hazardous sterile preparations (see Chapter 7).

Summary

Aseptic technique is a means of compounding sterile preparations without contaminating them. Proper use of the LAFW, strict aseptic technique, and conscientious work habits are the most important factors in preventing contamination. To ensure accuracy and completeness, the label and final product must be validated by a registered pharmacist before use.

References

1. Griffenhagan GB. The history of parenteral medication. *Bull Parenter Drug Assoc.* 1962; 16:129.
2. Howard-Jones N. The origins of hypodermic medication. *Sci Am.* 1971; 224:96–102.
3. Seibert FB. Fever producing substances found in distilled water. *Am J Physiol.* 1923; 67:90–104.
4. Masson AH. The early days of intravenous saline. *Pharm J.* 1976; 217:571–80.
5. Dudrick SJ. Rational intravenous therapy. *Am J Hosp Pharm.* 1971; 28:82–91.
6. Maki DG, Goldmann DA, Rhame FS. Infection control in intravenous therapy. *Ann Intern Med.* 1973; 79:867–87.
7. Deeb EN, Natsios GA. Contamination of intravenous fluids by bacteria and fungi during preparation and administration. *Am J Hosp Pharm.* 1971; 28:764–7.
8. Letcher K. In use contamination of intravenous solutions in flexible plastic containers. *Am J Hosp Pharm.* 1972; 29:673–7.
9. Curry CR, Quie PG. Fungal septicemia in patients receiving parenteral hyperalimen-tation. *N Engl J Med.* 1971; 285:1221–5.
10. McGowan JE. Six guidelines for reducing infections associated with IV therapy. *Am Surg.* 1976; 42:713–5.
11. Duma RJ, Latta T. What have we done—the hazards of intravenous therapy. *N Engl J Med.* 1976; 294:1178–80.
12. National Coordinating Committee on Large Volume Parenterals. Recommended methods for compounding intravenous admixtures in hospitals. *Am J Hosp Pharm.* 1975; 32:261–70.

13. National Coordinating Committee on Large Volume Parenterals. Recommended system for surveillance and reporting of problems with large-volume parenterals in hospitals. *Am J Hosp Pharm.* 1975; 32:1251–3.

14. National Coordinating Committee on Large Volume Parenterals. Recommendations for the labeling of large volume parenterals. *Am J Hosp Pharm.* 1978; 35:49–51.

15. National Coordinating Committee on Large Volume Parenterals. Recommended procedures for in-use testing of large volume parenterals suspected of contamination or of producing a reaction in a patient. *Am J Hosp Pharm.* 1978; 35:678–82.

16. National Coordinating Committee on Large Volume Parenterals. Recommended guidelines for quality assurance in hospital centralized intravenous admixture services. *Am J Hosp Pharm.* 1980; 37: 645–55.

17. National Coordinating Committee on Large Volume Parenterals. Recommended standards of practice, policies, and procedures for intravenous therapy. *Am J Hosp Pharm.* 1980; 37:660–3.

18. Barker KN, ed. *Recommendations of the NCCLVP for the Compounding and Administration of Intravenous Solutions.* Bethesda, MD: American Society of Hospital Pharmacists; 1981.

19. Hunt ML Jr. Training manual for intravenous admixture personnel, 4th ed. Chicago, IL: Baxter Healthcare Corp.; 1990.

20. American Society of Hospital Pharmacists. Aseptic preparation of parenteral products. Bethesda, MD: American Society of Hospital Pharmacists; 1985. Videotape and study guide.

21. American Society of Hospital Pharmacists. ASHP guidelines on quality assurance for pharmacy-prepared sterile products. *Am J Hosp Pharm.* 2000; 57:1150–69.

22. United States Pharmacopeial Convention Chapter 797 Pharmaceutical Compounding—Sterile Preparations. *United States Pharmacopeia 27th Ed/ National Formulary 22nd rev., First Supplement.* Official Date, January 1, 2004. On-line version www.uspnf.com. Accessed 04/01/04.

23. American Society of Health-System Pharmacists. *Manual for Pharmacy Technicians*, second edition. Bethesda, MD: American Society of Health-System Pharmacists; 1998.

24. Guideline for hand hygiene in health-care settings. *Morbidity and Mortality Weekly Report.* 2002;51(RR)16:1–44.

7 | Handling, Compounding, and Disposal of Cytotoxic and Hazardous Drugs

*Luci A. Power**

*The author acknowledges Douglas J. Scheckelhoff, who authored this chapter in the first edition of this text.

Introduction

Concern regarding the safety of workers handling cytotoxic drugs initially surfaced in the 1970s when reports of second cancers in patients treated with these agents were coupled with the discovery of mutagenic substances in nurses who handled these drugs and cared for treated patients.[1-3] The non-specific nature of the cytotoxic action of these drugs renders all cells at risk of DNA damage. This damage may be repaired by normal cell mechanisms or it may cause cell death or cell mutation, possibly leading to cancer.[4] Exposure to these drugs in the workplace has been associated with acute and short-term reactions. Anecdotal reports in the literature range from malaise and flu-like symptoms to hair loss, nail damage and mucosal sores.[5-8] Reproductive studies on health care workers have shown an increase in fetal abnormality, fetal loss and fertility impairment resulting from occupational exposure to these potent drugs.[9-12] Increased incidence of cancers for these exposed groups has been investigated with varying success.[13,14] The small number of individuals available for study presents a dilemma for the statistician.

To reduce the amount of exposure to workers, numerous groups promulgated guidelines to improve the methods in which these drugs were handled in the workplace. The Occupational Safety and Health Administration (OSHA), the National Institutes of Health (NIH), the Oncology Nursing Society (ONS), and the American Society of Health-System Pharmacists (ASHP) developed recommendations for the safe handling of these agents in numerous health-care settings.[15-18] While the guidelines differ in some respects, the general principles and goals are very similar: establish and maintain stringent work practices within a framework of engineering controls and personal protective equipment to reduce the amount of drug released into the environment during manipulation. Subsequently, this reduction in available drug will reduce the potential exposure to personnel as well.

Despite the implementation of these guidelines in the mid-1980s, continued research of areas where cytotoxics are manipulated shows both environmental contamination and worker contamination. Numerous studies conducted in Europe report contamination on drug vials, work surfaces, gloves and final product

that has been transferred to workers, validated by measurement of drug in the urine of workers who are both directly and superficially involved in the handling of these drugs.[19-28]

In 1999, a multi-center study [29] conducted in the United States and Canada documented surface contamination in both compounding and administration of hazardous drugs utilizing published safe-handling equipment, personal protection and work practices. While no single method of measuring and monitoring contamination and exposure has been found to be uniformly acceptable or useful,[30] the numerous positive findings along with the documented surface contamination require a reevaluation of the recommendations for the safe handling of hazardous drugs.[31]

Defining Hazardous Drugs (HDs)

Hazardous drugs include antineoplastic or cytotoxic agents, biologic agents, antiviral agents and immunosuppressive agents.

Federal Hazard Communication Standard (HCS)

The Federal Hazard Communication Standard (HCS) [32,33] defines a "hazardous chemical" to be any chemical which is a physical hazard or a health hazard. It further defines a "health hazard" to be a chemical for which there is statistically significant evidence based on at least one study conducted in accordance with established scientific principles that acute or chronic health effects may occur in exposed employees. The HCS further notes that the term "health hazard" includes chemicals, which are carcinogens, toxic, or highly toxic agents, reproductive toxins, irritants, corrosives, sensitizers, and agents that produce target organ effects.

Hazardous Drug Criteria

In 1990, ASHP selected the following criteria for determining the hazardous nature of a drug:[18] Drugs that may represent occupational hazards include any that exhibit the following characteristics:

1. Genotoxicity (i.e., mutagenicity and clastogenicity in short-term test systems);

2. Carcinogenicity in animal models, in the patient population, or both, as reported by the International Agency for Research on Cancer (IARC);

3. Teratogenicity or fertility impairment in animal studies or in treated patients; and

4. Evidence of serious organ or other toxicity at low doses in animal models or treated patients.

The National Toxicology Program[34] and the International Agency for Research on Cancer[35] (IARC), classify drugs according to carcinogenicity. Antineoplastic drugs, as well as, antibiotics and immunosuppressants are included in their lists of known or suspected human carcinogens.

NIOSH/NORA Group

In 2000, the National Institute for Occupational Safety and Health (NIOSH) in conjunction with the National Occupational Research Agenda (NORA) convened a group of individuals interested in occupational exposure to hazardous drugs. The resulting working group includes representation from government (OSHA, NIOSH, FDA), industry, pharmaceutical manufacturing, academia, membership organizations (such as ASHP and ONS) and union leaders whose members handle hazardous drugs. The goals of the working group are to assess existing information on occupational exposure, increase awareness of the risks to the affected workers, and determine appropriate plans of action to reduce these risks. In 2004, NIOSH issued a Hazardous Drug Alert, the result of this working group. A pre-publication version is available on the NIOSH website at: http://www.cdc.gov/niosh/docs/2004-HazDrugAlert/pdfs/2004-HazDrug Alert.pdf. In addition, NIOSH plans continuing research into the sources of contamination.

Recommendations

Policies and Procedures—Material Safety Data Sheets (MSDS)

Policies and procedures for the safe handling of hazardous drugs must be in place for all situations where these drugs are in use throughout a facility. A comprehensive safety program must be developed that deals with all aspects of the safe handling of hazardous drugs. A key element of this safety program is the Material Safety Data Sheet (MSDS) mandated by the HCS.[32] Employers are required to have an MSDS available for all hazardous agents located in the work place. A comprehensive safety program must include a process for monitoring and updating the MSDS database. When a hazardous drug is purchased for the first time, an MSDS must be requested and received from the manufacturer or distributor of this drug. The MSDS should define the appropriate handling precautions, including protective equipment, controls, and spill management associated with the drug.

Drugs that have been identified as requiring safe handling precautions, should be clearly labeled at all times during their transport and use. The Hazard Communication Standard applies to all workers, including those handling hazardous drugs at the manufacturer and distributor level. Appropriate controls should be in place to ensure safe distribution of these drugs. Cartons of such drugs transported from manufacturer or distributor should be labeled with an acceptable identifier to notify personnel receiving them to wear appropriate personal protective equipment when opening them. Sealing these drugs in plastic at the distributor level provides additional safety for workers who are required to unpack cartons. Examination of such cartons for any outward sign of damage or breakage is an important first step in the receiving process. Policies and procedures must be in place for handling damaged cartons or containers of hazardous drugs. These may include returning the damaged goods to the distributor following appropriate containment techniques. Any handling of damaged hazardous drugs must be done using appropriate protective controls, including gloves and respiratory protection. Staff engaged in this practice must be fit tested for the appropriate respirator and respirators must be available at all times.[36]

Label/Packaging from Point of Receipt

Hazardous drugs should be separated from other drugs. Drug packages, bins, shelves and all storage areas of hazardous drugs must bear distinctive labels identifying them as requiring special precautions. Segregation of hazardous drug inventory improves control and reduces the number of staff members potentially exposed to the danger. Hazardous drugs placed in inventory must be protected from potential breakage by storing in bins that have high fronts and on shelves that have guards to prevent accidental falling. The bins must also be appropriately sized so as to properly contain all stock. Care should be taken to separate inventory to reduce potential drug errors (e.g., pulling a look-a-like vial from an adjacent drug bin). As studies have shown that contamination on the drug vial itself is a consideration, all staff members must wear gloves when doing stocking, inventory control or when selecting drug packages for further handling. All transport of drug packages must be done in sealed containers to reduce contamination in the event of accidental dropping.

Environment

The compounding of hazardous drugs should be done in a controlled area, preferably centralized, where access may be limited to authorized personnel, trained in handling requirements. Due to the hazardous nature of these preparations, an environment where air pressure is negative to the surrounding areas is preferred. Positive pressure environments should be avoided due to the potential spread of contamination from poor technique or spills. Potentially contaminated air from compounding areas should be exhausted to the outside using appropriate ventilation techniques.

Only individuals trained in the administration of hazardous drugs should do so, and only in a controlled area. Access should be limited to those patients receiving therapy and essential personnel. Eating, drinking, and the presence of foodstuffs should all be avoided in areas where hazardous drugs are being handled.

Because much of the compounding and administration of hazardous drugs throughout the United States is done in outpatient or clinic settings with the patients and their family members proximal to the mixing area, care must be taken to minimize the contamination and to maximize the effectiveness of cleaning (decontamination) activities. Design of such areas must include surfaces that are readily cleaned and decontaminated. Avoid uphol-

stered and carpeted surfaces, as they are not readily cleaned. Several studies show floor contamination and ineffectiveness of cleaning practices on floors and surfaces.[22,29,37] Locating break areas and refreshment areas for staff, patients and others away from areas of potential contamination is critical in reducing unwanted exposure.

Ventilation Controls

Ventilation or engineering controls are devices designed to eliminate or reduce worker exposures to chemical, biological, radiological, ergonomic or physical hazards. Ventilation controls are also used to provide the critical environment necessary to compound sterile preparations (see Chapter 17).

In the early 1980s the Class II, Biological Safety Cabinet (BSC) was determined to reduce exposure to pharmacy staff compounding hazardous preparations when measured by the mutational response to the Ames test by urine of exposed subjects.[38,39] Studies in the 1990s, using analytical methods significantly more specific and sensitive than the Ames test, indicate that environmental and worker contamination occurs in work place settings despite the use of ventilation controls recommended in published guidelines, which include the use of the Class II, Biological Safety Cabinet (BSC).[19-24,26-29] The exact cause of contamination has yet to be determined. Studies have shown that there is contamination on the outside of vials received from the manufacturer or distributor;[22,25] that work practices required to maximize the effectiveness of the Class II BSC are unknown or neglected;[24,37] and that a possibility of vaporization of hazardous drug solutions exists which puts the effectiveness of the HEPA filter in providing containment in question.[39-43] Many studies of surface contamination have discovered deposits of hazardous drugs on the floor in front of the BSC indicating the escape of drug through the open front of the Class II BSC.[22,23,29]

Class II Biological Safety Cabinet (BSC) Concerns

It is imperative that workers understand and accept that the Class II BSC does not prevent the generation of contamination within the cabinet and its effectiveness in containing that contamination is technique dependent.

The Class II BSC, depending on the type, may have recirculating airflow within the cabinet and exhaust of contaminated air back into the work environment through HEPA filters.[44] The Class II BSC is designed with air plenums that are unreachable for surface decontamination; the plenum under the work tray collects room dirt and debris that mixes with hazardous drug residue when the BSC is operational.[18] Drafts and other laminar airflow equipment placed near the BSC can further damage the containment properties of the inflow air barrier resulting in contamination of the work environment.[45]

Recommendations for Use of Class II BSC

The use of a Class II BSC must be accompanied by a stringent program of work practices including, training, demonstrated competence, contamination reduction, ancillary devices (such as PhaSeal) and decontamination. Only Class II BSC with outside venting should be used for compounding hazardous drugs; type B total exhaust is preferred.

Class II BSCs are not recommended in traditional, positive pressure, clean rooms where the hazardous drug contamination may be spread from the open front to the surrounding areas.

Class III BSCs and Isolators (See Chapter 4)

An alternative ventilation control measure to the Class II BSC, the Class III BSC and/or isolator, has become increasingly popular as a way to avoid the complications of a traditional clean room and some of the disadvantages of the Class II BSC.[46-49] The totally enclosed design reduces the escape of contamination during the compounding process. The isolator is not sensitive to drafts and other laminar airflow equipment, including positive pressure environments. Many isolators produce less heat and noise than Class II BSCs.[46]

The isolator, as the Class II BSC, does not prevent the generation of contamination within it and its effectiveness in containing that contamination is still technique dependent. Contamination from the work area of the isolator may be brought into the room work environment through the "pass throughs" and on the surfaces of items placed in and removed from the isolators (final preparation). Appropriate arrangement of preparation into the pass through, coupled with wipe down of preparation before removal, is essential to reduce contamination of the workroom.[46] Recirculating isolators depend on HEPA filters, which may not be sufficient to remove contamination from the airflow. Isolators discharging contaminated air into the workroom through HEPA filters are no more effective than unvented Class II BSCs if the contamination vaporizes. Isolators used for compounding hazardous drugs must be at negative pressure to the surrounding areas to improve containment of contamination. Most isolators provide low-particulate environments for the protection of sterility of the preparations, not laminar airflow technology. Isolators should be more readily surface decontaminated than Class II BSCs.

Recommendations for the Use of Class III BSCs or Isolators

Only a ventilated cabinet designed to protect workers and adjacent personnel from exposure and to provide product protection may be used to compound sterile hazardous drugs.

Only Class III BSCs or isolators that are under negative pressure to surrounding areas should be used to compound sterile hazardous drugs.

The use of a Class III BSC or isolator must be accompanied by a stringent program of work practices including training, demonstrated competence, contamination reduction, closed system drug transfer devices (e.g., PhaSeal), and decontamination.

Decontamination of the Class III BSC or isolator must be done in a way that contains any surface contamination during the cleaning process. Gauntlets must not be removed, nor the cabinet accessed via pass-throughs or removable front panels, without completion of appropriate decontamination within the cabinet. Surface decontamination of final preparations must be done before placing sterile hazardous drugs into a transfer bag for removal from the cabinet.

After decontamination, clean gloves must be used to handle and label final preparations.

Ancillary Devices

Closed-system, Drug Transfer Devices

Closed-system, drug transfer devices are currently available for many injectable antibiotics. The ADD-Vantage[†] and Duplex[‡] are devices that allow the antibiotics to be transferred to the carrier solution in a closed system, avoiding contamination of the environment with active drug. A similar system that may offer increased environmental protection for hazardous drugs is a proprietary, closed-system drug transfer device known as PhaSeal.[§] This multicomponent system uses a double membrane to enclose a specially cut injection cannula as it moves into a drug vial, Luer Lock, or infusion set connector. The primary component, the "Protector," assembly fits snugly and permanently over a standard vial top and pierces the septum via a large bore air cannula, which serves to equalize pressure during compounding. An expansion chamber contains excess air pressure as reconstitution and withdrawal is completed, thus preventing escape of aerosols generated during reconstitution. The same double membrane is incorporated into the "Injector," "Adaptor," and "Connector." The Connector and Adaptor are used during drug administration. The Adaptor provides a dry connection for accessing an IV bag with an administration set. This allows retrograde priming to be done with little chance of generating contamination.

Several studies have shown reduction in contamination during both compounding and administration as compared to pre PhaSeal use.[50-53] Spivey and Connor used a visual fluorescent technique to demonstrate the effectiveness of PhaSeal.[54] Based on these data, the PhaSeal system appears to reduce environmental contamination with some hazardous drugs. However, the PhaSeal components cannot be used to compound all hazardous drugs. Certain drug vials will not accept the protective cap; PhaSeal provides no devices for drugs packaged in ampuls; and the Adaptor is un-vented and may not be used with glass containers.

[†]ADD-Vantage, Abbott Laboratories, North Chicago, IL.

[‡]Duplex, B. Braun Medical Inc., Irvine, CA.

[§]PhaSeal®, Carmel Pharma ab, Goteborg, Sweden. Distributed by BAXA, Denver, CO.

Many devices labeled as "chemo" adjuncts are currently available. Most utilize a filtered, vented spike to facilitate reconstituting and removing of hazardous drugs during the compounding process. It must be noted that none of these devices can be considered a closed-system transfer, and none has, to this point, been subjected to the rigorous testing that PhaSeal has to demonstrate its effectiveness in reducing environmental contamination. In 1984, Hoy and Stump[55] concluded that a commercial air-venting device reduced the release of drug aerosols during reconstitution of drugs packaged in vials. The testing was done only by visual analysis, however, not with the sensitivity or specificity of the analysis done of PhaSeal. In addition, the researchers concluded that the performance of the device was dependent on using the appropriate technique. Several drug manufacturers have labeled their vials against the use of a dispensing pin for fear that the spike may damage the vial septum, thus causing environmental contamination and possibly damaging the sterility of the vial.

Working in the BSC/Isolator

With or without ancillary devices, none of the available ventilation or engineering controls is perfect. Workers must recognize the limitations of the equipment and accommodate them with appropriate work practices.[18]

- Do not place unnecessary items in the work area of the cabinet or isolator where contamination from compounding may settle on them.

- Do not overcrowd the BSC/isolator.

- Transport bags must never be placed in the BSC/isolator during compounding to avoid inadvertent contamination of the outside surface of the bag.

- Decontaminate the work surface of the BSC/isolator before and after compounding with detergent or hypochlorite solution and neutralizer.

- Decontaminate all surfaces of the BSC/isolator with detergent or hypochlorite solution and neutralizer at the end of the batch, day or shift as appropriate to the workflow. Typically, a cabinet/isolator in use 24 hr per day would require decontamination two to three times a day.

- Wipe down the outside of the Class II BSC front opening and the floor in front of the

BSC with hypochlorite solution/neutralizer daily.

- Seal, then decontaminate surfaces of waste/sharps container before removing from the BSC/isolator.

- Decontamination is required following any spill in the BSC/isolator during compounding.

Personal Protective Equipment

Gloves

Gloves are essential for handling hazardous drugs. Gloves must be worn at all times when handling drug vials, including while performing inventory control procedures and when assembling hazardous drugs and supplies for compounding either a batch or a single dose.

During compounding in a Class II BSC, gloves and gowns are required to prevent skin surfaces from coming into contact with these agents. New studies on gloves indicate that many latex and non-latex materials are effective protection against penetration by most hazardous drugs.[56-59] Recent concerns about latex sensitivity have prompted testing of newer glove materials (see Chapter 19). Gloves made of nitrile, neoprene, and polyurethane have been successfully tested against a battery of antineoplastic drugs by several researchers.[58,59] Connor and Xiang[60] studied the effect of isopropyl alcohol on the permeation of latex and nitrile gloves exposed to antineoplastic agents. During the limited study period of 30 minutes, they found that the use of isopropyl alcohol for cleaning and decontaminating did not appear to affect the integrity of either material.

In most glove test systems, the glove material is static as opposed to the stressing and flexing that occurs to gloving material during actual use. In a study designed to examine permeation under static and flexed conditions, no significant difference in permeation was reported except in thin latex examination gloves.[61] A second study, however, detected permeation of antineoplastics through latex gloves during actual working conditions by using a cotton glove under the latex glove.[23] The breakthrough time for cyclophosphamide was only 10 minutes. The authors speculate that the cotton glove may have produced a wicking effect. Nonetheless, under actual working conditions, double gloving and wearing gloves no longer than 30 minutes is a prudent practice.

Permeability of gloves to the hazardous drugs has been shown to be dependent on drug, gloving material, thickness of gloves and exposure time. Powder-free gloves are preferred both to avoid contamination of the sterile processing area with powder particulates and to prevent absorption of contaminants by the powder resulting in the potential for increased dermal contact. Hands should be thoroughly washed before putting on gloves and after removing them. Care must be taken in removing gloves.

Several studies[22-24,26] indicate that contamination of the outside of gloves is common following compounding and that this contamination on the outside may be spread to other surfaces during the compounding process. Studies also indicate that this contamination may lead to dermal absorption by workers not actively involved in the compounding and administration of hazardous drugs.[22,62]

The use of two pairs of gloves is recommended for compounding. The outer glove should be removed once compounding has been completed and the final preparation wiped off. If an IV set is attached to the final preparation in the BSC or isolator, care must be taken to avoid contaminating the outside of the tubing. The inner glove is worn to affix labels and place the preparation into a sealable containment bag for transport. (Note: Transport bags must never be placed in the BSC during compounding to avoid inadvertent contamination of the outside surface of the bag.)

During batch compounding, gloves should be changed at least every 30 minutes. Gloves (at least the outer glove) must be changed whenever it is necessary to come out of and re-enter the BSC. For protection of the preparation, the outer glove should be sanitized when re-entering the BSC. Gloves must also be immediately changed if torn, punctured or contaminated. When wearing two pairs of gloves, one pair is worn under the gown cuff and the second pair placed over the cuff. When removing the gloves, the contaminated glove fingers must only touch the outer contaminated surface of the glove, never the inner surface. If the inner glove becomes contaminated then both pairs of gloves must be changed.

When removing any personal protective equipment, care must be taken to avoid putting contamination into the environment. Both the inner and outer gloves should be considered contaminated and glove surfaces must never touch the skin or any surface that may be touched by the unprotected skin of others. Gloves should be placed in a sealable plastic bag for containment prior to disposal.

Class III BSCs and isolators are equipped with attached gloves or gauntlets. These should be considered contaminated once the cabinet or isolator has been used for compounding hazardous drugs. Contamination from the gloves/gauntlets may be transferred to the surfaces of all items within the cabinet. Gloves/gauntlets must be surface cleaned after compounding is complete. All final preparations must be wiped off by staff, wearing clean gloves to avoid spreading the contamination. In one report on isolator use for handling hazardous drugs, the author notes that an additional pair of powder free, non-latex gloves is worn during compounding.[46]

Glove Recommendations

- Select powder-free, good quality gloves made of latex, nitrile, polyurethane, neoprene, or other materials that have been tested with hazardous drugs.

- Inspect gloves for visible defects.

- Wear double gloves for compounding.

- A single pair of good quality gloves should be sufficient for administration.

- Change gloves every 30 minutes during compounding, or immediately when damaged or contaminated.

- Change gloves after administering a dose of hazardous drugs or when leaving the immediate administration area.

- Remove outer glove after wiping down final preparation but before labeling or removing the preparation from BSC.

- In an isolator, gloves/gauntlets must be surface cleaned after compounding is complete and final preparation has been wiped down.

- Don fresh gloves to remove final preparation from pass through, label, and place in clean transport bag.

- Wash hands before gloving and after removing gloves. Remove gloves with care to avoid contamination.

- Contain and dispose of contaminated gloves as hazardous waste.

Gowns

The use of gowns or coveralls in the compounding of sterile preparations is to avoid inadvertent contamination of particulates from the clothes or skin of workers. Guidelines for the safe handling of hazardous drugs recommend the use of gowns for compounding in the BSC, administration, spill control and waste management to protect the worker from contamination by any residue generated during the handling process.[15-18]

Existing criteria for appropriate barrier protective gowns are that they provide adequate protection from hazardous drugs, are disposable, made of a lint-free, low-permeability fabric with a solid front, long sleeves, and tight fitting elastic or knit cuffs.[18] Washable garments, such as lab coats, scrubs and cloth gowns, absorb fluids and provide no barrier to hazardous drug absorption.

Recent studies into the effectiveness of disposable gowns in resisting penetration by hazardous drugs found variation in the protection provided by the commercially available materials. In an evaluation of polypropylene-based gowns, Connor found that polypropylene spunbond non-woven material alone and polypropylene-polyethylene copolymer spunbond provided little protection against penetration by a battery of aqueous and nonaqueous based hazardous drugs.[63] Various constructions of polypropylene (e.g., spunbond/meltblown/spunbond [SMS]) result in materials that are completely impermeable or only slightly permeable to hazardous drugs. Connor notes that these coated materials are similar in appearance to several other nonwoven materials but perform differently and that workers could expect to be protected from exposure for up to 4 hours when using the coated gowning materials. Harrison and Kloos reported similar findings in a study of 6 disposable gowning materials and 15 hazardous drugs.[64] Only gowns with polyethylene or vinyl coatings provided adequate splash protection and prevented penetration of the hazardous drugs.

In a subjective assessment of worker comfort, the more protective gowns were found to be warmer and thus less comfortable. These findings agree with an earlier study that found the most protective gowning materials were the most uncomfortable to wear.[65] Resistance has been reported to the use of gowns, especially by nurses during administration of hazardous drugs.[66] The lack of comfort could cause resistance to behavioral change.

Researchers have looked at gown contamination with fluorescent scans and HPLC and tandem mass spectrometry.[67,26] Industrial hygiene scans were conducted of nurses and pharmacists wearing gowns during compounding and administration of hazardous drugs.[66] Of a total of 18 contamination spots detected, 5 were present on the gowns of nurses after drug administration. No spots were discovered on the gowns of pharmacists after compounding.

In contrast, researchers using a more sensitive assay, placed pads in various body locations, both over and under the gowns used by the subjects during compounding and administration of cyclophosphamide and ifosfamide.[26] Workers wore short-sleeved nursing uniforms, disposable or cotton gowns and vinyl or latex gloves. More contamination was found during compounding than administration. Contamination found on the pads placed on the arms of preparers is consistent with the use of a Class II BSC. Remarkable is that one preparer had contamination on the back of the gown, indicating possible touch contamination with the BSC during removal of final product.

While existing guidelines do not contain a maximum length of time that a gown should be worn, Connor's work would support a 2–3 hour window for a coated gown. Contamination of gowns during glove changes must be a consideration. If the inner pair of gloves requires changing, a gown change should be considered. Gowns worn as barrier protection in the compounding of hazardous drugs must never be worn outside the immediate preparation area. Gowns worn during administration should be changed when leaving the patient care area and immediately if contaminated. Gowns are to be disposed of when removed to avoid being a source of contamination to other staff and the environment.

Gown Recommendations

- Select disposable gowns of material tested to be protective against hazardous drugs.

- Coated gowns must be worn no longer than 3 hours during compounding or changed immediately when damaged or contaminated.

- Non-coated gowns must be changed more frequently if used.

- Remove gowns with care to avoid contamination.

- Dispose of gowns immediately upon removal.

- Contain and dispose of contaminated gowns as hazardous waste.

- Wash hands after removing and disposing of gown.

Hazardous drug compounding in an enclosed environment, such as an isolator, may not require the operator to wear a gown. However, as the process of handling drug vials and final preparations, as well as accessing the isolator's pass-throughs, may present an opportunity for contamination, gown use should be considered. Coated gowns may not be necessary for this use.

Additional Personal Protective Equipment

Eye and face protection should be used whenever there is a possibility of exposure from splashing or uncontrolled aerosolization of hazardous drugs (e.g., containing a spill or damaged shipping carton). In these instances, a face shield, rather than safety glasses or goggles, is recommended due to the improved skin protection afforded by the shield.

Similar circumstances warrant the use of a respirator. All workers who may utilize a respirator must be fit tested and trained to use the appropriate respirator according to the OSHA Respirator Standard.[36] The appropriate size respirator must be available at all times. Surgical masks may be required in a controlled environment to add protection from contaminating the preparation. These masks, however, do not provide worker protection. An appropriate respirator will do both.

Shoe and hair coverings should be worn during the compounding process to minimize particulate contamination of the controlled work zone and the preparation. With the potential for hazardous drug contamination on the floor in the compounding and administration areas, shoe coverings are also recommended as contamination control mechanisms. As such, shoe coverings must be removed, while wearing gloves, when leaving the compounding area. Gloves should be worn and care must be taken when removing hair or shoe coverings to prevent contamination from spreading to clean areas. Hair and shoe coverings used in the hazardous drug areas must be sealed in plastic bags, along with used gloves, and discarded as hazardous waste.

Work Practices

Work practices for the compounding of injectable hazardous drugs differ somewhat with the use of a Class II BSC, Class III BSC or isolator. Universally, good organization skills are essential to minimize contamination and maximize productivity. All activities not requiring a controlled environment (checking labels, doing calculations, etc.) should be completed prior to accessing the BSC or isolator. All items needed for compounding must be assembled prior to beginning. This work practice should eliminate the need to exit the BSC or isolator once compounding has begun. One pair of gloves must be worn to assemble hazardous drug vials and supplies. These gloves should be carefully removed and discarded. Fresh gloves must be donned prior to aseptic manipulation.

Only essential supplies and drugs needed to compound the dose or batch should be placed in the controlled environment. Neither the BSC nor the isolator should be overcrowded to avoid extraneous contamination. Luer-locking syringes and connections should be used whenever possible for manipulating hazardous drugs as they are less likely to separate during compounding.

Spiking an IV set into a hazardous drug containing solution or priming an IV set with hazardous drug solution in an uncontrolled environment must be avoided. One recommendation is to attach and prime the appropriate IV set to the final container in the BSC or isolator prior to the hazardous drug being added. With newer closed-system transfer devices, such as the PhaSeal Adaptor, a "dry-connection" is achieved between the administration set and the hazardous drug final container. This allows the spiking of the container with a secondary set and priming done by a backflow of a primary, non-hazardous drug solution. This process may be done outside of the BSC or isolator thus reducing the potential of surface contamination settling on the IV set during the compounding process. A new IV set must be used with each hazardous drug

dose. The IV set must never be removed from a hazardous drug dose to prevent the residual fluid in the bag/bottle or tubing from being aerosolized during removal.

Transport bags must never be placed in the BSC or in the isolator work chamber during compounding to avoid inadvertent contamination of the outside surface of the bag. Final preparation must be wiped off and fresh gloves donned after compounding is complete and before labeling and placing the preparation into the transport bag.

Work Practices for the BSC

The Class II and III BSCs have vertical laminar flow, HEPA filtered air as their controlled aseptic environment. Before beginning an operation in a BSC, personnel should wash their hands; don an inner pair of appropriate gloves; if working in a Class II BSC, a coated gown, followed by a second pair of gloves. The work surface should be decontaminated with sodium hypochlorite and neutralizer or disinfected with alcohol, depending on when it was last decontaminated.

For the Class II BSC, the front shield must be placed to protect the face and eyes. The operator should be seated such that his/her shoulders are at the level of the bottom of the front shield. For either BSC, only those drugs and supplies needed to compound a dose or batch should be assembled to avoid leaving and reentering of the work area and reducing contamination on extraneous materials. IV bags and/or bottles may be hung from the bar, being careful not to place any sterile objects below them. All items must be placed well within the Class II cabinet away from the unfiltered air at the front barrier. Nothing should block the air grills of the BSC. The containment characteristics of the Class II BSC are dependent on the airflow through both the front and back grills. Clean air quality is lowest at the sides of the work zone, so manipulations should be performed at least 6 inches away from each sidewall in the horizontal plane. A small waste/sharps container may be placed along the sidewall toward the back of the BSC.

The use of a preparation pad in the Class II BSC has been found to possibly interfere with the airflow in one study [26] but was determined to be without consequences to the airflow in another.[68] The type of pad was not described by Minoia et al.[26] Peters[68] tested a flat, firm pad that did not extend into the air streams of the cabinet. The use of a large pad that might protrude into the front or rear airflows must be avoided. As the pad may absorb small spills, it may become a source of contamination for anything placed upon it. A preparation pad is not readily decontaminated and must be replaced and discarded after each batch and frequently during extended batch compounding. More information on the design and use of Class II BSCs is available from the NSF standard 49 [44] and the ASHP 1990 technical assistance bulletin.[18]

Work Practices for the Isolator

For work in an isolator, all drugs and supplies needed during the operation must be assembled and readied for placement in the airlock/pass-through. A technique described in the literature [69] involves the use of a tray that will fit into the airlock. A large primary zip-lock bag is placed over the tray. Labels and a second transport bag, which is used to contain the final preparation, are placed into the primary bag on the tray surface. Vials, syringes, needles and other disposables are placed on top of the sealed zip-lock. The enclosed tray is then taken into the main chamber of the isolator where the drug and supplies are used to compound the dose. The contaminated materials including the primary bag are removed using the closed trash system of the isolator. The dose is then labeled and placed into the second zip-lock for transport. This technique does not address contamination on the isolator gauntlets. Additional work practices may include cleaning off the gauntlets and final preparation after initial compounding and before handling the label and second zip-lock or using disposable gloves over the gauntlet and removing and discarding them after wiping off the final preparation. Care must be taken in transferring products out of the pass-through (airlock) and disposing of waste through the trash chute.

Aseptic Technique

Stringent aseptic technique, described by Wilson and Solimando[70] in 1981, remains the foundation of any procedure involving the use of needles and syringes in manipulating sterile dosage forms. This technique, when performed accurately, minimizes the escape of drug from vials and ampules. Needleless devices have been developed to reduce the risk of blood-borne pathogen exposure to health care workers. None of these devices has been tested for reduction of contamination. The appropriateness of these devices in the safe handling of hazardous drugs is unproven.

In reconstituting hazardous drugs in vials, it is critical to avoid pressurizing the contents of the vial that may cause the drug to spray out around the needle, aerosolizing the drug into the work area of the BSC or isolator. This may be accomplished by creating a slight negative pressure in the vial. Too much negative pressure however, can cause leakage from the needle when it is withdrawn from the vial. The safe handling of hazardous drug solutions in vials or ampules requires the use of a syringe that is no more than three quarters (75%) full when filled with the solution. This minimizes the risk of the plunger separating from the syringe barrel. Once the diluent is drawn up, the needle is inserted into the vial and the plunger is pulled back (to create a slight negative pressure inside the vial) so that air is drawn into the syringe. Small amounts of diluent should be transferred slowly as equal volumes of air are removed. The needle should be kept in the vial, and the contents should be swirled carefully until dissolved. With the vial inverted, the proper amount of drug solution should be gradually withdrawn while equal volumes of air are exchanged for solution. The exact volume needed must be measured while the needle is in the vial and any excess drug should remain in the vial. With the vial in the upright position, a small amount of air should be drawn through the needle and just to the hub of the syringe. The hub should be clear before the needle is removed.

If a hazardous drug is transferred to an IV bag, care must be taken to puncture only the septum of the injection port and avoid puncturing the sides of the port or the bag. After the drug solution is injected into the IV bag, the IV port, container, and set should be wiped with moist gauze. The final preparation should be labeled, including an auxiliary warning, and the injection port covered with a protective shield. Using clean gloves, place the final container into a sealable bag to contain any leakage.[18]

To withdraw hazardous drugs from an ampul, the neck or top portion should be gently tapped. After the neck is sprayed or wiped with alcohol, a 5-micron filter needle or straw should be attached to a syringe that is large enough that it will be not more than three quarters (75%) full when holding the drug. Then the fluid should be drawn through the filter needle or straw and cleared from the needle and hub. After this, the needle or straw is exchanged for a needle of similar gauge and length, any air and excess drug should be ejected into a sterile vial (leaving the desired volume in the syringe). Aerosols should be avoided. Then the drug may be transferred to an IV bag or bottle. If the dose is to be dispensed in the syringe, the plunger should be drawn back to clear fluid from the needle and hub. The needle should be replaced with a locking cap, and the syringe should be wiped with moistened gauze and labeled.

Training and Demonstration of Competence

All staff who will be compounding hazardous drugs must be trained in both the standard and stringent aseptic techniques necessary for working with sterile hazardous drugs. Once trained, staff must demonstrate competence by an objective method and competency must be reassessed on a regular basis.[71]

Decontamination

Decontamination may be defined as cleaning or deactivating. The use of alcohol for disinfecting the BSC or isolator will not deactivate any hazardous drugs and may result in the spreading of contamination rather than any actual cleaning.[22,72] Many drug manufacturers recommend the use of sodium hypochlorite bleach as an appropriate deactivating agent for many hazardous drugs.[73] Researchers have shown strong oxidizing agents, such as sodium hypochlorite bleach, are effective deactivators of many of the hazardous drugs.[74,75] SurfaceSafe is a commercially available product that provides a solution of sodium hypochlorite bleach with detergent on one towelette of a two-pack system. The second pack contains thiosulfate to neutralize the bleach and deactivate several of the drugs that do not oxidize readily (e.g., platinum-containing drugs). SurfaceSafe is designed for use in a Class II BSC but may also be used in a Class III cabinet or an isolator. The bleach is a disinfectant and reduces the need for alcohol.

Containment and Disposal

In 1976 the Environmental Protection Agency (EPA) enacted the Resource Conservation and Recovery Act (RCRA)[76]—to provide a mechanism for tracking hazardous waste from its generation to disposal. These regulations apply to drugs (pharmaceuticals), as well as chemicals discarded by pharmacies, hospitals, clinics and other commercial entities. RCRA includes lists of agents that are to be considered hazardous waste.[77]

The P-list and U-list include several drugs that, *regardless of concentration*, are designated as hazardous wastes if they are the sole active ingredient. This discussion will be limited to only those drugs that are compounded as sterile preparations. P-listed wastes are termed *acutely hazardous* and include epinephrine, nitroglycerine, and physostigmine. U-listed wastes are toxic, flammable, corrosive, or reactive. Pharmaceuticals on the U-list are generally toxic and include cyclophosphamide. In addition to the P and U lists, EPA also designates four characteristics of a hazardous waste: ignitability, toxicity, corrosivity, and reactivity.[78,79]

Any discarded drug that meets one of these criteria is considered a hazardous waste. RCRA allows hazardous drug waste to be further divided into trace and bulk-contaminated waste. As defined by the EPA, trace-contaminated materials are containers whose contents have been removed (e.g., no liquid in an IV bag or tubing) and the residue is no more than 3% of the capacity of the container. However, no *listed* hazardous waste may be considered trace. Many states are authorized to implement their own hazardous waste programs and these programs may be more stringent than the EPA. State and local regulations must be considered when establishing a hazardous waste policy for a given institution.

EPA also defines waste generation status by the total amount of hazardous waste generated per month.[80] Small and large quantity generators are determined by the amount of P and U listed wastes that are discarded on a monthly basis. Waste management requirements are more stringent for large quantity generators than for a "conditionally exempt small quantity generator" (CESQG). Most facilities using this chapter for guidance are more than likely to meet the criteria for a "large quantity generator" given the number of discarded pharmaceuticals containing high alcohol content (ignitability characteristic >24%), mercury preservatives (toxicity characteristic), as well as the chemotherapy agents.

Once hazardous waste has been identified, it must be collected and stored according to specific EPA and Department of Transportation (DOT) requirements.[76,81] Properly labeled, leak-proof and spill-proof containers of nonreactive plastic are required for areas where hazardous waste is generated. Hazardous drug waste may be initially contained in thick, sealable plastic bags before placing in approved containers. Needles and any glass fragments should be contained in small, puncture-resistant sharps containers to be placed into larger containers approved for temporary storage. Waste contaminated with blood or other body fluids must not be mixed with hazardous waste.

Transport of waste containers from satellite accumulation to storage sites must be done by individuals who meet OSHA mandated hazardous waste awareness training.[82,83] Hazardous waste must be properly manifested and transported by a federally permitted hazardous waste transporter to a federally permitted hazardous waste storage, treatment, or disposal facility.[80] A licensed contractor may be hired to manage the hazardous waste program. The waste generator, however, may be held liable for mismanagement of hazardous waste. Investigation of a contractor, including verification of possession and type of license, should be completed and documented before a contractor is engaged. More information on hazardous waste disposal is available at www.pharmecology.com.

Risk Assessment

A formal risk assessment of a worksite may not be available for most practitioners. An alternative is a performance-based, observational approach. Given the results of the numerous contamination studies, observation of current work practices at any given site will serve as an initial assessment of appropriate and inappropriate practices.

Summary

An effective safety program for the handling of hazardous drugs must encompass both prepa-

ration and worker protection. The newer mandates for ensuring the sterility of pharmacy-compounded injectable products may pose a risk to workers and the environment when hazardous drugs are involved. The use of positive pressure environments for preparation protection may compromise the effectiveness of the Class II biological safety cabinet and may result in widespread contamination from lapses in technique or occasional spills. A safety program must include policies and procedures, suitable ventilation controls, appropriate personal protective equipment and the use of proper work practices in handling hazardous drugs. Staff must be trained in the stringent technique necessary to handle hazardous drugs and must demonstrate their competence in a simulated environment. Evaluation of recommendations must be ongoing to maintain a safe and effective program.

References

1. Weisburger JH, Griwold DP, Prejean JD, et al. Tumor induction by cytostatics. The carcinogenic properties of some of the principal drugs used in clinical cancer chemotherapy; Recent results. *Cancer Res.* 1975;52:1–17.

2. Harris CC. The carcinogenicity of anticancer drugs: a hazard in man. *Cancer.*1976; 37:1014–23.

3. Falck K, Grohn P, Sorsa M, et al. Mutagenicity in urine of nurses handling cytostatic drugs. *Lancet.* 1979;1:1250–1.

4. Harris CC. Immunosuppressive anticancer drugs in man: their oncogenic potential. *Radiology.* 1975;114:163–6.

5. Ladik CF, Stoehr GP, Maurer MA. Precautionary measures in the preparation of antineoplastics. *Am J Hosp Pharm.* 1980;37:1184, 1186.

6. Crudi CB. A Compounding dilemma: I've kept the drug sterile but have I contaminated myself? *NITA.* 1980;3:77–8.

7. Crudi CB, Stephens BL, Maier P. Possible occupational hazards associated with the preparation/administration of antineoplastic agents. *NITA.* 1982;5:264–6.

8. Reynolds RD, Ignoffo R, Lawrence J, et al. Adverse reactions to AMSA in medical personnel. *Cancer Treat Rep.* 1982; 66:1885.

9. Hemminki K, Kyyronen P, Lindholm ML. Spontaneous abortions and malforma-

tions in the offspring of nurses exposed to anaesthetic gases, cytostatic drugs, and other potential hazards, based on registered information of outcome. *J Epidemiol Community Health.* 1985; 39:141–7.

10. Selevan SG, Linbohm ML, Hornung RW, et al. A study of occupational exposure to antineoplastic drugs and fetal loss in nurses. *New Engl J Med.* 1985;313 (19):1173–8.

11. Valanis B, Vollmer W, Labuhn K, et al. Occupational exposure to antineoplastic agents and self-reported infertility among nurses and pharmacists. *J Occup Environ Med.* 1997; 39:574–80.

12. Valanis B, Vollmer WM, Steele P. Occupational exposures to antineoplastic agents: self-reported miscarriages and stillbirths among nurses and pharmacists. *J Occup Environ Med.* 1999;41:632–8.

13. Skov T, Lynge E, Maarup B et al. Risks for physicians handling antineoplastic drugs. *Lancet.* 1990;2:1446. Letter.

14. Skov T, Maarup B, Olsen J, et al. Leukaemia and reproductive outcome among nurses handling antineoplastic drugs. *Br J Ind Med.* 1992;49:855–61.

15. Controlling occupational exposure to hazardous drugs. In: *OSHA Technical Manual* (OSHA Instruction CPL 2-2.20B CH-4). Washington: Directorate of Technical Support, Occupational Safety and Health Administration. 1995: Chap 21. Available at http://www.osha.gov/dts/osta/otm/otm_vi/otm_vi_2.html#2. Accessed October 7, 2003.

16. National Institutes of Health. Recommendations for the safe handling of cytotoxic drugs. 1992. Available at http://www.nih.gov/od/ors/ds/pubs/cyto/index.htm. Accessed October 7, 2003.

17. Brown KA, Esper P, Kelleher LO, et al. *Chemotherapy and Biotherapy Guidelines and Recommendations for Practice.* Pittsburgh, PA: Oncology Nursing Society; 2001.

18. ASHP technical assistance bulletin on handling cytotoxic and hazardous drugs. *Am J Hosp Pharm.* 1990;47:1033–49.

19. Ensslin AS, Pethran A, Schierl R, et al. Urinary platinum in hospital personnel occupationally exposed to platinum-containing antineoplastic drugs. *Int Arch Occup Environ Health.* 1994;65:339–42.

20. Ensslin AS, Huber R, Pethran A, et al. Biological monitoring of hospital pharmacy personnel occupationally exposed to cytostatic drugs: urinary excretion and cytogenetics studies. *Int Arch Occup Environ Health.* 1997;70:205–8.

21. Ensslin AS, Stoll Y, Pethran A, et al. Biological monitoring of cyclophosphamide and ifosfamide in urine of hospital personnel occupationally exposed to cytostatic drugs. *Occup Environ Med.* 1994; 51:229–33.

22. Sessink PJM, Boer KA, Scheefhals APH, et al. Occupational exposure to antineoplastic agents at several departments in a hospital: Environmental contamination and excretion of cyclophosphamide and ifosfamide in urine of exposed workers. *Int Arch Occup Environ Health.* 1992; 64:105–12.

23. Sessink PJM, Van de Kerkhof MCA, Anzion RB, et al. Environmental contamination and assessment of exposure to antineoplastic agents by determination of cyclophosphamide in urine of exposed pharmacy technicians: Is skin absorption an important exposure route? *Arch Environ Health.* 1994;49:165–9.

24. Sessink PJM, Wittenhorst BCJ, Anzion RBM, et al. Exposure of pharmacy technicians to antineoplastic agents: Reevaluation after additional protective measures. *Arch Environ Health.* 1997;52:240–44.

25. Kiffmeyer TK, Ing KG, Schoppe G. External contamination of cytotoxic drug packing: Safe handling and cleaning procedures. *J Onc Pharm Practice.* 2000;6:13.

26. Minoia C, Turci R, Sottani C, et al. Application of high performance liquid chromatography/tandem mass spectrometry in the environmental and biological monitoring of health care personnel occupationally exposed to cyclophosphamide and ifosfamide. *Rapid Commun Mass Spectrom.* 1998;12:1485–93.

27. Rubino FM, Floridia L, Pietropaolo AM, et al. Measurement of surface contamination by certain antineoplastic drugs using high-performance liquid chromatography: applications in occupational hygiene investigations in hospital environments. *Med Lav.* 1999;90:572–83.

28. DeMeo MP, Merono S, DeBaille AD, et al. Monitoring exposure of hospital personnel handling cytostatic drugs and contaminated materials. *Int Arch Occup Environ Health.*1995;66:363–8.

29. Connor TH, Anderson RW, Sessink PJM, et al. Surface contamination with antineoplastic agents in six cancer treatment centers in the United Sates and Canada. *Am J Health-Syst Pharm.* 1999;56:1427–32.

30. Baker ES, Connor TH. Monitoring occupational exposure to cancer chemotherapy drugs. *Am J Health-Syst Pharm.* 1996;53:2713–23.

31. Harrison BR. Exposure to hazardous drugs: time to reevaluate your program? [Editorial] *Am J Health-Syst Pharm.* 1999;56:1403.

32. Hazard Communication Standard. 29 C.F.R. part 1910–1200. Available at http://www.osha.gov/OshStd_data/1910.1200.html. Accessed October 7, 2003.

33. Hazard Communication-Final Rule. 29 C.F.R. part 1910, et al. Occupational Safety and Health Administration; *Federal Register* 59, no.27 (9 February 1994): 6/26–84.

34. U.S. Department of Health and Human Services (Public Health Service, National Toxicology Program, 2002). Report on carcinogens (10th ed). Available at http://ehis.niehs.nih.gov/roc/toc9.html. Accessed on October 7, 2003.

35. International Agency for Research on Cancer. Monographs database on carcinogenic risks to humans. 2002. Lyon, France: Available at http://www.iarc.fr/. Accessed on October 7, 2003.

36. U.S. Department of Labor. *Respiratory Protection Standard.* Washington, DC: Occupational Safety and Health Administration: 1984. 29 CFR 1910.134.

37. Kromhout H, Hoek F, Uitterhoeve R, et al. Postulating a dermal pathway for exposure to antineoplastic drugs among hospital workers. Applying a conceptual model to the results of three workplace surveys. *Ann Occup Hyg.* 2000;44:551–60.

38. Nguyen TV, Theiss JC, Matney TS. Exposure of pharmacy personnel to mutagenic antineoplastic drugs. *Cancer Res.* 1982;42:4792–6.

39. Anderson RW, Puckett WH, Dana WJ, et al. Risk of handling injectable antineoplastic agents. *Am J Hosp Pharm.* 1982;39:1881–7.

40. Connor TH, Shults M, Fraser TP. Determination of the vaporization of solutions of mutagenic antineoplastic agents at 23 and 36° C using a dessicator technique. *Mutat Res.* 2000;470:85–92.

41. Opiolka S, Schmidt KG, Kiffmeyer TK, et al. Determination of the vapor pressure of cytotoxic drugs and its effects on occupational safety [Abstract]. *J Oncol Pharm Practice.* 2000;6:15.

42. Kiffmeyer TK, Kube C, Opiolka S, et al. Vapor pressures, evaporation behavior and airborne concentrations of hazardous drugs: implications for occupational safety. *Pharmaceut J.* 2002;268:331–7.

43. Larson RR, Khazaeli MB, Dillon HK. A new monitoring method using solid sorbent media for evaluation of airborne cyclophosphamide and other antineoplastic agents. *Appl Occup Environ Hyg.* 2003;18:120–31.

44. National Sanitation Foundation (NSF) NSF/ANSI 49-2002. Class II (laminar flow) Biohazard Cabinetry. 2002. Ann Arbor, MI. Available at http://www.nsf.org/biohazard/bio_standards.html. Accessed on October 7, 2003.

45. Clark RP, Goff MR. The potassium iodide method for determining protection factors in open-fronted microbiological safety cabinets. *J Appl Biol.* 1981;51:461–73.

46. Tillet L. Barrier isolators as an alternative to a cleanroom. *Am J Health-Syst Pharm.* 1999;56:1433–6.

47. Mosko P, Rahe H. Barrier isolation technology: a labor-efficient alternative to cleanrooms. *Hosp Pharm.* 1999;34:834–8.

48. Rahe H. Understanding the critical components of a successful cleanroom and barrier isolator project. *Am J Health-Syst Pharm.* 2000;57:346–50.

49. Pharmaceutical Compounding – Sterile Preparations. United States pharmacopeia, 27th rev./national formulary, 22nd ed. (first supplement). Rockville, MD: United States Pharmacopeial Convention; 2004.

50. Gustavsson B. Evaluation of a technetium assay for monitoring of occupational exposure to cytotoxic drugs [Abstract]. *J Oncol Pharm Practice.* 1997;3:16.

51. Sessink PJM, Rolf ME, Ryden NS. Evaluation of the PhaSeal hazardous drug containment system. *Hosp Pharm.* 1999;34:1311–7.

52. Sessink PJM. How to work safely outside the biological safety cabinet [Abstract]. *J Oncol Pharm Practice.* 2000;6:15.

53. Connor TH, Anderson RW, Sessink PJ, et al. Effectiveness of a closed-system device in containing surface contamination with cyclophosphamide and ifosfamide in an I.V. admixture area. *Am J Health-Syst Pharm.* 2002;59:68–72

54. Spivey S, Connor TH. Determining sources of workplace contamination with antineoplastic drugs and comparing conventional IV drug preparation with a closed system. *Hosp Pharm.* 2003; 38:135–9.

55. Hoy RH, Stump LM. Effect of an air-venting filter device on aerosol production from vials. *Am J Hosp Pharm.* 1984; 41:324–6.

56. Connor TH. Permeability testing of glove materials for use with cancer chemotherapy drugs. *Oncology.* 1995;52:256–9.

57. Singleton LC, Connor TH. An evaluation of the permeability of chemotherapy gloves to three cancer chemotherapy drugs. *Oncol Nurs Forum.* 1999;26:1491–6.

58. Gross E, Groce DF. An evaluation of nitrile gloves as an alternative to natural rubber latex for handling chemotherapeutic agents. *J Oncol Pharm Practice.* 1998;4:165–8.

59. Connor TH. Permeability of nitrile rubber, latex, polyurethane, and neoprene gloves to 18 antineoplastic drugs. *Am J Health-Syst Pharm.* 1999;56:2450–3.

60. Connor TH, Xiang Q. The effect of isopropyl alcohol on the permeation of gloves exposed to antineoplastic agents. *J Oncol Pharm Practice.* 2000;6:109–14.

61. Colligan SA, Horstman SW. Permeation of cancer chemotherapeutic drugs through glove materials under static and flexed conditions. *Appl Occup Environ Hyg.* 1990;5:848–52.

62. Sessink PJM, Cerna M, Rossner P, et al. Urinary cyclophosphamide excretion and chromosomal aberrations in peripheral blood lymphocytes after occupational exposure to antineoplastic agents. *Mutat Res.* 1994;309:193–9.

63. Connor TH. An evaluation of the permeability of disposable polypropylene-based protective gowns to a battery of cancer chemotherapy drugs. *Appl Occup Environ Hyg.* 1993;8:785–9.

64. Harrison BR, Kloos MD. Penetration and splash protection of six disposable gown materials against fifteen antineoplastic drugs. *J Oncol Pharm Practice.* 1999;5:61–6.

65. Laidlaw JL, Connor TH, Theiss JC, et al. Permeability of four disposal protective-clothing materials to seven antineoplastic drugs. *Am J Hosp Pharm.* 1985;42:2449–54.

66. Valanis B, Shortridge L. Self-protective practices of nurses handling antineoplastic drugs. *Oncol Nurs Forum.* 1987;14:23–7.

67. Labuhn K, Valanis B, Schoeny R, et al. Nurses' and pharmacists' exposure to antineoplastic drugs: findings from industrial hygiene scans and urine mutagenicity tests. *Cancer Nurs.* 1998;21:79–89.

68. Peters, W. Containment capabilities of a Class II, Type A2 BSC using a chemo pad on the worksurface. NuAire, Inc., Minneapolis, MN. June 2, 2003.

69. Farris J. Barrier isolators and the reduction of contamination in preparation of parenteral products. *CleanRooms Life Sciences.* 2002; February S14–8 (Supplement).

70. Wilson JP, Solimando DA. Aseptic technique as a safety precaution in the preparation of antineoplastic agents. *Hosp Pharm.* 1981;15:575–81.

71. Harrison BR, Godefroid RJ, Kavanaugh EA. Quality-assurance testing of staff pharmacists handling cytotoxic agents. *Am J Health-Syst Pharm.* 1996;53:402–7.

72. Dorr RT, Alberts DS. Topical absorption and inactivation of cytotoxic anticancer agents in vitro. *Cancer.* 1992;70(suppl):983–7.

73. Johnson EG, Janosik JE. Manufacturers' recommendations for handling spilled antineoplastic agents. *Am J Hosp Pharm.* 1989;46:318–19.

74. Benvenuto JA, Connor TH, Monteith DK, et al. Degradation and inactivation of antitumor drugs. *Journal of Pharmacy Science.* 1993;82:988–91.

75. Hansel S, Castegnaro M, Sportouch MH, et al. Chemical degradation of wastes of antineoplastic agents: cyclophosphamide, ifosfamide and melphalan. *Int Arch Occup Environ Health.* 1997;69:109–14.

76. The Resource Conservation and Recovery Act of 1976. U.S. Code Title 42. Chapter 82, Sections 6901–6992k.

77. Smith CA. Rationale for inclusion of criteria for proper disposal of monograph pharmaceutical preparations based on the Resource Conservation and Recov-

ery Act. *Pharmacopeial Forum.* 1999;25(3) May/June:8309–12.

78. Characteristics of Hazardous Waste. 40 C.F.R. part 261.20–24. *Federal Register* (19 May 1980).

79. Characteristics of Hazardous Waste. Characteristic of Toxicity. 40 C.F.R. part 261.24. *Federal Register* (29 March 1990).

80. Protection of the Environment. Hazardous Waste Management System: General. Title 40, Volume d. 40 C.F.R. parts 260–268, 270. Revised July 1, 1996.

81. Hazardous Materials Table, Special Provisions, Hazardous Materials Communication. Department of Transportation. Title 49, Volume 2. 49 C.F.R. parts 172-172.123. Revised as of October 1, 2002.

82. Initial Training. 29 C.F.R. part 1910.120(e)(3)(i).

83. Emergency Response to Hazardous Substances Releases. 29 C.F.R. part 1910.120(q)(1–6).

8 | Factors Influencing Beyond-Use Dating of Compounded Sterile Preparations

*Caryn M. Bing**

*The author acknowledges Barbara T. McKinnon, who authored this chapter in the first edition.

Pharmacists should always assign beyond-use dates that accurately reflect the stability of the medication, combination of medications, or other components under the intended preparation, packing, shipping, storage, and administration conditions. To do this, the pharmacist must understand the chemical and physical factors that affect the sterility and stability of all components in a preparation. The pharmacist must also consider the contribution of environmental, operational, and personnel factors to the quality of a compounded preparation.[1]

The *expiration date* or shelf life assigned to a commercially available drug product reflects the longest time period during which 90 percent or more of the labeled active ingredient is available for delivery.[2] Expiration dates are applied to intact formulations from the manufacturer. When a product is reconstituted, diluted, and/or transferred into another container or administration device, the practitioner must establish an appropriate *beyond-use date* for the preparation. Beyond-use dating is usually shorter than the expiration date of the original product. Beyond-use dating must be based on professional experience and interpretation of reliable sources of information. The beyond-use dating must also reflect sterility considerations and the potential for microbial, physical, or chemical contamination during compounding.[3]

The beyond-use dating assigned to a preparation should be the maximum time period in which 90 percent or greater of a labeled active ingredient is measurable in the solution and container specified, under the stated storage or administration conditions.[1,4] These preparations should bear labels that specify their storage requirements, beyond-use dates, and latest time of day for use (when appropriate).[3,5]

The concentration or bioavailability of the active ingredients in a preparation can be affected by physical, chemical, and delivery system-related incompatibility or instability. *Incompatibility* refers to a physical or chemical phenomenon that reduces the concentration of the active ingredient(s). Examples include concentration-dependent precipitation and acid-base reactions.[4] *Physical or visual incompatibilities* are terms that describe visible changes in a preparation, such as precipitation, cloudiness or haziness, color change, viscosity change, cracking, and effervescence.

Instability usually refers to the chemical processes that result in a degradation or change in the active ingredients, including hydrolysis, oxidation, reduction, and photo degradation reactions. These changes are generally continuous and irreversible, and can form degradation products, which are therapeutically inactive and still exhibit toxicity. Examples include hydrolysis, oxidative, and other heat-catalyzed reactions. [2,3,4,6]

Common incompatibilities or instabilities often are classified as "physical" or "chemical," even though all incompatibilities are essentially chemical-based phenomena. In some cases, incompatibilities can be due to solubility changes or container interactions rather than to molecular changes in the active ingredient.

Physical Incompatibilities

Solubility

Drugs can be maintained in aqueous solution as long as their concentrations are below the saturation solubility. Supersaturated solutions are likely to precipitate. Drugs with poor water solubility are often formulated with water-miscible cosolvents such as ethanol, propylene glycol, and polyethylene glycol. For example, dilution of diazepam from the commercial dosage form may result in precipitation at some concentrations, while further dilution below the saturation solubility point can result in a stable preparation.[7-9] Other examples of drug formulations using a cosolvent include co-trimoxazole, digoxin, phenytoin, etoposide, and teniposide.[4]

pH Effect on Solubility

The solubility of drugs that are weak acids or weak bases is related to the pH of the diluent solution. Weak acids or weak bases that are insoluble in aqueous diluents are converted into salt to increase their solubility. Weak acids usually are made into salts of weak acids and strong bases (e.g., penicillin G potassium, pantoprazole sodium), while weak bases are made into salts of weak bases and strong acids (e.g., morphine sulfate, isoproterenol hydrochloride). As a rule, salts of weak acids and strong bases are physically and chemically incompatible with salts of weak bases and strong acids. Salts of weak acids and strong bases (e.g., ampicillin sodium) are generally less stable in acidic IV solutions (e.g., dextrose 5%) than in neutral or higher pH solutions (e.g., normal saline). Some drugs products are available in nonaqueous diluents that increase their solubility and stability (e.g., diazepam, digoxin, and phenytoin sodium injection). These drugs may undergo a "change of solvent" or pH effect in aqueous IV solutions, resulting in precipitation or chemical instability.

Solubility Issues in Parenteral Nutrition Solutions and TNAs

The complexity of parenteral nutrition formulations (e.g., amino acids, dextrose, fat emulsion, multiple mono- and divalent electrolyte salts, trace minerals, and vitamins) provides ample opportunity for the formation of insoluble salts. An FDA safety alert has been published on the hazards of precipitation associated with parenteral nutrition formulations. Medical personnel and patients or caregivers who administer parenteral nutrition formulations should be trained to visually inspect the preparation for precipitation or other evidence of degradation.[10]

Calcium-phosphate solubility issues

The risk of dibasic calcium phosphate salt formation and precipitation is well documented in the literature and stability references.[4,11-15] Although dibasic calcium phosphate is nearly insoluble in water, monobasic calcium phosphate is relatively soluble. The pKa is 7.2 for the equilibrium between dibasic and monobasic phosphate ions. Increases in pH will elevate dibasic phosphate ions, which increases the probability of dibasic calcium phosphate precipitation. Highly reactive salts (e.g., sodium bicarbonate and calcium chloride) should be avoided as additives, as they can also contribute to precipitate formation. Calcium phosphate precipitation also may be related to temperature. As temperature rises, particle movement increases the probability of a reaction between free calcium and dibasic phosphate ions. This effect may explain the reported occurrence of calcium phosphate precipitation in the lumen of central venous catheters and the parenteral nutrition solution tubing for infants in incubators.

Other factors include high concentrations of calcium and phosphate salts, increases in solution pH, increases in temperature, the addition of calcium before phosphate in the admixture process, lengthy time delays or slow infusion rates that increase exposure of the preparation to room temperature conditions, and use of the chloride salt of calcium. Low amounts of amino acids in the final preparation cut down on the buffer capability of the solution, which can also contribute to calcium phosphate insolubility.

Consider these factors that can improve solubility and enhance the stability of the preparation and individual components when determining an appropriate beyond-use date for parenteral nutrition solutions:

- Increased amino acid concentrations buffer the preparation.
- A lower pH reduces the dibasic phosphate salt available for precipitation with calcium.
- Lower storage (refrigerated) and administration temperature reduces the risk of precipitation.
- Use the more stable salts of calcium (gluconate or acetate rather than chloride) whenever possible.
- When using an automated compounding device, always follow the manufacturer's protocol for additives.
- Base the calculation of the calcium solubility on the volume of the preparation at the time the calcium is added, not on the final solution volume.
- For 2-in-1 solutions (no lipids added), keep the calcium concentration below 10 mEq/L and the phosphorus (phosphate) concentration below 30 mM/L to decrease the risk of precipitation.

Emulsion integrity issues with TNAs

3-in-1 or total nutrient admixtures (TNAs; dextrose, amino acids, and fat emulsions/lipids are combined in one container) require additional steps to ensure the stability of the resulting emulsion. First, the mixing order is critical. Lipids should never be added directly to dextrose before amino acids are added.

TNA emulsions are not stable below a final pH of 5, limiting their use in pediatric or neonatal parenteral nutrition solutions containing (highly acidic) cysteine hydrochloride.[14] Concentrations of divalent cations, such as calcium and magnesium, should be limited to avoid destabilizing the emulsion. Because no foolproof method has been found to predict TNA stability, the assigned beyond-use dates should be conservative based on all contributing factors.

Factors Affecting Stability

Many factors can affect the stability of medications. Table 8-1 provides examples of the most common factors and their causes.[1,4,16]

Solubility of large organic ions

Large organic anions and cations also may form precipitates or insoluble complexes. For example, heparin (a large anionic complex) may precipitate with cationic drugs such as aminoglycosides. Such precipitation depends on whether the solubility product of the heparin salt of the cationic drug is exceeded.

Therefore, precipitation is more likely to occur at high concentrations (if the drugs are not sufficiently diluted).

Sorption

Sorption occurs when drug is lost (from the solution to be administered) by adsorption to the surface or absorption into the matrix of the container material, administration set, or filter. The longer the contact time with the matrix, the more sorption and less availability of the drug in solution. Drugs that exhibit sorption properties include nitroglycerin, diazepam, vitamin A, dactinomycin, insulin, sufentanil, filgrastim, calcitriol, lorazepam, and aldesleukin. Beyond-use dating for these types of drugs is typically very short.

Table 8-1.

Common Factors Affecting Drug Stability

Factor	Incompatibility or Instability	Common Examples
Contact with metal (e.g., needles or components of devices)	Chemical reaction	Hydralazine, metronidazole (with aluminum)
Freezing temperature	Inactivation or denaturation	Heparin, filgrastim, erythropoetin
Large organic anions and cations	Precipitation or formation of insoluble complex	Heparin with aminoglycosides
Light (natural and room)	Accelerated chemical degradation reactions	Dobutamine, furosemide, cisplatin, hydroxyzine, carboplatin
Low temperature (refrigerated)	Crystallization or precipitation	5-fluorouracil, furosemide, acyclovir, metronidazole
Plastic containers, sets, in-line filters	Adsorption of lipophilic agents—especially important at low concentrations	Sufentanil, filgrastim, calcitriol, lorazepam, aldesleukin
PVC container permeability	Evaporation, with resultant over-concentration of solution	All PVC containers distributed in overwrap bags; small volume bags are most susceptible
Plasticizer content of containers and sets	Leaching carcinogenic plasticizer DEHP from PVC container	Paclitaxel, lipid emulsion, cyclosporine
Saturation solubility exceeded	Precipitation	Morphine sulfate, etoposide
Temperature above 8°C	Accelerated chemical degradation reactions	Ampicillin, others

Source: references 4, 16

Adsorption

When drugs are administered in small quantities or at low concentrations, a clinically relevant amount may be adsorbed and removed from solution. In these cases, adsorption plays an important role in determining the beyond-use dating. Drugs administered in larger concentrations or doses lose a smaller percentage of the total dose because of saturation of the binding sites on the container surface.

Absorption

Absorption into the matrix of plastic containers and administration sets, especially ones made of polyvinyl chloride (PVC), is a source of loss for lipid-soluble drugs (e.g., vitamin A). Phthalate plasticizers are used to make the plastic soft and flexible, but lipid-soluble drugs diffuse into them. Plastics that contain little or no phthalate plasticizers (e.g., polyethylene and polypropylene) do not readily absorb lipid-soluble drugs. Because of this difference in absorption potential, specialized containers or administration sets should be used for some solutions of highly susceptible medications (e.g., nitroglycerin, amiodarone). Short and/or small diameter administration sets can further reduce the surface area exposed for absorption.

Some lipid-soluble medications can cause the phthalate plasticizers to leach from the container or set into the solution. Concerns have been expressed about the extraction of the plasticizer d-2-ethylhexylphthalate (DEHP) by lipid emulsions.[17] To avoid the formation of toxic hydroperoxides,[18] lipid emulsions should be packaged in glass containers only. Repackaging them in plastic IV bags, which are relatively permeable to oxygen, should be avoided. TNAs can be packaged in plastic because the antioxidant from the amino acid product also protects the lipid emulsion; however, non-DEHP-containing bags are preferred, especially for pediatric or neonatal patients. PVC bags that utilize alternative plasticizers or ethylene vinyl acetate bags are available. Multiple-chamber container systems allow for the mixture of less stable or problematic preparations just prior to administration. These types of systems may be particularly helpful for advance preparation of multiple-days supply of TNA for patients in alternate site care.

Other Physical Incompatibilities

Other physical incompatibilities that can occur immediately or over time include:

- "Salting out" or precipitation of organic drugs in the presence of strong electrolytes.
- Complexation phenomena such as the formation of chelates of tetracycline with aluminum, calcium, iron, and magnesium.
- Color changes from chemical degradation to a colored decomposition product.
- Gas evolution (evident in reconstitution of ceftazidime).

Chemical Degradation

Drugs may undergo degradation by various chemical reactions. Although a few reactions produce visible changes, such as color and gas evolution, many chemical incompatibilities are not visually observable.[4]

Hydrolysis, Oxidation, and Reduction

Hydrolysis reactions involve the attack of labile bonds, by water, in dissolved drug molecules with resultant molecular changes. Hydrolysis rates increase exponentially with increases in ambient temperature.[3] Oxidation and reduction reactions involve exchange of electrons and valence changes in the drug molecules. To control oxidation reactions in parenteral products, manufacturers evacuate oxygen from glass containers and fill any head space with nitrogen. They may also adjust pH, add buffering agents to stabilize pH, add chelating agents such as ethylenediaminetetraacetic acid (EDTA), or add antioxidants such as sodium bisulfate.[4] When medications are diluted, the antioxidant, buffering, or antimicrobial properties may be lost.[3]

Photolysis

Photodegradation or photolysis is the catalysis of degradation reactions by light. Although various decomposition mechanisms may occur, all involve energy (light) which causes changes at chemical bonds and resultant changes to the chemical entity.[4] The more intense a light source is and the closer the photolabile drugs are to it, the greater is the rate of photodegradation.[6] Ultraviolet light is more destructive than visible light, and daylight has more damaging effects than fluorescent light on photolabile preparations.

In order to protect the integrity of photolabile drugs, they must be protected from light. Preparation containers and, when necessary, tubing, can be over-wrapped with foil or light blocking amber plastic. Protect the preparation from the initiation of compounding through the conclusion of administration.[4] Always be sure that the overwrap is properly labeled to facilitate the identity of the preparation.

Stability Related to Drug Delivery Systems

When assigning beyond-use dating to a compounded sterile preparation, always consider the potential impact of the container type and material, drug delivery system, and the environmental temperature during distribution, storage, and administration. While some practitioners may choose to extrapolate stability test results from one type of container to another, there are many examples of variation in stability data among container types.[1] For example, one study noted that Vitamin C (ascorbic acid) and Vitamin B1 exhibited more stability in TNA bags made from a multilayered plastic than in EVA bags.[19]

Delivery Systems

Large volume parenterals

Large volume parenteral admixtures are most often used to administer one or more medications or electrolytes over a longer time period or continuously. Multiple-ingredient preparations (such as parenteral nutrition), which must be infused over extended time periods, have a significantly increased potential for drug stability and compatibility problems due to the long contact time and exposure to ambient temperature and light conditions.

Higher concentration delivery systems

Intermittently administered medications are often prepared at greater concentrations than are typical for large volume infusions. For example, medications in small volume containers such as 25 to 150 ml bags or single elastomeric containers are more concentrated and generally infused over an appropriately short time period. Medications packaged in syringes are usually even more concentrated, and are often administered by IV push or syringe pump. Reservoirs of drugs used for controlled intermittent administration via ambulatory elec-

tronic pumps may be extremely concentrated, depending on the drug and patient's IV access. If more than one concentrated drug is combined in a syringe, small volume container, or reservoir, the potential for an incompatibility or other instability is increased due to high concentrations as well as prolonged contact time.

Y-site administration

For patients with limited venous access, a Y-site technique may be the only available method of administering additional medications. Y-site (and piggyback) drug delivery can reduce the potential for incompatibilities by decreasing the contact time of multiple ingredients and solutions.[20] Relatively few combinations of drugs are so chemically unstable that Y-site administration is precluded.[4] A study simulating the Y-site administration of 106 drugs into nine different TNA formulations revealed 23 that were incompatible with one or more components of the TNA; six resulted in precipitates, and seventeen caused disruption of the TNA emulsion.[21] Naturally, practitioners should ensure that the Y-site route will not affect either the administered drug or the contents of the primary container.

Other container issues

The major manufacturers of parenteral solutions packaged in PVC containers have established maximum usage times after removal from the commercial over-wrap. Table 8-2 summarizes the manufacturer recommendations.[1] The primary consideration is aqueous evaporation through the PVC, resulting in decreased volume of the solutions and alteration of additive concentration. Once additives are placed in these containers, the beyond-use date should be the shorter of the drug stability dating or the solution manufacturer's maximum recommended time for use after removal from the over-wrap and storage at room temperature.

Ready-to-use products

A number of commercial premixed products can be purchased as ready-to-use (RTU) solutions. Consult the product labeling for all commercial premixed and frozen medications for the recommended maximum storage time and conditions (before and after removal of protective over-wrap and/or thawing). Most of these RTU products contain additional ingredients that help to stabilize or preserve the active drugs.

Table 8-2.

Manufacturer Storage Recommendations for Plain Solutions in PVC After Removal from Protective Over Wrap

Manufacturer/Brand	Volume	Maximum Storage Time
Abbott/Lifecare[a]	25 mL	21 days
Abbott/Lifecare[a]	>25 mL	30 days
Baxter/Viaflex[b]	≤50mL	15 days
Baxter/Viaflex[b]	≥100mL	30 days

[a]Manufacturer letter to C. Bing. Abbott Hospital Products Division Medical Department, November 1999.

[b]Manufacturer letter to C. Bing. Baxter Healthcare Corporation I.V. Systems Delivery, November 1999.

Do not extrapolate the product expiration dating assigned to these commercial formulations to extemporaneously compounded sterile preparations.[1]

Environmental Temperatures

Clinical setting

Always consider the effects of temperature on medications in the clinical setting. While most preparations are stored under refrigeration (or even frozen), they are usually warmed to room temperature prior to administration. Depending on the infusion duration, the preparations can be exposed to ambient temperatures for prolonged periods. Portable infusion devices (such as ambulatory pumps or elastomeric devices) may expose drugs to near-body temperatures, and some drugs instilled into the reservoirs of implantable pumps remain at body temperature (37 °C) for up to 60 days. Always consider the stability of the preparation at its expected delivery temperature and period of use when determining the beyond-use date.

Cumulative room temperature storage time will also affect the preparation's stability. For example, sterile preparations may be stored in the pharmacy refrigerator, removed from the refrigerator and warmed to room tempera-

ture prior to delivery to the patient care unit, and then, if not administered immediately, returned to the refrigerator. In some cases, the preparation may even be returned to the pharmacy to be re-issued for another patient. The beyond-use date that applies to either the refrigerated or room temperature storage conditions may no longer be valid under such circumstances. When assigning a beyond-use date, the pharmacist must determine the expected stability of the preparation under actual or anticipated storage conditions. When accepting an unused preparation for potential redispensing, consult credible references[1,4] to determine if the labeled beyond-use dating is still valid and if the preparation is suitable for another patient.[3]

Alternate site care settings

The continued increase of medication infusions in the home care, ambulatory, and long term care settings has increased the need for extended beyond-use dating. Longer dating helps to minimize costs related to deliveries, and can reduce waste. For multiple dose intermittent infusions via an ambulatory infusion device, the drugs should be stable for a minimum of 24 hours at or above room temperature. When medications have limited room temperature stability, administration via a device that combines the drug with the diluent at administration time is a more common and practical choice.

Sterility Limitations

Even under the best aseptic processing conditions, microorganisms might inadvertently contaminate sterile preparations. Therefore, refrigerated storage of sterile preparations that are not intended for prompt administration will inhibit microbial growth. Preparations intended for prompt administration after compounding may be retained at room temperature.

When evaluating the sterility-associated risk level, consider a preparation's ability to support microbial growth. Although clinical infections related to microbial contamination of infusion solutions are identified less frequently than other causes of infusion-related infections (e.g., catheter related), contamination of batch-compounded preparations can lead to epidemic infections.[22,23] The recognition of the risk of microbial contamination or excessive endotoxins led to the development of USP Chapter 797, which outlines the guidelines for assigning sterility-based beyond-use dating.[3] Table 8-3 summarizes the guidelines for beyond-use dating (in the absence of additional preparation sterility testing) for completed compounded sterile preparations at each of the preparation risk levels outlined in USP <797>. These guidelines presume that the sterile preparation processes meet the criteria outlined in USP <797> for that risk level to ensure sterility of the compounded sterile preparation, as well as documented evidence that the preparation is chemically stable for the labeled time period.

Preparations as Culture Media

Practitioners should also consider the potential for a compounded sterile preparation to support microbial growth if inadvertently contaminated. Total nutrient admixtures and lipids (and lipid complexes) may be more likely to foster microbial growth.[24-30] Isotonic solutions, such as dextrose 5% and normal saline, may also provide an adequate media for the survival of microorganisms in the presence of nutrient agents.

Total Parenteral Nutrition

After reports of protein hydrolysate contamination with both bacteria and fungi, parenteral nutrition solutions gained a reputation of being prone to contamination.[31-33] Actually, the crystalline amino acid solutions currently in use are poor growth media for bacteria. Most strains either die or show minimal growth.[33,34]

Poor bacterial survival has been attributed to the low pH and hypertonicity of amino acid

and dextrose solutions. However, *Pseudomonas* and *Escherichia coli* can withstand the pH and osmolarity of higher concentration parenteral nutrition formulations. Dilution of the dextrose (as for peripherally infused formulations) improves the survival of *Staphylococcus aureus*, *Streptococcus faecalis*, and *P. aeruginosa*.[33,34]

Fungi, particularly *Candida albicans*, proliferate in standard crystalline amino acid-based solutions.[33] Numerous cases of fungal sepsis associated with parenteral nutrition have been reported.[35-38]

Because of the potential for fungal proliferation within a brief period (24 hr), parenteral nutrition solutions should be refrigerated immediately after preparation. Prolonged refrigerated storage has been reported with no bacterial contamination. Each organization (pharmacy) should validate the compounding process to ensure that the beyond-use dating assigned to these medium risk, multicomponent compounded sterile preparations is appropriate. For these solutions, stability of components is also an important consideration for beyond-use dating. Significant losses of tryptophan and other amino acids have been reported.[39] End-preparation sterility testing is recommended to validate extended beyond-use dating that exceeds published guidelines and standards.[40]

TNAs

TNAs that combine fat emulsion with dextrose and amino acids have become widely used in both inpatient and home infusion care. The risk of microbial contamination during administration may be reduced because of fewer manipulations of the parenteral nutrition container and tubing. However, these admixtures may provide better growth media for pathogenic micro-

Table 8-3.

USP <797> Storage and Beyond-Use Dating Conditions for Compounded Sterile Preparations [3]

Condition	Low Risk	Medium Risk	High Risk
Controlled room temperature	≤ 48 hours	≤ 30 hours	≤ 24 hours
Refrigeration (2°C–8°C)	≤ 14 days	≤ 7 days	≤ 3 days
Frozen (below -20°C)	≤ 45 days	≤ 45 days	≤ 45 days

organisms. *Staphylococcus epidermidis, C. albicans*, and *E. coli* can survive in TNAs.

Because TNAs cannot be filtered through a bacterial-retentive 0.22-micron filter, growth of even a few microorganisms could harm the patient. 1.2-micron filters should be used in line for TNAs; they will removes *C. albican* but not *S. epidermidis* or *E. coli.*

Growth of most microorganisms was significantly better in TNAs than in standard parenteral nutrition solutions without lipid emulsion.[34] However, in a study with inoculum sizes that approximated touch contamination, bacterial and fungal growth were limited to less than l log in 24 hours. About 48 hours was required to reach stationary phase growth in TNAs.[41] In light of these studies, the recommended maximum TNA infusion (administration) duration is 24 hours at room temperature.[41,42] TNA infusion hang times of 12 to 18 hours are commonplace in the home care and ambulatory patient population.

Lipid Emulsions

Lipid emulsions provide an excellent medium for the growth of gram-positive, gram-negative, and fungal species at room temperature,[43] and after refrigeration. In one report, lipid emulsions supported bacterial and fungal growth at the same level as trypticase soy broth.[44] Although the Centers for Disease Control recommended a 12-hr hang time for lipid emulsions because of concerns about infection,[45] a subsequent study found no differences in microbial contamination or infection complications in a clinical setting between bottles hanging for less 12 hours and those with a hang time of 24 hours.[30] A lipid emulsion hang time (at room temperature) of up to 24 hours an accepted clinical practice.

IV Immune Globulins

The increasing use of intravenous immune globulins (IVIGs) (which are generally expensive medications) in ambulatory and home infusion presents some unique challenges for assigning beyond-use dating. Although some preparations are available as ready to infuse solutions, most IVIG preparation labeling recommends administration within a few hours after reconstitution. This has restricted the ability to provide these infusions in an alternate site of care, or has resulted in the reconstitution of these medications outside of the pharmacy IV preparation area (such as in a patient's home by a nurse). Fortunately, studies have demonstrated that properly reconstituted solutions remain chemically stable for 1 month at 37 °C,[46] and that they do not support bacterial and fungal growth at refrigerated, room, or body temperatures.[47] Practitioners should exercise judgment in assigning a realistic beyond-use date to these preparations consistent with the logistics and capabilities of the site of care.

Ambulatory Infusion Devices and Reservoirs

Preparations infused via ambulatory infusion devices (including portable pumps and disposable multi-day infusors) are often exposed to body temperatures and ambient temperatures that exceed "controlled room temperature" for periods up to a week. Unless the filtration of a particular drug is contraindicated, bacterial retaining filters should be added to or integral with the administration sets. In light of USP <797> guidelines for sterility-based beyond-use dating, practitioners should validate the preparation and storage process to ensure that these multi-day infusions do not harbor or promote bacterial or fungal growth. USP <797> also recommends that the chemical and physical stability of these preparations be confirmed from the literature or via direct testing.[3]

Multidose Vials

Preservatives help to maintain the sterility of multidose vials (MDVs) by inhibiting growth of any inadvertently introduced microorganism. As with all parenteral medications, strict aseptic technique should be practiced, including the wiping of the rubber septum of vials with 70% isopropyl alcohol and use of sterile needles or needle-less adapters for each entry. Time limits on using multidose vials after opening them have been investigated. Of primary concern is the potential contamination of vials that could lead to nosocomial sources of infection.[48] As a matter of conservative practice, many organizations discard MDVs no later than 30 days after opening. USP <797> requires MDVs to be refrigerated after opening (unless otherwise specified by the manufacturer), and, provided that the labeled storage conditions have been adhered to, discarded 30 days after the vial has been opened (unless otherwise specified by the manufacturer).[3] Some organizations have established specific policies requiring separately labeled vials for each patient, which can minimize the potential for spreading infections between patients due to improper technique.

Determination of Beyond-Use Dates

Whenever possible, beyond-use dating should be in accordance with the product's approved labeling or with reliable, published stability data. When these data are not available or applicable to the specific administration conditions and container, then a theoretical beyond-use dating must be arrived at. USP <797> recommends that, in the absence of published information or analytical studies, beyond-use dating periods not exceed 30 days.[3]

Manufacturer Information

In some instances, it is not possible to adhere to the product-approved labeling and guidelines. For example, a higher concentration of drug may be prescribed, a different diluent may be required, or a patient may require a preparation for longer periods (e.g., home delivery). Ideally, pharmacists should consult the product literature or obtain written information from the manufacturer to establish appropriate beyond-use dating. Be sure to communicate the deviations from the package insert when requesting stability information, including the strength, diluent, fill volume, and container type (e.g., PVC bag, plastic syringe, and elastomeric infusion device).

Published Stability Information

Published stability information, if carefully applied, can help to determine a theoretical beyond-use date for a given product. References on drug stability include the *Handbook on Injectable Drugs*,[4] *Remington's Pharmaceutical Sciences*,[49] *Extended Stability for Parenteral Drugs*,[1] and published research studies.

Applying published stability data can introduce inaccuracies if the characteristics of the preparation to be compounded differ greatly from the characteristics of the reported products. Do not assume equivalency of data for differing characteristics (e.g., composition, concentrations of ingredients, fill volume, and container type and material). Additionally, consider the conditions during in-home use (e.g., homes without air conditioning in a hot climate.) Informational resources used to establish beyond-use dates, should be reliable, referenced, and respected. "Word of mouth" and historical precedent are not acceptable references under any circumstances. Beyond-use dates predicted from published resources should not extend beyond the realistic and practical patient care needs and operational capabilities of the pharmacy.

Pharmacists should maintain a record of resources used for establishing beyond-use dates and develop policies and procedures for their appropriate assignment. A referenced table or chart of accepted beyond-use dates for commonly prepared products may be a helpful, saving time internal resource that ensures consistency in an organization.

Preparation-Specific Experimental Studies

Preparation-specific experimental studies are the only valid evidence of stability from which beyond-use dating should be predicted. The greater one's doubt about the accuracy or applicability of available stability data, the greater the need to establish beyond-use dating experimentally. For example, failure of one preparation to support bacterial and fungal growth under specific conditions should not be extrapolated to other preparations unless specific and reliable data are available. Experimental studies should always be considered for high-risk sterile preparations compounded from nonsterile ingredients.

Semiquantitative procedures, such as thin-layer chromatography, may be acceptable for some preparations. However, quantitative stability-indicating assays (e.g., high-performance liquid chromatography) are more appropriate for critical preparations. Examples include drugs with

1. A narrow therapeutic range.

2. Minimal supporting evidence of an appropriate beyond-use dating period.

3. A significant margin of safety that cannot be verified for the proposed theoretical period.

Beyond-use dates not specifically referenced in the product's approved labeling should be limited to 30 days.[3]

Summary

Beyond-use dating has important cost and safety implications. Preparations with longer dates may allow more efficient batch compounding in pharmacies, less frequent deliveries for home care practitioners, and recycling of unused preparations in hospitals. Batch compounded preparations may be subjected to greater quality control checks.

Beyond-use dates for compounded sterile preparations must be based on stability and sterility considerations. Both physical and chemical breakdowns are possible. Solubility-related problems may occur from changes in pH, temperature, and drug structure. In addition, drug adsorption to and absorption within preparation containers must be considered. Chemical degradation due to hydrolysis, oxidation, reduction, or photolysis can also quickly deteriorate a preparation. Moreover, the method and environment of drug administration can affect the drug's stability.

Sterility is separate from but as important as stability. Although a preparation may be stable for an extended period, its sterility also must be a factor in assigning a beyond-use date. The potential for bacterial growth has been widely studied and verified. With an increased use of TPN, TNA, IVIG, and other sterile preparations non-acute care settings (requiring extended usage and administration time), this issue takes on increasing importance. After considering physical, chemical, and delivery system effects, a pharmacist may still have to limit beyond-use dating. While manufacturers and published references may provide sufficient information regarding extended stability, the pharmacist may need to conduct or contract for separate stability studies using accepted compendial methods.

References

1. Bing C, ed. *Extended Stability for Parenteral Drugs.* 2nd ed. Bethesda, MD: American Society of Health-System Pharmacists; 2003.

2. Stella VJ. Chemical and physical bases determining the instability and incompatibility of formulated injectable drugs. *J Parenter Sci Technol.* 1986;40:2142–63.

3. Pharmaceutical compounding - Sterile preparations. In: United States pharmacopeia, 27th rev./national formulary, 22nd ed. Rockville, MD: United States Pharmacopeial Convention; Available at www.uspnf.com by subscription. Accessed April 4, 2004.

4. Trissel LA. *Handbook on Injectable Drugs.* 12th ed. Bethesda, MD: American Society of Health-System Pharmacists; 2003.

5. ASHP Guidelines on Quality Assurance for Pharmacy-Prepared Sterile Products. *Am J Health-Syst Pharm.* 2000:57:1150–69.

6. Newton DW. Physicochemical determinants of incompatibility and instability of drugs for injection and infusion. *Am J Hosp Pharm.* 1978:35:1213–22.

7. Newton DW, Driscoll DF, Goudreau JL, et al. Solubility characteristics of diazepam in aqueous admixture solutions: theory and practice. *Am J Hosp Pharm.* 1981;38:179–82.

8. Mason NA, Cline S, Hyneck ML, et al. Factors affecting diazepam infusion: solubility, administration-set composition, and flow rate. *Am J Hosp Pharm.* 1981;38:1449–54.

9. Morris ME. Compatibility and stability of diazepam injection following dilution from intravenous fluids. *Am J Hosp Pharm.* 1978;35:669–72.

10. Food and Drug Administration. Safety alert: Hazards of precipitation associated with parenteral nutrition. *Am J Hosp Pharm.* 1994;51:1427–8.

11. Driscoll DF, Newton DW, Bistrian BR. Precipitation of calcium phosphate from parenteral nutrient fluids. *Am J Hosp Pharm.* 1994;51:2834–6.

12. Robinson LA, Wright BT. Central venous catheter occlusion caused by body-heat mediated calcium phosphate precipitation. *Am J Hosp Pharm.* 1982;39:120–1.

13. Niemiec PW, Vanderveen TW. Compatibility considerations in parenteral nutrient solutions. *Am J Hosp Pharm.* 1984;41:893–911.

14. Wells P. *A Guide to Total Nutrient Admixtures.* Chicago, IL: Precept Press; 1992.

15. Trissel LA. *Calcium and Phosphate Compatibility in Parenteral Nutrition.* Houston, TX: TriPharma Communications; 2001.

16. Lima HA. Drug stability and compatibility: special considerations for home care.

Infusion. 1996;2:11–6.

17. U.S. Food and Drug Administration. Safety assessment of di(2-ethylhexyl) phthalate (DEHP) released from PVC medical devices. Available at www. fda.gov/Cdrh/ost/dehp-pvc.pdf. Accessed on April 4, 2004.

18. Helback HJ, Moltehnik DA, Ames BN. Toxic hydroperoxides in intravenous lipid emulsions used in preterm infants. *Pediatrics.* 1993;91:83–7.

19. Dupertix YM, Morch A et al. Physical characteristics of total parenteral nutrition bags significantly affect the stability of vitamins C and B1: a controlled prospective study. *J Parenter Enteral Nutr.* 2002;26(5):310–16.

20. Leissing NC, Story KO, Zaske D. Inline fluid dynamics in piggyback and manifold drug delivery systems. *Am J Hosp Pharm.* 1989;46:89–97.

21. Trissel LA, Gilbert DL et al. Compatibility of medications with 3-in-1 parenteral nutrition admixtures. *J Parenter Enteral Nutr.* 1999;23(2):67–74.

22. Bozzetti F, Bonfanti G, Regalie E, et al. Catheter sepsis from infusate contamination. *Nutr Clin Pract.* 1990;5:156–9.

23. Kastango ES. The cost of quality for sterile products. *Int J Pharm Compd.* 2002; 6:404–7.

24. Miller WA, Smith GL, Latiolais CJ, et al. A comparative evaluation of compounding costs and contamination rates of intravenous admixture systems. *Drug Intell Clin Pharm.* 1971;5:51–60.

25. DeCicco M, Chiaradia V, Veronese A, et al. Source and route of microbial colonization of parenteral nutrition catheters. *Lancet.* 1989;2:1258–61.

26. Takagi J, Kalidi N, Wolk RA, et al. Sterility of total parenteral nutrition solutions stored at room temperature for seven days. *Am J Hosp Pharm.* 1989;46:973–7.

27. Bronson MH, Stennett DJ, Egging PK. Sterility testing of home and inpatient parenteral nutrition solutions. *J Parenter Enter Nutr.* 1988;12:25–8.

28. Dolvin BJ, Davis PD, Holland TA. Contamination rates of 3-in-1 total parenteral nutrition in a clinical setting. *J Parenter Enter Nutr.* 1987;1:413–5.

29. Sitges-Serra A, Jaurrieta E, Pallares R, et al. Clinical experience with fat containing TPN solutions. In: *Advances in clinical nutrition.* Johnson I, ed. Boston, MA: MTP Press; 1983:207–12.

30. Ebbert ML, Farraj M, Hwang LT. The incidence and clinical significance of intravenous fat emulsion contamination during infusion. *J Parenter Enter Nutr.* 1987;11:425.

31. Freeman JB, Lemire A, MacLean LD. Intravenous alimentation and septicemia. *Surg Gynecol Obstet.* 1972;135:708–12.

32. Goldmann DA, Martin WT, Worthington JW. Growth of bacteria and fungi in total parenteral nutrition solutions. *Am J Surg.* 1973;126:314–8.

33. Rowlands DA, Wilkinson WR, Yoshimura N. Storage stability of mixed hyperalimentation solutions. *Am J Hosp Pharm.* 1973;30:436–8.

34. Scheckelhoff DJ, Mirtallo JM, Ayers LW, et al. Growth of bacteria and fungi in total nutrient admixtures. *Am J Hosp Pharm.* 1986;43:73–7.

35. Meunier-Carpentier F, Kiehn TE, Armstrong D. Fungemia in the immunocompromised host. *Am J Med.* 1981;71: 363–70.

36. Henderson DK, Edwards JE, Montgomerie JZ. Hematogenous Candida endophthalmitic in patients receiving parenteral hyperalimentation fluids. *J Infect Dis.* 1981;143:655–61.

37. Klein JJ, Watanakunakorn C. Hospital-acquired fungemia. *Am J Med.* 1979;67:51–8.

38. Montgomerie JZ, Edwards JE. Association of infection due to Candida albicans with intravenous hyperalimentation. *J Infect Dis.* 1978;137:197–201.

39. Laegeler WL, Tio JM, Blake MI. Stability of certain amino acids in a parenteral nutrition solution. *Am J Hosp Pharm.* 1974;31:776–9.

40. Parr MD, Bertch KE, Rapp PR. Amino acid stability and microbial growth in total parenteral nutrition solutions. *Am J Hosp Pharm.* 1985;42:2688–91.

41. Gilbert M, Gallagher SC, Eads M, et al. Microbial growth patterns in a total parenteral nutrition formulation containing lipid emulsion. *J Parenter Enter Nutr.* 1986;10:494–7.

42. Brown DH, Simkover RA. Maximum hang times for IV fat emulsions. *Am J Hosp Pharm.* 1987;44:282–4.

43. Melly MA, Mend HC, Schaffer W. Microbial growth in lipid emulsions used in parenteral nutrition. *Arch Surg.* 1975;110: 1479–81.

44. Kim Ch, Lewis DE, Kumar A. Bacterial

and fungal growth in intravenous fat emulsions. *Am J Hosp Pharm.* 1983;40: 2159–61.

45. Guidelines for the Prevention of Intravascular Catheter-Related Infections. MMWR Recommendations and Reports, August 9, 2002/51(RR10);1–26. http:// www.cdc.gov/mmwr/preview/mmwr html/rr5110a1.htm. Accessed 07/09/ 04.

46. Freidi HR. Methodology and safety considerations in the production of an intravenous immune globulin preparation. *Pharmacotherapy.* 1987;7(2):36–40S.

47. Pfeifer RW, Siegel J, Ayers LA. Assessment of microbial growth in intravenous immune globulin preparations. *Am J Hosp Pharm.* 1994;51:167–69.

48. Moi S, Thornton JP. Time limit on multidose vials after initial entry. *Hosp Pharm.* 1991;26:805–6.

49. Avis KE and Levchuk JW. Parenteral preparations. In: *Remington: The Science and Practice of Pharmacy.* 20th ed. Gennaro AR, ed. Baltimore, MD: Lippincott Williams & Wilkins; 2000:780–806.

9 | Labeling Sterile Preparations

*Patricia J. Kuban**

*The author acknowledges Douglas J. Scheckelhoff, who wrote this chapter in the first edition.

A properly compounded sterile preparation, must be labeled accurately and completely to facilitate appropriate and safe administration to the patient. Checking the accuracy of the compounded sterile preparation's label independently against the original physician's order/prescription and the ingredients used to compound the preparation is an intregal part of the pharmacist's verification process prior to release of the preparation. In addition, the sterile preparation's primary and auxiliary labels serve as communication tools regarding proper handling, storage, administration, and drug information for the person administering the drug to the correct patient. Therefore, the terminology used on the label should be descriptive but still appropriate to the knowledge of the user with the use of abbreviations minimized. All labels should be legible and affixed to the final container in a manner enabling them to be read both before and while the sterile preparation is being administered. If a container is to be hung, each label must be positioned so that it is right side up during administration. Light-resistant bags, for photosensitive drugs, and other overwraps should not limit the visibility of the label.

Small containers may require unique methods of affixing the label. For medium-sized syringes, labels often are "flagged" so that syringe markings are not covered or obstructed. Labels are often "flagged" for compounded sterile preparations dispensed in small vials and ophthalmic bottles. Very small syringes can be sealed in a larger bag or overwrap, which is then labeled. If the syringe might be removed from the bag some time before administration, a second, smaller label on the syringe should give key information (e.g., drug name, concentration, beyond-use date, and route). Based on the sterilization method, e.g., steam, final labeling with all required labeling components may need to occur post-sterilization.

The exact information on a label varies based on the preparation type and the patient's location/setting, not the ASHP[1] or USP[2] compounded sterile preparation risk-levels. Effective in 2004, there are official USP required labeling elements for all compounded sterile preparations regardless of where the patient is receiving the preparation.[2] General label content is similar, but slight variations exist[1,3] in addition to the USP standard for patient specific labeling in institutional and home care settings as well as for compounded sterile batch preparations. This chapter will review general labeling guidelines, the USP labeling requirements for sterile preparations, both required and optional patient specific labeling elements as specified by ASHP[1,4-7] and JCAHO,[8,9] batch labeling elements, and additional labeling strategies that can be utilized to help prevent medication errors and facilitate proper disposal of returned preparations to ensure compliance with the Health Insurance Portability and Accountability Act (HIPAA) privacy regulations.

General Labeling Guidelines

In order to ensure proper labeling, the following guidelines should be followed:

- Drug labeling is required if the compounded sterile preparation is not administered immediately or if it is administered by someone other that the person who prepared the medication.[8]

- The label conforms to all applicable federal, state and local laws and regulations.

- Medication labels are typed or electronically printed in a standardized format to ensure accurate and complete labeling. The label is legible, easily read, and free from erasures and strikeovers.

- The appropriate primary and auxiliary labels are firmly affixed to the container.

- The metric system of measures should be used instead of the apothecary system.

- Numbers, letters, coined names, unofficial synonyms, and prohibited abbreviations[9] are not used to identify medications with the exception of approved letter or number codes for investigational drugs.

- All medications with illegible or worn labels are properly and safely destroyed.

- A uniform, systematic labeling method is used. One order or drug preparation batch is filled and labeled at a time.

- During the hours the pharmacy is open, dilutions and labeling are done in a pharmacy. Within the pharmacy, only a pharmacist or authorized pharmacy technician under the direction and supervision of a pharmacist, may label and dispense medications, make labeling changes, or transfer medications to different containers.

USP Labeling Requirements for Compounded Sterile Preparations

With the introduction of the new United States Pharmacopeia's (USP) Chapter <797>, there exists a minimum labeling standard for compounded sterile preparations that applies to all health care settings,[2] not just health care institutions and pharmacies. Figure 9-1 illustrates a sample label. The parts of the label are described below; the numbers in parentheses correspond to information on the label.

Names and amounts or concentrations of ingredients (1)

The name of each drug, preferably generic, should be clearly shown. This includes the names of all drug products or ingredients added or used to prepare the finished preparation, including admixture solutions and their corresponding volumes. The trade drug name or commonly known name of the preparation can be included if it can reduce the potential for error. Although the amount or volume of admixture solution, e.g., dextrose or sodium chloride, usually is unimportant in the patient's therapy, it may be a consideration in certain clinical settings. The admixture solution itself; however, definitely affects the compounded sterile preparation's stability and beyond-use dating. Preservative-free ingredients, admixture solutions, and diluents should be used in compounding sterile preparations given by the intrathecal or intravitreal routes and to neonatal patients. In some cases it may be appropriate to label ophthalmic sterile preparations with the concentration not only of the active ingredients, but also the preservatives. Moreover, the amount and units of measure should be standard and easily understood.

Total volume of the preparation (2)

Total volume is usually expressed in the metric system, e.g., milliliters (mls) or liters. For IV piggybacks and continuous infusions, this measurement allows tracking the patient's total fluid intake. If the volume of the admixture solution is not significantly different from the total volume, these measurements are used interchangeably (e.g., antibiotic solutions). For larger volume solutions with multiple additives, the actual or calculated total volume should be used (e.g., TPN solutions). For syringes and vials that are overfilled, both the overfill volume and the volume of the prescribed medication dose should be clearly shown on the label.

Beyond-use date (3)

This date is the last date that the sterile preparation can be used by the patient and should be consistent within each health care setting. Beyond-use dating should be based on known stability information and sterility considerations. The specific beyond-use date of a preparation should be based on published

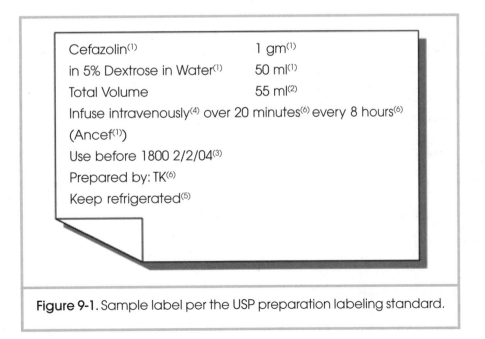

Cefazolin[1]   1 gm[1]

in 5% Dextrose in Water[1]   50 ml[1]

Total Volume   55 ml[2]

Infuse intravenously[4] over 20 minutes[6] every 8 hours[6]

(Ancef[1])

Use before 1800 2/2/04[3]

Prepared by: TK[6]

Keep refrigerated[5]

Figure 9-1. Sample label per the USP preparation labeling standard.

data, appropriate testing, or USP-NF standards. The methods used to assign actual beyond-use dates are discussed in Chapter 8.

Appropriate route(s) of administration (4)

Even though the route of administration may be implied by the dosage form (e.g., IV bag implies IV or intravenous administration unless labeled otherwise), the appropriate route(s) of administration should be placed on the preparation's label. Especially when a container is used outside the normal pattern or a dosage form has multiple uses, the route must be clearly stated to prevent medication errors. Often, drugs can be given only by certain routes or the amount/concentration is route specific and, therefore, may be dangerous otherwise. Preparations used for irrigation, cardioplegia, intrathecal and epidural injections, and peritoneal dialysis should be clearly marked and distinctively labeled (by size, shape, and the use of auxiliary labels).

Syringes should be clearly labeled with the intended route of administration (e.g., IV push, pump or gravity, epidural or intrathecal, intravitreal, or intramuscular). In some cases, the ramifications of giving a particular drug or dose by an unintended route can be fatal (e.g., IV dose given intrathecally). Patient-controlled analgesia (PCA) containers also should be clearly marked since they may be the same for IV and epidural PCA, but the concentration of drug differs.

Storage conditions (5)

Storage instructions can be put on the primary label or added as an auxiliary label. Preparations must be stored in accord with the conditions stated on the label to ensure the preparation's sterility and stability. This can include, but is not limited to, whether the preparation should be refrigerated, kept at room temperature, protected from light, or not shaken. If the sterile preparation requires refrigeration, it should be separated from food to avoid contaminating the outside of the container.

Other information for safe use (6)

Other information, including cautionary statements, for the safe use of the preparation can be put on the primary label or added as auxiliary labels. This information should include the initials of the responsible pharmacist who prepared or checked the preparation and com-

plete directions for the proper clinical administration of the compounded sterile preparation, including device specific settings and instructions. In addition, hazardous drugs[10] should have appropriate precautionary labels to facilitate safe handling, use, and disposal. For facilities that ship preparations to recipients outside there own facility, including patients, disposal instructions for out-of-date or unused units should be included.[2]

Patient Specific Labeling

In addition to the above USP minimum labeling standards, patient specific compounded sterile preparations have additional requirements when used in institutional and/or home care settings. Accurate labels not only help staff efficiently deliver preparations, but also supply needed information to staff or patients/caregivers to safely administer the correct medication to the correct patient.

Labels in Institutional Settings

Figure 9-2 illustrates a sample label used in an institutional setting. The parts of this label are described below; the numbers in parentheses correspond to information on the label.

Required Labeling

Patient name and identification number (1)

A patient name on a label defines the dose as ordered for the patient. Exclusion of a name may indicate that the preparation can be used on other patients and may lead to errors. Moreover, both the first and last names of the patient should be identified. A middle initial can be helpful if two patients have the same first and last names. A medical record number and/or account number also identifies each patient in most hospital computer systems and can serve as a second unique patient identifier. This number is critical to drug administration in hospitals that use bar code technology based on each patient's medical record or account number.

Patient location (2)

Location information within a treatment facility ensures that the drug gets to the correct patient. Transfer or discharge of patients also

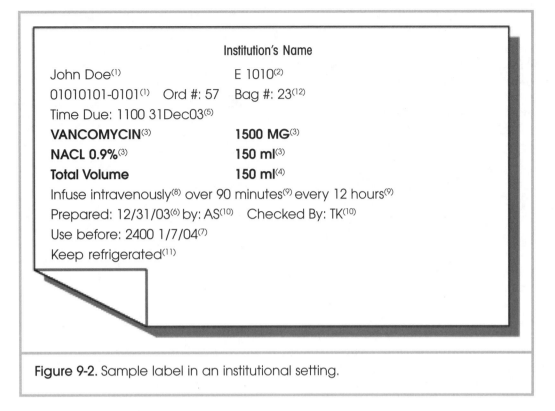

Institution's Name

John Doe[1]   E 1010[2]

01010101-0101[1]   Ord #: 57   Bag #: 23[12]

Time Due: 1100 31Dec03[5]

VANCOMYCIN[3]   **1500 MG**[3]

NACL 0.9%[3]   **150 ml**[3]

Total Volume   **150 ml**[4]

Infuse intravenously[8] over 90 minutes[9] every 12 hours[9]

Prepared: 12/31/03[6] by: AS[10]   Checked By: TK[10]

Use before: 2400 1/7/04[7]

Keep refrigerated[11]

Figure 9-2. Sample label in an institutional setting.

should be tracked so that label information is updated. If the data are not relayed or used, delays in therapy and unnecessary work can result.

Name and amount of drug(s) added and name of admixture solution (3)

This section is similar to item (1) on the USP label; however, it includes the names and amounts or concentrations of the drugs added to the compounded sterile preparation in addition to the name of the admixture solution used in compounding the sterile preparation. Identification of the admixture solution makes the label more complete and accurate. Diluent information often is not listed on the label when sterile water for injection is required to reconstitute drugs.

Approximate final total volume of admixture solution (4)

This section is the same as item (2) on the USP label. The total volume should be listed for all preparations, including intermittent and continuous IV admixtures, critical care infusions, total parenteral nutrition fluids, irrigations, dialysate fluids, and small volume sterile preparations, such as syringes.

Time and date of scheduled administration (5)

In institutions, the scheduled administration time is generally referred to as the "due" time and is expressed in military time, e.g., 1300 is used to express 1:00 pm. This information notifies the nursing staff of the administration schedule maintained in the pharmacy. Nurses can make a professional decision about when to begin administration based on whether the patient is scheduled for a test or procedure out of the patient care area as well as the number of patients the individual nurse is assigned. However, if both pharmacy and nursing schedules are the same, errors will be minimized.

If nurses follow the scheduled administration time and date printed on the label, admixtures will not be used out of sequence. When admixtures are in improper sequence, the "oldest" one (with the earliest expiration) may not be administered; its expiration or beyond-use date may then be passed, creating waste. Institution specific standardized administration times also reduce confusion and waste and prevent omitted doses.

Time and date of compounding (6)

The time and date of compounding are needed to determine actual beyond-use times for recycling preparations. In addition, JCAHO requires the date prepared for all compounded IV admixtures and parenteral nutrition solutions and a beyond-use time for all preparations with beyond-use periods less than 24 hours.[8] This information may be contained on the label, even if it is not stated clearly. For example, the scheduled administration time may indicate when a drug was prepared based on that sterile preparation's batch or fill-list period.

Beyond-use date (and time, if applicable) (7)

This section is similar to item (3) on the USP label. Traditionally in an institutional setting, the expiration or beyond-use date assigned to a preparation can be the actual time that it is deemed unusable for the patient or a standard time in which it should be returned to the pharmacy (e.g., 24 hours). After its return, the pharmacist can determine if the preparation should be recycled or discarded. Methods used to assign actual beyond-use dates are discussed in Chapter 8. For compounded sterile preparations with beyond-use periods less than 24 hours, a beyond-use time is also required.[8]

Route of administration (8)

This section is the same as item (4) on the USP label.

Administration instructions (9)

This section is similar to item (6) on the USP label; however, it includes all directions needed for proper clinical administration of the preparation to a patient in an institutional setting. For intermittent doses, administration instructions should include the duration and, sometimes, rate of administration. If the preparation requires activation or some other manipulation prior to patient administration, this information should also be included on the primary label or added as an auxiliary label (e.g., break seal and mix prior to administration). For continuous infusions, administration instructions generally include the rate and possibly a stop time. The rate should not be included for a continuous infusion if the drug is being titrated because the rate may change without the pharmacy's knowledge and without a notation on the label. This situation could result in a medication error. In these cases, "infuse as directed" or "titrate" may be more appropriate.

Initials of persons who prepare and check IV admixture (10)

The identity of the preparer and/or pharmacist who releases the preparation should be noted on the label or in a dispensing record in the pharmacy. State boards of pharmacy often require the initials of the responsible pharmacist to be on the label. This information is helpful when questions arise about the preparation.

Storage conditions (11)

This section is the same as item (5) on the USP label since storage instructions can be put on the primary label or added as an auxiliary label. This information can remind nurses to refrigerate, protect from light, or not shake a preparation prior to patient administration. In fact, since refrigeration of compounded sterile preparations usually is the standard, this information should be highlighted for emphasis.

Auxiliary Labeling

Auxiliary labeling provides supplemental instructions and/or precautions similar to item (6) on the USP label, without the space limitations of pre-formatted or computerized labels. Auxiliary labels have an added advantage of highlighting the information since the label looks different. Auxillary labels also help staff follow the manufacturer's recommendation and/or the pharmacy's guidelines for storage of all medications prior to distribution. Figure 9-3 illustrates sample auxiliary labels.

The same auxiliary labels should be used each time a particular sterile preparation is dispensed; otherwise, the user may question the importance or validity of the information. Auxiliary labels often are used for information about

- Light protection (e.g., "Protect from light").
- Final filters (e.g., "Use in-line filter").
- Rate precautions.
- Storage conditions (e.g., "Refrigerate" or "Do not refrigerate" or "Do not shake").
- Drug concentration.
- Routes of administration (e.g., "For the eye" or "Not for IV use" or "For irrigation only").
- Other information for safe use (e.g., "Break seal and mix prior to administration," "Caution chemotherapy," or "STAT").

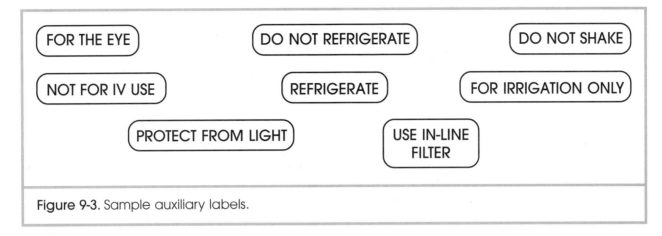

Figure 9-3. Sample auxiliary labels.

All information for the safe use of the preparation is now required as part of the labeling, which can be either on the primary label or on auxiliary labels.

Optional Labeling

Bottle or bag sequence number (12)

The sequence number of the container may be important, depending on the type of drug or number of doses ordered. The total doses given also should be tracked by the nurse who administers the drug since bags might be given out of sequence or doses might be lost.

Labels in Home Care Settings

Labels used in home care are similar to those used in institutions but have some unique requirements. Because the preparation is an outpatient prescription, it must meet state board of pharmacy requirements. Moreover, the label must be understood by a lay person since the user may be the patient, a family member, or other caregiver. The label also should contain few abbreviations or other confusing terminology. Patient and/or caregiver training should include reading the container's label(s) immediately prior to administration to ensure the right patient, drug, dose, route, and time of drug administration.[2] The label should serve as an adjunct to other written and verbal instructions given to the patient and/or caregiver regarding the compounded sterile preparation.

Figure 9-4 illustrates a sample label used in the home care setting.[5,9] The parts of this label are described below; the numbers in parentheses correspond to information on the label.

Required Labeling

Prescription number, date filled, prescribing physician, and authorized refills (1)

This information typically is required by state boards of pharmacy, but it also is used by the dispensing pharmacy to reference the original order.

Patient name and address (2)

The patient's full name should be printed as part of the prescription label. Although the address is optional, it may simplify delivery procedures and ensure efficient delivery of the correct medication, equipment, device or supplies to the correct patient or patient's representative.

Directions to the patient for use of the medication (3)

This section is similar to item (9) on the institutional label; however, should be easy for the patient or care giver to understand. Clear instructions should be included regarding required manipulations of the sterile preparation, e.g., measuring, reconstituting, or adding other ingredients as well as setting up needed tubing or filters for proper drug administration. Directions should include the route of administration, rate of administration, frequency of administration, and any special precautionary handling or storage requirements (e.g., "Caution chemotherapy," "Refrigerate," or "Do not shake"). If the drugs are to be administered with an infusion device, the device settings should also be included on the label.[5]

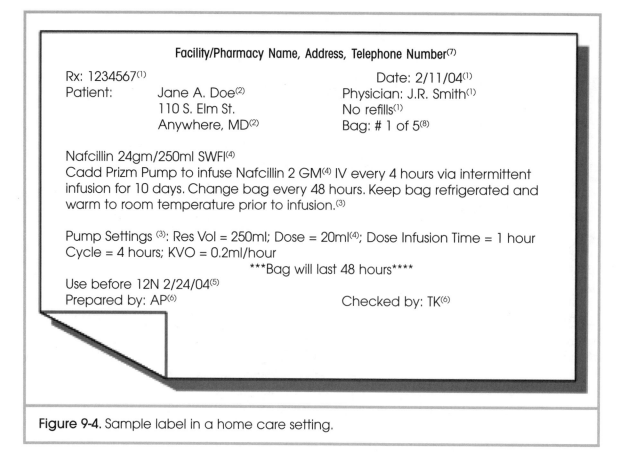

Figure 9-4. Sample label in a home care setting.

Name and amount or strength of drug added and name and volume of admixture solution (4)

This section is similar to items (3) and (4) on the institutional label; however, the admixture may contain more than one dose. In this situation, the label should indicate both the amount of drug in one dose and the appropriate volume for that amount as well as the total amount of drug or nutrient within the preparation container (e.g., bag, bottle, cassette, syringe, or vial). The total volume of the preparation should be clearly indicated on the label. The label format should be well designed to avoid misinterpretation of dosage information when multiple doses of a drug are aseptically compounded in one container.

Beyond-use date (5)

This section is the same as item (3) on the USP label. The beyond-use date used in home care settings usually is the actual beyond-use date established for the preparation so that a multiple day supply of the preparation can be dispensed and delivered. Beyond-use dates often are maximized for practical reasons,

such as the patient's distance from the pharmacy. Beyond-use dating of compounded sterile preparations used in ambulatory infusion pumps worn close to the body must take into account that these drugs are administered at temperatures warmer than room temperatures. Methods used to assign actual beyond-use dates are discussed in Chapter 8. Since patients typically are more stable at home than in an institution, their medications are less likely to change, requiring return to the pharmacy. Furthermore, these preparations will not be recycled even if returned unused because they are compounded outpatient prescriptions and were stored at home.

Initials of persons who prepare and check IV admixture (6)

Similar to the institutional setting, state boards of pharmacy often require that the initials or name of the responsible pharmacist appear on the label. Furthermore, this information is helpful when questions arise about product preparation.

Name, address, and telephone number of the compounding facility/pharmacy (7)

This information typically is required by state boards of pharmacy and provides an easy mechanism for the patient to contact the dispensing pharmacy when questions arise about product preparation, delivery, storage, administration, and disposal.

Auxiliary Labeling

This section is similar to the auxiliary labeling described on the institutional label; however, the federal transfer labeling must be included, as with any outpatient prescription, and must be easily understood by the user. Other information may also be required by individual state laws or regulations.

Optional Labeling (8)

As in the institutional setting, the bottle or bag sequence number can help to track the specific number of doses ordered and/or the total number of doses administered (e.g., bag 1 of 7).

Batch Labeling

Batch compounded sterile preparations require additional labeling elements beyond the USP labeling because these preparations are compounded in anticipation of an actual physician's order or prescription. Figure 9-5 illustrates a sample label used for batch preparations. The parts of this label are described below; the numbers in parentheses correspond to information on the label.

Required Labeling

Name of preparation (1)

The commonly known name of a preparation is useful, especially for one with multiple ingredients, so that it can be readily identified.

Name and amount of drug added (2)

The names and amounts of drugs added to a solution should be all inclusive. Additives, such as preservatives and buffering agents, also should be listed.

Admixture solution or diluent used (3)

Admixture solutions or diluents, such as normal saline, 5% dextrose, and sterile water for injection may affect how a final preparation is used, especially whether the preparation contains preservatives.

Total volume of solution (4)

The total volume may be simply stated as a common metric volume for the final preparation (e.g., milliliters) or as a concentration that includes both the amount of drug and the total volume in which it is contained. Use of the abbreviation for cubic centimeters (cc) rather

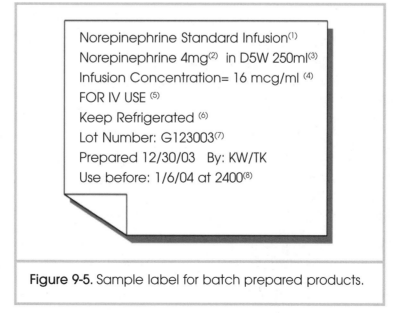

Norepinephrine Standard Infusion[1]
Norepinephrine 4mg[2] in D5W 250ml[3]
Infusion Concentration= 16 mcg/ml [4]
FOR IV USE [5]
Keep Refrigerated [6]
Lot Number: G123003[7]
Prepared 12/30/03   By: KW/TK
Use before: 1/6/04 at 2400[8]

Figure 9-5. Sample label for batch prepared products.

than ml for milliliters is discouraged by JCAHO.[9]

Route of administration (5)

Route of administration can be specific (e.g., "for irrigation") or general (e.g., "for injection") if the preparation can be used safely for more than one route.

Storage conditions (6)

Storage requirements should reflect preferred conditions before and/or after the preparation is opened or administered to the patient.

Lot number or control number (7)

A lot or control number tracks a preparation back to its batch preparation documentation sheet (see Chapter 14). These numbers usually are generated internally, based on some logic, and should be readily traceable to information on how the preparation was made and tested. The date of preparation and either a specifically assigned drug preparation number or daily sterile compounding sequence number are usually included in the numbering logic.

Beyond-use date (8)

This section is the same as item (3) on the USP label. Beyond-use dating should be based on known stability information and sterility considerations. If the beyond-use dating is based on storage conditions other than room temperature, they also should be listed (e.g., refrigeration and freezing).

Auxiliary and Optional Labeling

Since batch-prepared products are relabeled with patient specific information prior to dispensing, auxiliary labels should not be used. Any pertinent auxiliary or optional information should be incorporated into the batch label if possible. Use of auxiliary labels may lead to errors if old labels are not removed prior to dispensing of the relabeled preparation. The one exception is auxiliary labels that are pertinent to the patient specific preparation and are correctly positioned on the preparation's final container enabling them to be be read both before and at the point of patient administration after the preparation has been relabeled with patient specific information.

Additional Labeling Strategies

Labels should clearly present information, be easy to read, and reduce the risk of medication errors. In this age of various marketing strategies, pharmacy staff and manufacturers get very creative when it comes to unique labeling options. The overall question; however, is whether they are effective in enhancing patient safety.

Use of Color on Labels

The use of color on labels to reduce the risk of errors has been met with mixed reviews. Color differentiation has been used successfully to highlight preparation information and make various label features or components stand out (e.g., drug concentration).[11] Color labels have also been employed in workflow design (e.g., making STAT preparations print on a different color label to facilitate efficient and timely pharmacy preparation and delivery as well as nursing administration to the patient). In these examples, color itself is not used as a standard code to classify or identify the therapeutic drug class.

On the other hand, the Institute of Safe Medication Practices (ISMP) warns that color-coding should be used with extreme caution as under this system, people identify a color with a function.[11] This practice from both pharmaceutical vendors and individual health care facilities can contribute to medication errors. Therefore, it is not a prudent practice to rely solely on a standard color to classify or identify drug categories, even high-risk medication categories. People need to carefully read the exact drug name, strength, and dose they are preparing, dispensing, and/or administering.

Tall Man Letters

In an effort to reduce medication errors, the FDA Office of Generic Drugs' voluntarily asked manufacturers of 16 look-a-like generic drug name pairs to use "tall man" letters (e.g., DAUNOrubicin, DOXOrubicin) to differentiate the selected look-a-like drug names on their labels.[12] In addition, to manufacturers phasing in these changes, some pharmacies use "tall man" characters to distinguish between similar or look-a-like drug names on compounded sterile preparation labels. To date, the field effectiveness of the "tall man" lettering strategy is unknown[13]; however, Grasha found tall man lettering "reduced drug selection errors by 35% in a simulated pharmacy dispensing environment."[14]

Specialty Labels

HIPAA privacy regulations enacted in April 2003, state that patient confidentially of protected health information[15] must be maintained. Some label companies have designed new label formats that ensure patient privacy/ confidentiality whereby the portion of the label that contains the patient's name and other identifying information can be peeled off or removed prior to destruction of any sterile preparation. This design allows for the patient information component of the label to follow the institution's or business's confidential waste stream and the actual sterile preparation to follow the appropriate general or hazardous waste stream as dictated by the drug entities and volumes involved. Even if specialty designed labels are not used, patient confidentiality and privacy need to be ensured.

Summary

Accurate and complete labeling of sterile preparations in any setting is critical to quality assurance and is a USP requirement for all compounded sterile preparations regardless of where the patient is receiving the preparation[2]. The information on the label must be legible, accurate, easy to understand, uniform, and appropriately displayed. Minor differences exist in the label information for patient specific institutional and home care settings as well as for sterile batch preparations. Patient specific labeling information for compounded sterile preparations should include, but not be limited to

- Patient name and identifier (either a patient identification number or prescription number).

- Patient location.

- Names and amounts or concentrations of all ingredients, including drugs, admixture solutions, and diluents.

- Total volume of the compounded sterile preparation.

- Beyond-use date (and time if applicable).

- Appropriate route(s) of administration.

- Storage conditions

- Other information for safe use, including

  - specific administration instructions or directions for use

  - time and date of scheduled administration

  - responsible pharmacist's initials

  - date of preparation

  - warning or precautionary statements, when appropriate

  - any additional information to ensure the safe use of the compounded sterile preparation

These labeling requirements can be met on either the primary label or on auxiliary labels. Unique labeling techniques and strategies should continue to be studied, utilized, and evaluated for effectiveness in preventing potentially significant toxicities and medication errors as well as ensuring patient privacy of protected health information. The goal of any labeling strategy utilized for compounded sterile preparations should be based on facilitating appropriate and safe drug administration to the patient.

References

1. American Society of Health-System Pharmacists. ASHP guidelines on quality assurance for pharmacy-prepared sterile products. *Am J Health-Syst Pharm.* 2000; 57:1150–69.

2. Pharmaceutical compounding - Sterile preparations. In: United States pharmacopeia, 27th rev./national formulary, 22nd ed. Rockville, MD: United States Pharmacopeial Convention; Available at www.uspnf.com. Accessed April 1, 2004.

3. Brzozowski DF, Hale KM, Segal R, et al. Pharmacist opinions about compliance with recommendations for intravenous admixture practices. *Am J Hosp Pharm.* 1987;44:2077–84.

4. American Society of Health-System Pharmacists. ASHP guidelines on preventing medication errors with antineoplastic agents. *Am J Health-Syst Pharm.* 2002; 59:1648–68.

5. American Society of Health-System Pharmacists. ASHP guidelines: minimum standards for home care pharmacies. *Am J Health-Syst Pharm.* 1999;56:629–38.

www.ashp.org/bestpractices/practicsettings/Practice Settings Guidelines Min.Std. Accessed December 17, 2003.

6. American Society of Health-System Pharmacists. ASHP guidelines:minimum standard for pharmaceutical services in ambulatory care. *Am J Health-Syst Pharm.* 1999;56:1744–53. www.ashp.org/bestpractices/practicesettings/Practice Settings Guidelines Min.Std. Accessed December 17, 2003.

7. American Society of Hospital Pharmacists. ASHP technical assistance bulletin on pharmacy-prepared ophthalmic products. *Am J Hosp Pharm.* 1993;50:1462–3.

8. *2004 Comprehensive Accreditation Manual for Hospitals, Automated.* Joint Commission on Accreditation of Healthcare Organizations. Medication Management Standard and Rationale for MM.4.30. Available at www.jcaho.org. Accessed December 17, 2003.

9. 2004 National Patient Safety Goals. Available at www.jcaho.org/accredited+organizations/patient+safety/04+npsg.

Accessed March 12, 2004.

10. National Institute for Occupational Safety and Health. *Reducing occupational exposures to hazardous drugs in healthcare.* Pre-publication Alert, June 7, 2004. Available at www.cdc.gov/niosh/docs/2004-HazDrugAlert/pdfs/2004-HazDrugAlert.pdf.

11. A spectrum of problems with using color. *ISMP Medication Safety Alert.* 2003;8(issue 23);1–2.

12. U.S. Food and Drug Administration Center for Drug Evaluation and Research. Name Differentiation Project. www.fda.gov/cder/drug/MedErrors/nameDiff.htm. Last updated May 8, 2002. Accessed December 19, 2003.

13. Let us know if "tall man" letters have been effective. *ISMP Medication Safety Alert.* 2003;8(issue 19):3.

14. For every problem a solution; for every solution a problem. *ISMP Medication Safety Alert.* 2004;9(issue 2):2.

15. Giacalone RP, Cacciatore, GG. HIPAA and its impact on pharmacy practice. *Am J Health-Syst Pharm.* 2003;60:433–42.

10 | Documentation of Compounded Sterile Preparations

Philip J. Schneider

Documentation is a record of activities. In the case of compounding sterile preparations, documents tell how a drug was processed and what quality attributes it possesses. This documentation helps to ensure that a system is in place to compound preparations properly and also serves as a checklist for compounding procedures. Documentation must be performed precisely, unfailingly, consistently, quickly, and in sufficient detail to permit another individual to duplicate the compounding process exactly.

Uses of Documentation

Outside Organizations

Sterile preparation records may be inspected by many organizations including State Boards of Pharmacy, third-party payers, the Joint Commission on Accreditation of Healthcare Organizations, the Drug Enforcement Agency, and the Food and Drug Administration. These organizations use documentation records when determining payments, granting licensure, and, possibly, justifying continued accreditation of certain programs. Standards of practice including the United States Pharmacopeia Chapter 797[1] and ASHP Guidelines on Quality Assurance for Pharmacy-Prepared Sterile Products[2] also provide recommendations for documentation of environmental and equipment quality, personnel training and technique, compliance with compounding procedures and both the products used and final preparation compounded.

Legal Situations

If a patient pursues litigation related to a compounded sterile preparation, an attorney may subpoena the pharmacy's quality-assurance records and other relevant documents. These records would also be reviewed by the organization's attorney as well as its malpractice insurance carrier. In this situation, the quality of documentation may prevent a costly lawsuit or judgment.

Workload Justification

Besides serving as a record of past actions, documentation of goods and services provided by the pharmacy can be used to develop workload statistics and productivity ratios. This information can subsequently support a formal request for adding staff, equipment, or workspace or for reallocating these same resources elsewhere.

Quality Improvement

If problems are discovered with compounded sterile preparations, all documentation should be double checked as soon as possible. Whenever the quality of a compounded sterile preparation is questioned, the following documents should be reviewed:

- Original prescription
- Batch record
- Results of quality-control tests
- Calibration and setup procedures for involved equipment
- Environmental quality-control results for the time of compounding
- Validation and training records for involved personnel

Results of the investigation then should be used in a continuous quality-improvement process to

1. Identify problems.
2. Take action to improve problem areas.
3. Evaluate the effectiveness of the action taken.

Documented Information

Documentation can be brief or extensive as long as important facts are not omitted. Forms, worksheets, and computer software can prompt the user to document all essential information. Computerized labels, no-carbon forms, or addressographs may save time by avoiding duplicate data entries (e.g., patient names and locations). Documentation should occur *when* and *where* the work is completed or while it is in progress.

Documentation errors must be handled carefully to avoid the appearance of a coverup. Correction fluid should never be used on pharmacy records; a single line should be drawn through the mistake, and the word "error" with the person's initials should be written by it.

Medication-related Records

Maintenance of all medication-related records (including prescription documents and medication orders for hospital and home care patients) must follow the mandates established by federal and state laws. Prescription records must be readily retrievable for the number of years required by the State Board of Pharmacy; however, records may need to be retained longer for other purposes (e.g., 5 years for Medicare). Often, no-carbon or faxed copies of physician's orders are sent to institutional pharmacies. These copies do not have to be kept for long term, however, as long as the original is in the patient's medical record and all other documents (e.g., patient medication profile and batch record) are filed.

Records for controlled substances and investigational drugs require special handling. Inventories and prescriptions for controlled substances may be kept separately or have the letter "C" stamped in the lower right corner for easy retrieval. Narcotic order forms must be stored for at least 2 years; state laws vary. A perpetual inventory is usually maintained for both controlled substances and investigational drugs. A biennial controlled substance inventory is also required.

The statute of limitations for litigation is 2 years for adults. For pediatric patients, however, litigation may be initiated until the child reaches the age of majority. Therefore, many hospitals and home care organizations utilize microfiche or compact disk files for long-term storage of their records.

The records that should be maintained for at least 2 years include[3]

- patient profiles
- medication records
- purchase records
- biennial controlled substance inventories
- policies and procedures for cytotoxic waste
- lot numbers of components used in compounded sterile preparations

Batch Compounding Records

As discussed in Chapter 14, batch preparation records must be maintained. For routinely compounded preparations, a set of master production records helps to ensure that all associated activities can be reproduced with a high degree of uniformity. While compounding, these records document that the preparation meets established specifications. Master compounding records contain the model requirements for the batch formula and compounding directions. Specifications for selection and handling of equipment are critical; substitution of a different item, such as a filter with a different pore size, can have serious consequences.

Batch compounding records show that each significant step prescribed for the compounding of a preparation was completed. Furthermore, signatures of the employees who performed and checked the procedures authenticate that the compounding was done correctly. Control records confirm that specifications for the preparation were met, based on analytical determinations of the process and the final preparation. Environmental monitoring records show the conditions that existed during the compounding of the preparation. Records of quarantine and a copy of the label for each final preparation should be maintained.

Pharmacy Quality Improvement Records

Records of the quality of pharmacy activities should be filed for an adequate time, consistent with organizational policies.[2] These documents include the

- organization's policies and procedures
- logs of refrigerator and freezer temperatures
- certification of laminar airflow workbench(s), biological safety cabinets, and cleanrooms
- results of environmental monitoring

Personnel Training, Certification, and Recertification Records

Orientation and training of new pharmacists and technicians who compound sterile preparations must be documented. Some State Boards of Pharmacy now review training records during their routine annual pharmacy inspections.[4] It is not adequate simply to state that an employee passed an initial evaluation period. Specific training about aseptic technique, use of a ISO Class 5 (Class 100) environment, appropriate garb and personal hygiene, and storage and handling of drugs and supplies should be documented.

Employees should also be trained in the setup, calibration, and use of all compounding devices and equipment; this training should be recorded for each type of equipment used. The completion of an acceptable validation procedure should be documented before employees are certified to compound sterile preparations for patients. Personnel records also should include documentation of employee health procedures (e.g., annual physical and tuberculin skin test) and an offer to provide vaccination against hepatitis B.

At appropriate intervals, employees should be recertified to verify that they follow good technique and current institutional procedures. For example, an annual recertification could include:

- Written test covering aseptic technique, use of a ISO Class 5 environment, and environmental monitoring procedures.

- Evaluation of aseptic technique with media fills (process validation) followed by immediate feedback.

- Recertification records should be maintained in an employee's personnel file.

Summary

Documentation is an important and essential part of any sterile preparation compounding program. Documentation records may be used to justify third-party payments, to prevent or provide a basis for legal action, to justify workload, and to discover errors in policies and procedures. At a minimum, documentation should be collected for all activities related to medication supply and use, batch compounding procedures, quality improvement programs, and personnel training.

References

1. Pharmaceutical compounding - Sterile preparations. In: United States pharmacopeia, 27th rev./national formulary, 22nd ed. Rockville, MD: United States Pharmacopeial Convention; Available at www.uspnf.com. Accessed April 1, 2004.

2. American Society of Hospital Pharmacists. ASHP guideline on quality assurance for pharmacy-prepared sterile products. *Am J Health-Syst Pharm.* 2000;57:1150–69.

3. Model State Pharmacy Act and Model Rules of the National Association of Boards of Pharmacy. Fall 2002. Available at http://WWW.NABP.NET/FTPFILES/NABP01/MODELACT02-03_REV.PDF.

4. Section 1751.5. Training of Staff, Patient and Caregiver. *2004 Lawbook for Pharmacy.* Available at http://www.pharmacy.ca.gov/pdfs/lawbook_2004.pdf.

11 | Handling of Sterile Commercial Products and Preparations Within the Pharmacy

E. Clyde Buchanan*

*The author acknowledges Barbara T. McKinnon, who authored this chapter in the first edition of this text.

This chapter covers pharmacy's responsibility for sterile commercial products and compounded preparations beginning when products are first received and continuing through compounding and waste disposal. To ensure both preparation quality and public safety, correct storage and handling procedures are necessary every step of the way.

This chapter does not cover selection and quality control of non-sterile components and raw materials (see Chapter 2); nor does it discuss the handling of hazardous drugs and materials (see Chapter 7). And it does not cover the delivery of compounded preparations either within the institution or outside the institution, for example in home care (see Chapter 12).

Receipt of Sterile Commercial Products

Sterile Components

Components are comprised of active and inactive ingredients, intermediate containers (e.g., a syringe used to transfer a drug from one containter to another), final containers and closures. A procedure should specify the visual inspection of commercially available drug products, sterile ready-to-use containers, and devices (e.g., syringes and needles) upon receipt in the pharmacy. All items must be free from defects, within the manufacturer's expiration dating, and suitable for their intended use.[1] Expired, inappropriately stored,

or defective products should not be used; defective drugs and devices should be promptly reported via the MedWatch program to the Food and Drug Administration (FDA).[2]

For handling of non-sterile components and raw materials see Chapter 2.

USP Storage Conditions

Intravenous solutions, sterile commercial products, and sterile supplies should be stored according to manufacturer labeling or USP product monographs to preserve stability of ingredients.[3] Most sterile products are aqueous solutions for which hydrolysis is the most common chemical degradation reaction. In general, the rate of a chemical reaction increases exponentially for each 10^0 C increase in temperature.[4] Thus, storage of a beta-lactam antibiotic solution for one day at controlled room temperature will have an equivalent hydrolytic effect of approximately 3 to 5 days in cold temperatures.[5] Cold temperatures may cause harm as well, for example refrigeration may cause precipitates and freezing may break an emulsion or denature proteins.[4] USP limits for storage temperatures are listed in Table 11-1.

Recommended storage conditions are usually stated on a product's label and may include a specified temperature range or a designated place (e.g., "refrigerate"). Supplemental instructions (e.g., "protect from light") should also be followed carefully. If a preparation must be protected from light and is in a clear

Table 11-1.

USP Storage Conditions[3]

Condition	Centigrade Temperature Range	Farenheit Temperature Range
Freezer	-25 to -10 degrees	-13 to 14 degrees
Cold	Not exceeding 8 degrees	Not exceeding 46 degrees
Refrigerator	2 to 8 degrees	36 to 46 degrees
Cool	8 to 15 degrees	49 to 59 degrees
Controlled room temperature	20 to 25 degrees (excursions are allowed between 15 to 30 degrees)	68 to 77 degrees (excursions are allowed between 59 and 86 degrees)
Warm	30 to 40 degrees	86 to 104 degrees
Excessive heat	Above 40 degrees	Above 104 degrees

or translucent container enclosed in an opaque outer covering, this covering should not be removed until the contents are to be used.

In the absence of specific instructions, a sterile product should be stored at controlled room temperature[4] away from excessive or variable heat, cold, and light, e.g., away from heating pipes and fluorescent lighting fixtures.

Clarifying Controlled Room Temperature

Since controlled room temperature may range from 15° C to 30° C, such storage may not be adequate for certain temperature-sensitive drugs.[6] Clinically important changes can result from only a 5° C variation in room temperature over the shelf life of a preparation.[7] Alterations in temperature-related drug stability could potentially compromise a pharmacist's interpretation and assignment of beyond-use dates to compounded preparations. Therefore, USP has further defined controlled room temperature[3]:

> Controlled room temperature . . . encompasses the usual . . . working environment of 20° C to 25° C (68° to 77° F) . . . that results in a mean kinetic temperature calculated to be not more than 25 degrees; and that allows for excursions between 15 and 30 degrees C (59° and 86° F) . . . in pharmacies, hospitals, and warehouses.

Monitoring Storage Conditions

To ensure that the potency of a sterile commercial product is retained through its expiration date, pharmacy personnel must monitor drug storage areas. Controlled temperature areas like refrigerators, freezers, and incubators should be monitored at least once daily and the results should be documented on a temperature log (see Chapter 18). A continuous temperature recording device or a thermometer with adequate accuracy and sensitivity may be used if properly calibrated at reasonable intervals.[5]

On each working day, pharmacy personnel should verify that the recording device is working and that temperatures are within the desired range. The temperature-detecting mechanism should be carefully placed so that it accurately reflects the unit's temperature. The pharmacy personnel must also monitor conditions that cause temperature fluctuations such as frequent or extended opening of refrigerator doors.

Inventory Control

Inventories of commercial drugs and solutions should be inspected periodically to ensure that they are not damaged, soiled, expired, or otherwise unsuitable. Moreover, all storage areas should be monitored to ensure that temperature, light, humidity, and ventilation remain within manufacturer and compendial requirements.[5] To permit adequate floor cleaning and avoid water damage, drugs and supplies should be stored on shelves above the floor. Drugs should be stored no closer that 18 inches from the ceiling, so as not to interfer with the fire-control sprinkler system.

Temperature Excusions

Temperature may be a particular problem in large warehouse areas with garage-type doors opening to the outside. For such facilities, a temperature log may help to ensure that appropriate storage conditions are met. If temperature fluctuations exceed acceptable limits, drug supplies must be relocated.

Product Integrity

Before use, each drug, ingredient, and container should be visually inspected for damage, defects, and expiration date.[5] Products that have exceeded their expiration dates should be removed from active storage areas. Organizations with computerized perpetual inventory capabilities might generate a monthly report that can be used to retrieve products about to expire. Although "just-in-time" ordering has decreased the problem of excessive inventory and expired drugs for some organizations, little-used inventory locations still must be checked carefully.

Partially Used Packages

Opened commercial drug packages (e.g., multidose vials) for subsequent use are properly stored under restricted access conditions in the compounding facility Such packages cannot be used when visual inspection detects unaurhorized breaks in the container, closure, and seal; when the contents do not possess the expected appearance, aroma, and texture; when the contents do not pass identification tests specified by the compounding facility; and when either the beyond-use or expiration date has been exceeded.[5]

Product Recall

When a commercial product is recalled, a mechanism must be in place for tracking and retrieving it from specific patients. A batch record, with lot numbers and expiration dates, can greatly facilitate a product recall (see Chapter 13). Additionally, computerized inventory management systems may help large organizations to determine quickly whether the pharmacy has the recalled product in stock.

Transport Into Controlled Areas

When products and supplies are transported from relatively uncontrolled areas (e.g., main pharmacy or warehouse) into the controlled area (anteroom or cleanroom), caution is needed to prevent contamination of the controlled area. Access to the controlled area should be limited to designated, qualified personnel.

Supplies

In the anteroom, all supplies should be removed from shipping cartons and wiped with a disinfecting agent (e.g., 70% isopropyl alcohol) while being transferred to a clean, sanitized cart. Individually pouched supplies need not be wiped because the pouches can be removed just before the supplies are transported into the cleanroom.[5]

Although some frequently used supplies can be decontaminated and stored on shelving in the anteroom, an excessive accumulation can lead to dust collection. Objects that shed particles like pencils, cardboard boxes, paper towels, cotton items, and reference books should not be taken into the cleanroom.[5]

Carts

Carts used to bring supplies from a storage area should not be rolled beyond the anteroom; carts used in the cleanroom should not be rolled outside of it or the anteroom unless they are cleaned and disinfected before returning.[5] To maintain this segregation, carts can be designated as "clean" or "dirty."

Clean carts stay in the cleanroom and anteroom only, and supplies from the storage area are conveyed on dirty carts. In the anteroom, a demarcation line on the floor denotes how far a dirty cart can travel. At the line, supplies are decontaminated and transferred to a clean cart.

This process minimizes the ingress of particulate and microbial contamination from carts and packaging materials (see Chapter 3).

Handling Products in the Cleanroom

Supplies to be used in the cleanroom are accumulated and decontaminated by wiping or spraying the outer surface with 70% isopropyl alcohol or removing the outer wrap just before being introduced into the laminar air-flow workbench or isolator. Such supplies are limited to the operation at hand and are arranged so that a clear, uninterrupted path of HEPA-filtered air will bathe all critical sites at all times during aseptic compounding.[1] After compounding is complete, a closure is usually placed on the preparation to enable detection of tampering later on. Used syringes, ampules, vials and other supplies are removed with a minimum of exit and re-entry into the laminar air-flow workbench or isolator to minimize the risk of introducing contamination into the ISO Class 5 (Class 100) workspace.

Storage of Compounded Preparations

When time and personnel availability permit, compounding manipulations in the ISO Class 5 workspace are separated from post-compounding quality inspection before sterile preparations are dispensed. Once inspected by a pharmacist, sterile preparations should be refrigerated until they are used, if the preparation permits.[5] However, sterile preparations intended for administration *promptly* after compounding may be retained at room temperature prior to delivery. When sterile preparations are known to have been exposed to temperatures warmer than the warmest labeled limit for more than 4 hours such preparations should be discarded, unless appropriate documentation or direct assay data confirm their continued stability.[5] Personnel should note the storage temperature when placing the preparation into or removing the preparation from the storage unit in order to monitor any temperature abberations.

Although there is always some risk that microorganisms may contaminate sterile components during compounding, refrigerated storage inhibits microbial growth.[5] Exposure to room temperatures or greater increases the risk of microbial growth. Risk level categories should be considered prior to compounding. ASHP[1] assigns strerile preparations to risk levels according to time before administration and storage temperature (Table 11-2).

According to USP,[5] for low-risk preparations, in the absence of passing a sterility test, the storage periods cannot exceed the following time periods before administration: the sterile preparation is stored for not more than 48 hours at controlled room temperature; for not more than 14 days at a cold temperature or for not more than 45 days in solid frozen state at -20 degrees centigrade or colder.

For medium-risk preparations, in the absence of passing a sterility test, the storage periods cannot exceed the following time pe-

riods before administration: the sterile preparation is stored for not more than 30 hours at controlled room temperature; for not more than 7 days at cold temperature and for not more than 45 days in solid frozen state at -20 degrees centigrade or colder.[5]

For high-risk preparations, in the absence of passing a serility test, the storage periods can not exceed the following time periods before administration: the sterile preparation is properly stored for not more than 24 hours at controlled room temperature; for not more than 3 days at cold temperature and for not more than 45 days in solid frozen state at -20 degrees centigrade or colder.[4] (See Table 11-3 for a summary of USP storage periods before use.)

Table 11-2.

Assignment of Preparations to Risk Level 1 or 2 According to Time and Temperature Before Completion of Administration[1]

		Number of Days in Storage	
Risk Level	Room Temperature (15° C to 30° C)	Refrigerator (2° C to 8° C)	Freezer (-20° C to -10° C)
1	Completely administered within 28 hr	Not greater than 7 days	Not greater than 30 days
2	Storage and administration exceed 28 hr	Greater than 7 days	Greater than 30 days

Note: ASHP provides this table to assist pharmacists in determining which risk level conditions pertain to the preparations they are compounding.

Table 11-3.

USP Sterile Preparation Storage Conditions Before Administration[5]

	Room Temperature	Cold Temperature (2–8 degrees centigrade)	Frozen (Less than 20 degrees centigrade)
Low risk preparations	Not longer than 48 hours	Not longer than 14 days	Not longer than 45 days
Medium risk preparations	Not longer than 30 hours	Not longer than 7 days	Not longer than 45 days
High risk preparations	Not longer than 24 hours	Not longer than 3 days	Not longer than 45 days

Note: USP provides this information to help pharmacists set maximum storage periods for sterile preparations for which there is no sterility test.

Redispensed Sterile Preparations

The pharmacist is solely responsible for determining whether a sterile preparation not administered as originally intended can reused for a different patient or under alternate conditions. All sterile preparations that are not used as originally intended must be returned to the pharmacy for appropriate disposition, which may include redispensing, but only if adequate continuing quality can be fully ensured.[5] The following may prove such assurance:

- the sterile preparation was maintained under continuous refrigeration and protected from light, if required;

- no evidence of tampering or any readying for use outside the pharmacy exists; and

- there is sufficient time remaining until the originally assigned beyond-use time and date will be reached.

Thus, initial compounding and thaw times should be documented and reliable measures should have been taken to prevent and detect tampering. Compliance with all procedures associated with maintaining product quality is essential. The sterile preparation must not be redispensed if there is not adequate assurance that preparation quality and packaging intergrity (including connections of devices, where applicable) were continuously maintained between the time the sterile prepartion left the pharmacy and time that it was returned to the pharmacy.[5] The presence of microbial contamination in sterile liquids cannot be detected visually, but any haze, color change, cloudiness, surface film, particulate or flocculent matter, or gas formation is sufficient reason to suspect possible contamination.[4]

Waste Management

Preparation Materials

After compounding is completed, used syringes, bottles, vials, and other supplies should be removed. Exit and reentry into the laminar-airflow workbench should be minimized, however, to decrease the dragging of contamination into this ISO Class 5 workspace.[5] Disposal of packaging materials should be performed at least daily to enhance sanitation and avoid accumulation.[1]

Needles must be left on syringes that are disposed of carefully to prevent possible injuries. The used needle/syringe should be placed in a puncture-resistant ("sharps") container that can be permanently sealed. Needles and syringes used for patient drug administration should never be recapped. They should be discarded as an intact unit, along with IV catheters or other sharp objects. Sharps containers should be sealed and properly discarded when they are no more than three-quarters full.

In 1976 the Environmental Protection Agency (EPA) enacted the Resource Conservation and Recovery Act (RCRA)[8] to provide a mechanism for tracking hazardous waste from its generation to disposal. These regulations apply to drugs, as well as chemicals discarded by pharmacies, hospitals, clinics, and other commercial entities. Drugs that are not on the RCRA "P-list" or "U-list" or are not ignitable, corrosive, reactive or toxic are not considered hazardous and, with the exception of controlled drugs, may be disposed of through the municipal sewer system.[9] However, state and local regulations must be considered when establishing a pharmaceutical waste policy for a given institution.

EPA also defines waste generation status by the total amount of hazardous waste generated per month.[10] Most facilities using this guide are not likely to meet the criteria for a "conditionally exempt small quantity generator" (CESQG) given the number of discarded pharmaceuticals containing high alcohol content (ignitability characteristic >24%); mercury preservatives (toxicity characteristic); as well as chemotherapy agents. Non-hazardous IV solutions (e.g., dextrose 5% in water or 0.9% sodium chloride) may be discarded into the municiple sewer system.

Needles and any glass fragments should be contained in small, puncture-resistant sharps containers to be placed into larger containers approved for temporary storage. Clean paper or plastic packaging and empty glass and plastic bottles may be discarded in the municiple waste stream. Waste contaminated with blood or other body fluids must not be mixed with hazardous waste. Transport of waste containers from satellite accumulation to storage sites must be done by individuals who meet OSHA mandated hazardous waste awareness training.[11,12]

Hazardous Materials

See Chapter 7 for a complete discussion of the containment and disposal of hazardous drugs and related materials.

Expired Drugs

Expired drugs should be segregated from other inventory so that they are not inadvertently dispensed. Certain drugs may be returned to the manufacturer for credit. Generally, expired drugs are handled in one of four ways:

1. Expired controlled substances must be removed from perpetual inventory. In some cases, they may be returned to the manufacturer. A listing of the drugs waiting to be returned is sent to the manufacturer, who prior has been requested to issue Drug Enforcement Agency (DEA) Form 222 to the pharmacy. This form must accompany the returned controlled drugs.

2. Open drug containers and unused compounded doses are usually not returnable for credit; controlled substances must be destroyed. In some states, a state board of pharmacy inspector must view this destruction of controlled substances. Alternatively, expired opened controlled substances may be sent to the DEA for disposal. Non-controlled, non-hazardous drugs must be discarded as waste and therefore stored, transported and disposed of in the proper way,[9] usually by a licensed waste contractor.

3. Expired hazardous drugs must be properly labeled and disposed of in puncture-proof containers. These containers must be sent to a licensed hazardous waste incinerator or licensed hazardous waste dump via a licensed hazardous waste contractor. Pharmacists should check with state agencies to make sure transporters and disposal facilities have the necessary licenses and permits.[9]

4. Unopened expired drugs other than controlled substances or hazardous materials should be delivered to a reverse distributor or to a waste contractor for proper disposal. Typically, expired large-volume, harmless IV fluid containers are emptied into the sewer system before disposal to reduce their weight. Non-hazardous drugs should not be discarded with hazardous drugs.

Summary

Storage and handling of pharmacy-compounded sterile preparations is of critical importance. Beginning with the components themselves, proper procedures for receipt, storage, and control must be established.

Once a final preparation has been compounded, it must be appropriately transported within and delivered from the aseptic compounding area. Furthermore, storage conditions for final preparations differ from those of the original components.

Finally, waste management of used supplies and drug preparations must be adequately defined. Strict procedures must ensure that pharmaceutical wastes are handled appropriately so as to protect the handler and the environment in legal fashion.

References

1. American Society of Health-System Pharmacists. ASHP Guidelines on quality assurance for pharmacy-prepared sterile products. *Am J Health-Syst Pharm.* 2000;57:1150–69.

2. U.S. Food and Drug Administration. The FDA safety information and adverse event reporting system. Available at www.fda.gov/medwatch. Accessed October 23, 2003.

3. General notices. Storage temperature and humidity. In: United States pharmacopeia, 27th ed./national formulary, 22nd rev. Rockville, MD:United States Pharmacopeial Convention. Available at www.uspnf.com. Accessed January 24, 2004.

4. Stability considerations in dispensing practice. In: United States pharmacopeia, 27th ed./national formulary, 22nd rev. Rockville, MD: United States Pharmacopeial Convention. Available at www.uspnf.com. Accessed January 24, 2004.

5. Pharmaceutical compounding – sterile preparations. United States pharmacopeia, 27th ed./national formulary, 22nd rev (first supplement). Rockville, MD: United States Pharmacopeial Convention. Available at www.uspnf.com. Accessed April 1, 2004.

6. Nahata MC. Standard room temperature needed for stability and compatibility studies. *Am J Hosp Pharm.* 1993;50:912–3.

7. Newton DW, Miller KW. Room temperature and drug stability. *Am J Hosp Pharm.* 1994; 51:406–9.

8. Resource Conservation and Recovery Act of 1976. Public Law 42, U.S. Code, Chapter 6901–692k.

9. Young D. Improper discard of toxic drugs hurts environment, leads to fines. *Am J Health-Syst Pharm.* 2001;58:1576–8.

10. Hazardous Waste Management System: General. 40 C.F.R. parts 260–8, 270.

11. Initial Training. 29 C.F.R. part 1910.120(e)(3)(i).

12. Emergency Response to Hazardous Substances Releases. 29 C.F.R. Part 1910.120(q)(1–6).

12 | Maintaining the Integrity of Compounded Sterile Preparations Outside the Pharmacy

Caryn M. Bing*

*The author acknowledges Douglas J. Scheckelhoff, who authored this chapter in the first edition.

While compounded sterile preparations are within the confines of a cleanroom, storage and other handling conditions can be largely controlled. Since sterile preparations must be transported for use in various patient care settings, their handling outside the pharmacy also must be considered. Efforts must focus on the acceptability of the sterile preparation for patient use (including stability of ingredients and sterility) and also on the reduction of waste and preparation costs. Key factors to consider include the transfer of the sterile preparation from the sterile compounding area, storage conditions during transport and in the patient care setting, and methods for return, recycling, and disposal.[1-9] USP chapter <797> states that pharmacy is responsible for ensuring that compounded sterile preparations maintain their quality until administration to the patient.[7] All personnel (including couriers and other non-pharmacy staff) who package, handle, transport, and store compounded sterile preparations outside the pharmacy must be appropriately trained so that this expectation is met.

Delivery Methods

Hospital Campuses

Within the hospital facility or hospital campus, compounded sterile preparations can be delivered by health care personnel or by automated means. Many hospitals also use the centralized pharmacy to provide compounded sterile preparations for on-campus ambulatory services and long-term care sites. Procedures and systems to ensure proper training of delivery personnel, product security, and timeliness of delivery remain the responsibility of the pharmacy.

With the extensive use of polyvinyl chloride (PVC), ethylvinyl acetate (EVA) and other durable containers for compounded sterile preparations, rapid turn around time can be readily offered by using pneumatic tube systems for delivery. However, some medications and compounded sterile preparations are not suitable for this method of transport. In the absence of uniform standards related to delivering medications by pneumatic tube systems, and considering the variety of features and capabilities of different brands of these systems, organizations have developed their own guidelines for acceptable use of pneumatic tube

systems. Special "do not tube" labels can be affixed to the medication labels to ensure that these medications are handled properly when they are issued and when they are returned to the pharmacy. Figure 12-1 summarizes some representative guidelines for the transportation of compounded sterile preparations by this method. Syringes also may require special handling to prevent the plunger from depressing and causing leakage into the tube container or system. Padding specifically designed for use in pneumatic tube cartridges can minimize this potential problem.

Home Care and Off-Premises Settings

Additional steps to safeguard the integrity of compounded sterile preparations are required when providing these services for home care patients and off-premises care settings (including long-term care facilities, physicians' offices, and remote site ambulatory clinics). Both the distance from the compounding pharmacy and the drug's stability affect how a preparation is transported for delivery.[4]

Temperature control during off-premises delivery of compounded sterile preparations is critical. The pharmacy must provide appropriate packaging that will maintain temperatures near the midpoint of the specified acceptable storage range during transit and under expected environmental conditions.

The pharmacy should develop and follow written procedures for packaging. Additional precautions (e.g., double bagging, special labeling) should protect the courier, patient, and caregiver from leakage of any hazardous substances. The courier, patient, and caregiver should be trained to recognize and respond appropriately if there is an accidental spill.

Certain preparations require special packaging for transport to the home care and off campus settings. If the container is fragile or susceptible to jarring (e.g., preloaded syringe, glass containers, very full flexible plastic parenteral container), it should be packaged to protect its integrity. Fragile containers may be placed in a hard plastic or cardboard tube, wrapped in bubble packs, or cushioned in clean shipping pellets.

Transport containers and procedures should be evaluated under the most reasonably expected extreme conditions (summer heat, winter cold, significant traffic delays) and documented to ensure that they do provide effective

1. Do not attempt to exceed the weight or size limitations of the tube cartridge (as established by the tube system vendor). This can cause the tube system to fail, or result in breakage, damage, or leaking of the contents.

2. If a sterile preparation container is breakable (such as a glass IV bottle, ampule, vial, or some fragile/brittle plastic bags), or if it could be inadvertently opened or activated by the tube transit process (such as a syringe), ensure that it is adequately secured and/or padded in the tube cartridge.

3. Many tube systems have a security feature that facilitates transporting compounded sterile preparations of controlled substances with a security release code. In these circumstances, appropriate measures can be taken to minimize the risk of diversion. In the absence of this capability, controlled substances should not be sent via pneumatic tubes.

4. When a sterile preparation's ingredient cost is very high, is difficult to procure, and/or the compounding process is extensive or difficult, the organization should avoid the risk of losing the preparation through an unsecured transport process.

5. Do not transport hazardous, potentially infectious, explosive (e.g., freshly prepared CO_2 generating compounds) or flammable materials via this method. This includes sterile preparations such as chemotherapy, cytotoxic medications (e.g., ganciclovir), caustic agents, radiopharmaceuticals, blood, or blood products.

6. Always avoid the risk of altering the active ingredient or diluent system of compounded sterile preparations via the pneumatic tube process. The tube system process can denature or inactivate the ingredients (including, immune globulins, colony stimulating factors, monoclonal antibodies, interferons), crack emulsions (lipids, total nutrient admixtures), and generate foam that will affect the measurement of the dosage (as happens with many protein compounds). If any ingredient in a compounded sterile preparation includes a "do not shake" or similar warning, then the preparation should probably be transported via another method.

Figure 12-1. Suggested guidelines for compounded sterile preparation and delivery via pneumatic tube systems.[14,15]

temperature control and protection of the contents. These evaluations should be repeated any time the containers or procedures are changed. Postdelivery temperature checks can ensure that packaging materials (ice packs, coolers, bubble packs, etc.) maintain adequate control. Temperature sensors can be included inside shipments using common carriers to ensure that the contents arrive within accepted storage parameters.

When commercial carriers are used, the pharmacy is responsible for their selection. Before using a carrier, the pharmacy should provide a written statement of shipping requirements, delivery schedules, transit time duration, handling, and external temperature control, then obtain the carrier's assurance for fulfilling them. Temperature sensitive medications should never be delivered without assurance that they are received as intended. Good business and risk management practices include obtaining a signature upon delivery, and NOT leaving medications "on the doorstep." Some carriers request special packaging and labeling before they will handle hazardous chemicals or biomedical waste.

Delivery personnel should know the shipping requirements for each package. Ingredient labels generally provide temperature storage parameters; if preparations are boxed or labels are otherwise concealed, apply an exterior label directing the recipient to open the package immediately and refrigerate the preparations as labeled.

Storage Methods

Institutional Setting

In the hospital and long-term care facility setting, responsibility for storing compounded sterile preparations shifts from the pharmacy to other health care providers on a patient care unit. Compounded sterile preparations should be issued in limited quantities and organized in the refrigerators so that nursing staff avoid the practice of assembling multiple doses for a patient hours before scheduled medication administration.

As part of the hospital or long-term care facility unit inspection process, temperatures of patient care unit medication refrigerators should be monitored and documented daily.[7] If IV solutions are removed from the refrigerator long before administration time (e.g., at the beginning of a shift), the beyond-use dating for room temperature storage conditions must be followed. This costly and wasteful practice reduces the ability to recycle unused medications within a hospital.

Specialized drug delivery systems

Drug delivery systems that are stable at room temperature (e.g., ready-to-use medications in administration containers) or those that are reconstituted immediately before administration can eliminate the need for refrigeration. The pharmacy must be aware of the beyond-use-dating and storage requirements for these medication systems (see Table 12-1). After removal of a PVC bag from its overwrap, the bag (and any medication container that becomes attached to it) has a very limited (2–4 weeks) room temperature shelf life.[4]

Home Care Setting

In the home setting, compounded sterile preparations are usually stored in the patient's own refrigerator. Patients or caregivers should be instructed to designate a shelf, drawer, or other area segregated from food to avoid contamination of the outside of the container. Compounded sterile preparations should be supplied with an overwrap (such a sealable plastic bag) to protect the container from other items in the refrigerator and help organize multiple doses. When the quantity and volume of preparations dispensed are likely to tax the capacity of patient's own refrigerator, a separate refrigerator should be considered. Some home infusion providers give the patient a small refrigerator to store a one to two week supply of parenteral nutrition preparations. Patients should be instructed to store medications (such as short stability additives) and supplies not requiring refrigeration in a secure, temperature and humidity controlled area.

Table 12-1.

Manufacturer Storage Recommendations for Plain Solutions in PVC After Removal from Protective Overwrap

Manufacturer/Brand	Volume	Maximum Storage Time
Abbott/Lifecare[a]	25 mL	21 d
Abbott/Lifecare[a]	>25 mL	30 d
Baxter/Viaflex[b]	≤50 mL	15 d
Baxter/Viaflex[b]	≥100 mL	30 d

[a]Manufacturer letter to C. Bing. Abbott Hospital Products Division Medical Department, November 1999.

[b]Manufacturer letter to C. Bing. Baxter Healthcare Corporation I.V. Systems Delivery, November 1999.

NOTE: Consult product labeling for all commercial premixed and frozen medications for recommended storage time and conditions after removal of protective overwrap.

Appropriate temperature control in the home is important while the preparation is being administered. Labels should specify the storage requirements and the beyond-use-dating on each dosage unit of a compounded sterile preparation. Patients should be trained to check preparations for beyond-use dating and to verify refrigerator temperatures daily. They also should be trained to contact the pharmacy before administration of a medication if a refrigerator malfunctions or there are suspicions of improper storage conditions.

Each time pharmacy or home health personnel visit a patient's home they should confirm that drug storage is adequate with regard to temperature control, cleanliness, separation of food and drug items, and avoidance of improper preparation use (e.g., a single-dose vial used as a multiple-dose container). Improperly stored, soiled, expired, or visibly defective preparations should be removed. Home visits should also assess compliance with waste disposal procedures. When home visits are not conducted directly by the pharmacy, the pharmacy staff should provide telephone instruction, reassessment, and reinforcement of medication storage conditions and procedures to the patient or caregiver.

Return Methods

Discontinued or changed orders and "extra" or duplicate doses are often returned to the pharmacy by normal delivery methods. When these items can be legally returned to the pharmacy, they should be retrieved as quickly as possible to maximize their recycling potential. If these preparations are left unrefrigerated for pickup when the next scheduled pharmacy delivery is made, many hours may be lost. Based on the cost of these items, an active retrieval mechanism may reduce both effort and waste.

Recycling Methods

Hospitals

Sterile preparations that are returned to the hospital pharmacy may be recycled if the pharmacist knows how they were stored and handled outside the pharmacy. Room temperature beyond use dating should be used if the pharmacist is uncertain about the storage and transportation conditions of the preparation.

Recycling decisions should be based on beyond use dating and preparation risk levels. Preparations with very short stability characteristics usually are labeled with an actual beyond use date and time, and are generally not subject to recycling decisions. Other longer-stability parameter preparations typically are labeled with the room temperature "standard" expiration date (e.g., 24 hr) in hospital settings. If the standard expiration date is used, the pharmacist must decide if the returned preparation may be recycled according to its actual beyond use date (based on stability, infection control guidelines, storage conditions, etc.—see Chapter 8). Preparations should only be used in time frames that are consistent with published data and the compounded sterile preparation's established risk level category.[2,4,7,9]

If a preparation is recycled, this fact should be noted on the label. Therefore, if the IV is returned again, its true preparation time is still identifiable to the pharmacist who must decide on suitability for recycling.

Home Care and Long-Term Care

Compounded sterile preparations returned from the home and long-term care environment usually are not recycled since their storage and handling cannot be directly controlled or evaluated the pharmacy. Many state boards of pharmacy prohibit reuse or reissuance of compounded sterile preparations once they have left the control of the pharmacy.[10]

Reuse of intact items that have not been repackaged (e.g., intact vials or prefilled syringes) may be acceptable when allowed by law and regulation if the packaging is tamper evident, the items are stable at room temperature, and the pharmacist has confidence that controlled temperatures were maintained while the item was in the patient home or long-term care facility.

Waste Disposal Methods

A variety of methods are employed for disposal of waste pharmaceuticals. Important concerns include prevention of diversion or accidental ingestion. Heightened awareness of improper drug disposal and the impact on the environment is an important issue for pharmacy.[11-13]

Institutional Setting

Disposal methods vary based on the type of preparation and regulations governing the hospital. For example, since chemotherapy waste is considered hazardous, it usually must be incinerated. The process must meet regulatory requirements specific for destruction of hazardous materials (relative to incineration temperature and duration).

Many drugs that require disposal are not hazardous, and may or may not be considered as regulated waste. Disposal methods are often prescribed by the landfill where the waste is sent. Since landfill regulations and restrictions are strict and can significantly increase disposal costs, many hospitals treat all drug waste as hazardous materials disposed of by incineration.

Home Care Setting

Patients receiving hazardous drugs (e.g., chemotherapy) in the home should be instructed on proper waste disposal. A separate area in the home should be identified for storage of hazardous waste, and all family members should be instructed on the potential dangers of contact with this waste. When needles or other sharps are used, the patient should receive a sharps container designated for disposing of used supplies.

A schedule for hazardous waste or sharps container removal should be developed and agreed on by both the pharmacy and the patient. Patients should contact the home care pharmacy if waste is not removed according to this schedule.

Summary

The pharmacy retains responsibility for establishing methods to ensure the integrity of compounded sterile preparations after they leave the pharmacy. The pharmacist must ensure that policies, procedures and resources guarantee proper delivery, storage, return, and recycling of these preparations as well as the destruction of any preparation waste or hazardous materials.

References

1. American Society of Hospital Pharmacists. ASHP technical assistance bulletin on handling cytotoxic and hazardous drugs. *Am J Hosp Pharm.* 1990;47:1033–49.
2. American Society of Hospital Pharmacists. ASHP guidelines on quality assurance for pharmacy-prepared sterile products. *Am J Health-Syst Pharm.* 2000; 57:1150–69.
3. Birdwell SW, Meyer GE, Scheckelhoff DJ, et al. Survey of wastage from intravenous admixture in U.S. hospitals. *Pharmacoeconomics.* 1993;4:271–7.
4. Bing C, ed. *Extended Stability for Parenteral Drugs*, 2nd ed. Bethesda, MD: American Society of Health-System Pharmacists; 2003.
5. Billeter M, Nowak MM, Rapp RP, et al. Waste of IV admixtures in the ADD-vantage system and a traditional minibag system. *Am J Hosp Pharm.* 1990;47: 1598–1600.
6. Mitchell SR. Monitoring waste in an intravenous admixture program. *Am J Hosp Pharm.* 1987;44:106–11.
7. Pharmaceutical compounding. In: United States pharmacopeia, 27th rev./national formulary, 22nd ed. Rockville, MD: United States Pharmacopeial Convention; 2004.
8. Salberg DJ, Newton RW, Leduc DT. Cost of wastage in a hospital intravenous admixture program. *Hosp Form.* 1984;19: 375–8.
9. Trissel, LA. *Handbook on Injectable Drugs,* 12th ed. Bethesda, MD: American Society of Health-System Pharmacists; 2003.
10. National Association of Boards of Pharmacy. Model State Pharmacy Practice Act and Model Rules of the National Association of Boards of Pharmacy. Fall 2002. Available at www.nabp.net.
11. Smith CA. Managing Pharmaceutical Waste—What Pharmacists Should Know. *Journal of the Pharmacy Society of Wisconsin.* 2002;(Nov/Dec):17–22.
12. Young D. News: Improper discard of toxic drugs hurts environment, leads to fines. *Am J Health-Syst Pharm.* 2001;58:1576–8.
13. Saljoughian M. Disposal of hazardous pharmaceutical waste. *U.S. Pharmacist.* 2004; 29:HS224.
14. Peak A. Delivering medications via a pneumatic tube system (letter.) *Am J Health-Syst Pharm.* 2002;59:1376.
15. Peak A. Delivering medications via a pneumatic tube system. *Hosp Pharm.* 2003;38:287–90.

13 | Compounding and Sterilization of Batch Preparations

Philip J. Schneider*

*The author acknowledges Barbara T. McKinnon, who authored this chapter in the first edition of this text.

The term "extemporaneous compounding" describes the preparation of drugs or solutions that have no commercially available equivalents. For sterile preparations, this term is associated with high-risk batch compounding activities (e.g., intermediate pooling of ingredients, batch mixing in open reservoirs, or use of nonsterile ingredients or components). Examples of extemporaneous compounding include the compounding of (1) injectable morphine from nonsterile powder or tablets and an appropriate diluent and (2) nutritional solutions from nonsterile components.

Compounding Techniques

Batch compounding is a useful technique to compound many dosage units efficiently and with dose-to-dose uniformity. Before initiating a program, pharmacists should consider what preparations are needed and what method is most appropriate. Table 13-1 lists a few preparations that are typically compounded using a batch compounding technique.

Requirements for facility design, operator and process validation, garb, testing of compounded preparations, and the environment must be met for the risk level of the preparation (see Chapter 1). If the pharmacy cannot comply with the requirements for high-risk compounding, an alternative approach should be considered. For example, for IV catheter flushes, commercially available prefilled syringes can be used instead of batch compounded urokinase syringes. Similarly, preservative-free commercial morphine products, in various concentrations, may reduce the need for extemporaneously compounding morphine preparations from powdered morphine.

Various compounding methods are available, ranging from the compounding of a single dose of morphine from nonsterile tablets to the compounding of a 200 liter batch of parenteral nutrition preparation in an open tank. The precautions specific to each method should be recognized.

Syringe Compounding

Syringes may be used as a final dosage form for repackaged medications or as a processing step in the reconstitution of powdered ingredients. If syringes are used to repackage a commercially available sterile injectable solu-

Table 13-1.

Common Batch Compounded Preparations

- Antibiotic unit doses in syringes, minibags, or manufacturers' piggybacks
- Standardized parenteral nutrition solutions
- Injections repackaged into unit dose syringes
- Repackaged respiratory therapy solutions
- Ophthalmic solutions
- Epidural morphine solutions
- Cardioplegia solutions

tion, the solution must be compatible with the materials of the syringe and plunger. Beyond-use dating assigned for these preparations should be based on potency testing or the recommendations published in the literature.[1]

Syringes are convenient closed containers for reconstitution of small quantities of nonsterile powdered components. These reconstituted preparations must be sterilized through a 0.22-micron filter and then transferred into a sterile sealed container before dispensing. A post-use filter integrity test should be performed for preparations compounded from nonsterile components.

Mass Reconstitution

Reconstitution of parenteral drugs is time consuming. Efficiency can be increased by reconstituting several vials in bulk and then refrigerating or freezing them. For this technique, a reconstitution device can be used. The device consists of a spring-loaded syringe attached to one end of a two-way valve; tubing, with a spike on one end, is attached to the other end of this valve. The spike on the tubing is attached to the solution container.

As the plunger of the syringe is pulled back, solution from the container enters the syringe. As the plunger is pushed in, solution is forced out of the spring-loaded syringe and through the needle attached to the two-way valve. The plunger can be adjusted to deliver any volume of diluent and then locked to that position. Once the syringe is adjusted and the plunger is pushed in to expel the solution, the plunger automatically returns to the same place. This procedure allows the same volume of diluent to enter the syringe repeatedly.

Some advantages of mass reconstitution are accuracy, control, and speed.[2] Applications of this technique include

- Mass reconstitution of multiple vials of powdered drugs for injection.

- Dispensing of reconstituted, bulk-packaged antibiotics into multiple minibags.

- Reconstitution of lyophilized medications supplied as manufacturers' piggybacks.

Pharmacy compounding pumps also are useful for mass reconstitution. They make the operation both easier and more precise when properly calibrated.

Pooling

"Pooled" preparations are made by combining sterile ingredients in a sterile closed system, by aseptic transfer, before subdivision into patient units. These preparations have a higher risk level than similar preparations made by aseptic transfer without this intermediate pooling. The risk is greater because contamination of the pooled preparation could cause contamination of more than one patient dose. Pooling may be convenient and save time.

For example, for parenteral nutrition solutions, an electrolyte pool may be made in a sterile closed container. The total quantity of each required electrolyte is multiplied by the total number of units to be compounded. The total volume of all additives required for one patient unit is then calculated. Incompatible additives, such as calcium and phosphate, are excluded. Base solutions of dextrose and amino acids are made first, and then the calculated volume of additives for each patient unit is aseptically transferred from the electrolyte pool. Calcium or phosphate is added last.

The pool technique decreases the number of entries into each container and may save time. To avoid potential error, calculations should be double checked.

Open Reservoir Mixing

Open reservoir mixing combines either sterile or nonsterile ingredients using an open-system transfer or an open reservoir before ter-

minal sterilization or subdivision into units. These preparations are defined as Risk Level 3 in the ASHP Guidelines on Quality Assurance for Pharmacy-Prepared Sterile Products[3] or high risk CSPs by the USP in Chapter 797.[4]

Requirements for processes, facilities, and final assessment of preparations are more demanding in the Risk Level 3/high risk category than in the Risk Levels 1/low risk level CSPs and Risk Levels 2/medium risk level CSPs. Personnel must be specially trained and thoroughly knowledgeable about ISO Class 5 (Class 100) critical area technology and design. Even a sterile, commercially available product cannot be considered sterile after it is manipulated in an open reservoir. Maintenance of an ISO Class 5 environment and the use of specialized compounding garments do not guarantee sterility when a preparation is exposed to the environment.

The critical aspect of compounding that involves nonsterile components or equipment is the sterilization of the nonsterile preparations. This process requires more effort than simply manipulating a sterile product and not introducing contamination. Use of an appropriate, validated sterilization process is essential for Risk Level 3/high risk level products.

Batch Sterilization

The sterility of a preparation is defined as the absence of viable microorganisms. On a practical basis, absolute sterility cannot be demonstrated because of limitations in testing. For this reason, the term "sterility assurance" defines the probability that a lot of a preparation is sterile. Sterility assurance can be established only by adequate sterilization and validated aseptic processing.[5]

Terminal sterilization should be used for preparations compounded with nonsterile components or equipment. Sterilization may be accomplished in the final sealed container by autoclaving.[5] If heat sterilization capabilities are not available or if heat-labile drugs or container-closure systems preclude it, preparations may be sterilized by filtration and processed aseptically.[4] The suitability of sterilization procedures for a particular purpose should be validated.[4]

Sterilization by Filtration

A sterilizing filtration process should remove

microorganisms from the solution. The filter must have a rated pore size of 0.22 micron or smaller.[6] The pharmacist may rely on vendor certification for commercially available, presterilized, ready-to-use filter devices. This certification indicates their appropriateness for human use in sterile pharmaceutical applications. Manufacturer certification includes microbial retention testing with *Pseudomonas diminuta*, at a minimum concentration of 10^7 organisms/cm^3, as well as testing for membrane and housing integrity, nonpyrogenicity, and extractables.[5]

When relying on vendor certification, pharmacists should ensure that the testing conditions (e.g., duration of filtration, rate, temperature, and product pH, viscosity, and osmolarity) are representative of the intended parameters of use. For filtration apparatus assembled in the pharmacy, validation should be established experimentally.[5]

During sterilization by filtration, microbial contamination of the filtrate should be prevented. The sterilized preparation should be filtered into pre-sterilized containers under aseptic conditions. Pharmacy personnel involved in such high-risk compounding should have sufficient knowledge, training, and experience to perform their tasks correctly and safely and to ensure quality.

Filter selection

The pharmacist should select the appropriate filter size, based on the volume of solution to be filtered and the particulate load so that a single filter can process the entire batch. Filters should not have to be replaced during the filtration process. The selection of a filter should be based on the characteristics of the filter and of the solution. Filters and their housing apparatus must be physically and chemically compatible with the solution and be capable of withstanding the processing temperatures and pressures. When filters are selected, four characteristics should be considered:

- Pore size
- Compatibility
- Fluid volume
- Particulate load

Reference 7 offers a more in depth discussion of filter selection.

Pore size. Pore size determines the size of the particles retained by the sieving action of the membrane filter. Some particles smaller than the pore can be retained by entrapment within the membrane. To achieve clarification, particles that measure about 5 microns or more must be removed.

Sterilization requires a filter with a maximum rated pore size of 0.22 micron. Although this process is not absolute, it carries a certain probability of success called the sterility assurance level (SAL). The SAL for sterilizing a solution with a 0.22-micron filter is normally accepted as 1:1000. In other words, no more than 0.1% of the originally present microorganism remains.[7,8]

Compatibility. Membrane filters are compatible with most pharmaceutical solutions. In general, the filters are polymers that are inert and contain few additives. The inherent charge on some filters can lead to loss by adsorption of susceptible molecules, such as proteins and polypeptides. Therefore, great care must be exercised when choosing filters for biological products. Moreover, solvents in pharmaceutical solutions mainly alcohols, glycols, and dimethylformamide can cause swelling and even dissolution of the filter polymer.[7]

Fluid volume. To provide a practical flow rate of a solution, a filter with the appropriate surface area must be used (i.e., the larger the volume of solution, the greater the amount of filter membrane surface area is required). In the pharmacy, the volume of solution ranges from a few milliliters to a few liters; a disk filter of 25- or 47-mm diameter often is suitable. If many liters of a viscous solution have to be filtered, a cartridge filter with more surface area may provide an appropriate flow rate.[7]

Particulate load. Most pharmaceutical solutions are compounded under controlled conditions, and the load of particles is low. Some preparations may have a large load (e.g., an impure research drug). If the filtration is intended to sterilize the filtrate, the process should be completed without changing the filter. Some preliminary experimentation may be needed to determine the rate of clogging. When the particulate load is high, one or more prefilters (e.g., depth filters) are used upstream of the sterilizing filter to remove most particulates. This process may be completed in two or more individual steps with sterile, disposable filter units. If the particulate load is relatively low (e.g., glass particles in a sterile solution after an ampul is opened), a 5-micron membrane filter may be used.[7]

Filter integrity

Sterilization filters should be checked for integrity at the time of use. Integrity of commercially available, sterile, self-contained filter devices may be tested at the conclusion of filtration. Integrity testing is performed by assessing the resistance of the filter to a substance being forced through it. Greater resistance can be detected if air is forced through a wet filter membrane (the airlock principle). For a simple integrity test, an attempt should be made to force a large syringe of air through the wet filter membrane. If the membrane is intact, the air will not pass through it.

Filter integrity kits, suitable for pharmacy use, are commercially available for testing the bubble point of small disk filters. A pressure gauge attached to a three-way stopcock quantifies the pressure held by the filter. This test must be performed with a large-caliber syringe because a small-caliber syringe, such as a tuberculin, may generate excessive pressure.[5]

Quantitative integrity testing (e.g., bubble point or pressure hold) should be performed with pharmacy-assembled filtration apparatus.[5] Bubble point is integrity testing with a more definite endpoint. When a source of nitrogen or compressed air is used to apply pressure gradually upstream of a water-wet disk membrane filter, air bubbles suddenly appear downstream in the transparent tubing or water reservoir in an open flask or other container (Figure 13-1). The pressure that is causing bubbles is the bubble point, which is a reliable indicator of the largest pores in a membrane filter. The bubble point is approximately 50 psi for a water-wet, 0.22-micron polysulfone filter and approximately 30 psi for a 0.45-micron filter (Figure 13-2). These values vary with the manufacturer and polymer. Specific values are available from manufacturers.[7]

The bubble point has been correlated with the retention of microorganisms by the filter. This point is related to

the logarithm of the reduction value (LRV) for the microbial population in the filtrate (Figure 13-3).[9] The LRV is an expression of the filter's efficiency at removing microbes. It is calculated as the ratio of the concentration of

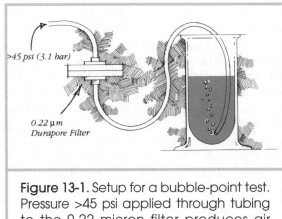

Figure 13-1. Setup for a bubble-point test. Pressure >45 psi applied through tubing to the 0.22 micron filter produces air bubbles in the water reservoir downstream from the filter. (Reproduced, with permission, from Millipore Corporation, Bedford, MA.)

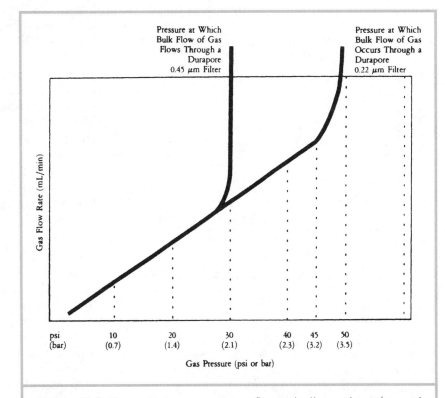

Figure 13-2. Gas pressure versus gas flow rate through water-wet polysulfone membrane filters with 0.45 or 0.22 micron pores. (Reproduced, with permission, from Millipore Corporation, Bedford, MA.)

microorganisms in the unfiltered solution to that in the filtrate, expressed as the logarithm to base 10.

As the pore size decreases, the bubble point increases so that fewer bacteria can pass through the filter. At 0.45 microns, only some smaller bacteria can pass. At 0.22 microns, or a bubble point of approximately 50 psi, bacteria are completely removed. Therefore, some microorganisms are removed when a pharmaceutical solution passes through a membrane filter larger than 0.22 microns, but sterilization is unlikely.[7] Certain drug preparations may lower the bubble point of the filter, resulting in air passing through it at a lower pressure than expected. If the test is questionable, the preparation should be resterilized. Table 13-2 describes a sample procedure for filter integrity testing of small disk filters.

The bubble-point test must be modified for cartridge filters because they have a much higher surface area than disk filters. This

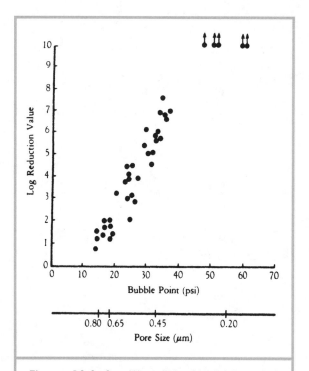

Figure 13-3. Scatter plot of bubble point (or pore size) versus bacterial reduction. Bacterial reduction is the logarithm of the reduction in the bacterial count achieved by filtering a standardized suspension of Pseudomonas diminuta. (Reproduced, with permission, from Millipore Corporation, Bedford, MA.)

modification or pressure-hold test is based on air diffusion through the water in pores of the thoroughly water-wet membrane.[10] Air pressure is applied upstream of the cartridge filter until a designated pressure, usually about 80% of the bubble-point pressure, is shown on an expanded-scale gauge. This pressure is shut off. Its loss over a period is a measure of the diffusive airflow through the water in the membrane pores. The filter manufacturer states the maximum allowable loss in pressure.[7]

Sterilization by Heat

By using saturated steam under pressure, thermal sterilization is carried out in a chamber called an autoclave. Preparations or components are terminally sterilized when they are processed in the autoclave to achieve a 10^c microbial survivor probability. This probability assures only one chance in a million that viable microorganisms are still present in the sterilized preparation. With heat-stable items, the approach often is to "overkill" to exceed the critical time necessary to achieve the 10^{-6} microbial survivor probability. For preparations that may be damaged by excessive heat exposure, the development of sterilization cycles depends on knowledge of the microbial burden of the preparation.

The D value is the time in minutes required to reduce the microbial population of a specific solution by 90% or one log cycle at a specific temperature. For example, if the D value of a biologic indicator (e.g., *Bacillus stereothermophilus* spores) is 1.5 min at 121° F, its lethality can be described as 8D when treated for 12 min. This D value can be applied to preparations with a known initial bioburden. If the microbial burden of a preparation before sterilization is 10^2, a lethality input of 8D is needed to achieve a probability of 10^{-6} survival.[5]

Sterilization cycles should be validated to ensure that the survival of the most resistant microorganisms is no greater than 10^{-6} under specified operating conditions and parameters (e.g., sterilization time and temperature, size and nature of load, and chamber loading configuration). The validation and monitoring of heat sterilization should be in writing along with specific critical parameters, such as necessary temperatures, pressures, and use of commercially available biologic indicators. Monitoring data from each cycle should be recorded to ensure that the processes are per-

Table 13-2.

Procedure for Postuse Filter Integrity Testing of Small Disk Filters

1. The following items should be assembled: filter integrity test kit containing a 10-ml syringe, three-way stopcock, and small pressure gauge (30 psi minimum); sterile 0.22-micron filter appropriate for solution to be sterilized; and sterile water for injection.

2. The preparation should be compounded as usual, using aseptic technique, and filtered through the presterilized filter membrane into a sterile container.

3. The filter membrane should be aseptically disconnected and connected to a syringe containing at least 10 ml of sterile water for injection. The filter membrane should be flushed with the sterile water for injection to remove traces of drug that could alter the bubble-point test.

4. The syringe should be disconnected; the three-way stopcock should be connected to the syringe tip.

5. The pressure gauge should be attached to the perpendicular connection of the three-way stop-cock.

6. Then 10 ml of air should be drawn up in the syringe, and the filter should be reconnected to the three-way stopcock.

7. Pressure should be applied (about 50 psi for a 0.22-micron filter) with the syringe plunger and held for 15 sec. The expected bubble point of each filter membrane is available from the manufacturer.

8. Integrity of the filter housing and membrane is proven by retention of air and steady pressure in the syringe. Failure of integrity is indicated by airflow through the filter.

9. If failure occurs, connections should be checked for leaks and the above steps should be repeated. With any filtration failure, the preparation should not be released for patient use. It must be resterilized and packaged in a new container, and the filter integrity test must be repeated. When this test is repeated, the volume of sterile water for injection flush should be increased to remove all traces of drug.

---

formed properly and that all critical parameters are within specified limits during compounding.[4] Autoclaving must be reserved for items that can be penetrated by water vapor. Therefore, dry sealed containers, oils, and waxes may not be suitable for sterilization via autoclaving.

Heat sterilization is complex and should not be used in hospitals that do not have the proper equipment and validated expertise. A very complete technical monograph on the topic of moist heat sterilization has been published by the Parenteral Drug Association.[11]

Sterilization by Gas

Gas sterilization may used be instead of heat when the preparation to be sterilized cannot withstand high temperatures or moisture. The active ingredient used in gas sterilization is ethylene oxide. Disadvantages of this agent are its highly flammable nature (unless mixed with suitable inert gases), its mutagenic properties, and the possibility of toxic residues in treated materials, particularly those containing chloride ions.

Preparations to be sterilized must be dry because moisture may inactivate ethylene oxide. Items that might dissolve and retain ethylene oxide, such as oils and waxes, should not be sterilized using this method. Generally, gas sterilization is carried out in a pressurized chamber similar to a steam autoclave. Facilities using ethylene oxide should provide adequate poststerilization degassing to (1) enable microbial survivor monitoring and (2) minimize exposure of operators to the potentially harmful gas.

Validation of this sterilization procedure requires monitoring of temperature, humidity, vacuum/positive pressure, and ethylene oxide concentration. All critical process parameters within the chamber must be adequate during the entire cycle. Validation generally is performed by using biologic indicators such as *Bacillus subtilis*. These indicators also should be used to monitor routine runs. Ethylene oxide is limited in its ability to diffuse gas to the innermost product areas that require sterilization. Package design and chamber loading patterns must provide minimal resistance to gas diffusion.[5]

Sterilization by Radiation

The proliferation of heat-sensitive medical devices and concerns about ethylene oxide safety have resulted in many applications of radiation sterilization.[5] It can be used for many drug substances and final dosage forms. The advantages of this sterilization include low chemical reactivity, low measurable residues, and fewer variables to control.

The two types of ionizing radiation are radioisotope decay (gamma radiation) and electron beam. In both types, the radiation dose should be established to yield the required degree of sterility assurance (within the range of minimum and maximum doses set) so that the properties of the article being sterilized are acceptable. Validation of this sterilization procedure includes

- Establishing compatibility of the preparation to be sterilized.

- Establishing a preparation loading pattern and completion of dose mapping in the sterilization container (including identification of minimum and maximum dose zones).

- Demonstrating delivery of the required sterilization dose.

For electron-beam irradiation, validation also must include online control of the voltage, current, conveyor speed, and electron-beam scan.[4]

Summary

Batch compounding can be used for preparations such as antibiotic minibags or syringes, parenteral nutrition solutions, and epidural morphine solutions. Processes classified as batch compounding include syringe repackaging, mass reconstitution, pooling of multiple ingredients, and open reservoir mixing. Each method requires a high level of quality assurance, because these preparations may be used as multiple doses for one patient or as single doses for many patients.

Quality assurance testing also should guarantee the sterility, non-pyrogenicity, and potency of these batch compounded preparations (see Chapter 21). Depending on the characteristics of the preparation, sterilization can be performed by filtration, by heat or chemical means, or by radiation.

References

1. Trissel LA. *Handbook on Injectable Drugs*, 12th ed. Bethesda, MD: American Society of Hospital Pharmacists; 2002.
2. Hunt ML Jr. Training manual for intravenous admixture personnel, 4th ed. Chicago, IL: Baxter Healthcare Corp.; 1990.
3. American Society of Health-System Pharmacists. ASHP guidelines on quality assurance for pharmacy-prepared sterile products. *Am J Health-Syst Pharm.* 2000; 57:1150–69.
4. Pharmaceutical compounding—sterile preparations. In: United States pharmacopeia, 27th rev./national formulary 18th ed. Rockville, MD: United States Pharmacopeial Convention; 2004. Available at www.uspnf.com. Accessed 04/01/04
5. Sterilization and sterility assurance of compendial articles. In: United States pharmacopeia, 27th ed/national formulary, 22nd rev. Rockville, MD: United States Pharmacopeial Convention; 2004. Available at www.uspnf.com. Accessed 04/01/04.
6. Leahy TJ, Sullivan MJ. Validation of bacterial-retention capabilities of membrane filters. *Pharm Technol.* 1978;2 (Nov):65–75.
7. McKinnon BT, Avis KE. Membrane filtration of pharmaceutical solutions. *Am J Hosp Pharm.* 1993; 50:1921–36.
8. Office of Compliance, Division of Manufacturing and Product Quality. Guidelines on sterile drug products produced by aseptic processing. Rockville, MD: Food and Drug Administration; 2002.
9. Fifield CW, Leahy TJ. Sterilization filtration. In: Block SS, ed. *Disinfection, Sterilization, and Preservation.* Philadelphia, PA: Lea & Febiger; 1983: 1478.

10. Emory SF. Principles of integrity-testing hydrophilic microporous membrane filters, part II. *Pharm Technol.* 1989;13 (Oct):36–46.

11. Technical monograph no. 1. Industrial most heat sterilization in autoclaves. *PDA J Pharm Sci Technol.* 2003;57 (suppl.):1–155.

14 | Batch Compounding Documentation

*Philip J. Schneider**

*The author acknowledges Barbara T. McKinnon, who authored this chapter in the first edition of this text.

Batch compounding involves the compounding of multiple sterile components, in a single discrete process, by the same individuals during one limited period.[1] The term "batch compounding" often has been associated with compounding of units for multiple patients, but a batch also may be compounded for one patient. For example, hospital pharmacists may compound a batch of identical cardioplegic solutions for multiple patients, while home care practitioners may compound a batch of parenteral nutrition solutions for a single patient's use over several days. Careful documentation of raw materials, preparative processes, product evaluations, and environmental tests is necessary to maintain control of quality.

Batch compounding can be an efficient method of compounding commonly used sterile preparations. Advantages include:

- Cost savings in labor, drugs, and supplies.
- Savings in resources and time.
- More consistent and reliable service to patients and customers.
- Finished product testing and other quality-control monitoring.

If batch compounding is not properly managed, the health and safety of many patients can be threatened.

Master work sheets and batch compounding records can help to establish and maintain a quality-assurance program for batch compounded sterile preparations.

Master Work Sheets

A standardized record of compounding or "master work sheet" should be developed for routinely compounded batch preparations. To keep consecutive batches nearly identical, all compounding activities should be reproduced uniformly by following this master worksheet.[2] It includes:

- Master formula.
- Records of quality checks of components.
- Specifications for necessary equipment and supplies.
- Checks of preparative procedures.
- Compounding directions.

- Sample of the preparation labeling.
- Results of in process testing.
- Result of evaluation of final preparation.

Each time the preparation is compounded, a batch record is generated to document its preparation, control, and distribution. The master work sheet is the permanent record of the compounding and control of all batches of one particular preparation.[2]

Although a sheet is not needed for all compounded sterile preparations, it should be developed for batch-compounded sterile preparations and all "high risk" preparations (USP High Risk /ASHP Risk Level 3 preparations—see Chapter 1).[1] For example, master work sheets should be established for (1) standardized parenteral nutrition solutions compounded as a batch in anticipation of orders, (2) cardioplegic solutions, and (3) batches of ophthalmic solutions used by multiple patients.

Master Formula

A specific formula must be developed to address desired attributes of the preparation (e.g., final concentrations of ingredients, final pH, and osmolarity). The required diluents, preservatives, and other excipients, antioxidants, chelating agents, and buffers also should be addressed. The formula should be reviewed by a pharmacist to determine if the preparation meets formulation and stability requirements as well as physiologic norms for solution osmolarity and pH appropriate for the intended route of administration.

Master formulas should list all preparations clearly by name, concentration, and total quantity (weight or volume required). A complete listing of names and quantities of all batch ingredients, including excipients, is necessary. An identifying code for each product (e.g., NDC code number) can minimize errors.

All calculations required in compounding should be specified in the master formula. For example, the method for increasing the volume of a formula to allow for overfill should be indicated. An overfill factor may be specified so that calculations of required excess amounts are handled consistently for each ingredient. Similarly, directions should specify how to handle existing overfill when preparation additives are measured.

The *theoretical* yield of the master formula, in either weight or volume (as appropriate), should be specified for high risk preparations.[1,3] The acceptable *actual* yield also should be set; if it is not met, the cause should be investigated.

Component Quality Checks

Commercially available sterile components

When commercially available sterile components are used (e.g., drug products, ready-to-use containers, and devices), they should be routinely inspected. If they are expired, defective, unsuitable for the intended use, or inappropriately stored, these components should not be used. Defective components should be promptly reported to the Food and Drug Administration[4] and identified by name, lot number, and expiration date. Ingredients used to compound sterile preparations should be stable, compatible, and appropriate, according to the manufacturer, United States Pharmacopeial (USP) guidelines, or relevant scientific references.[1-3]

Nonsterile components

When nonsterile drug components are used, they should meet USP standards. Certificates of analysis, from reputable manufacturers of bulk drug substances, can establish that each lot received by the pharmacy meets specifica-

tions.[3] If the material is USP/NF, or reagent grade, the minimum assay of the manufacturer may be assumed. Specifications can include color, appearance, assay requirements, purity, and heavy metal content.[5]

After receiving each lot of bulk drug substance, a designated pharmacy person should inspect the lot and document any visual evidence of deterioration, unacceptable quality, and wrong identity. Documentation also should verify that components have been assayed by the manufacturer to meet specifications (Figure 14-1).

Bulk drug substances that are stored properly in the pharmacy should retain their quality until the manufacturer's labeled expiration date. Substances without a labeled expiration date should be

- Dated on receipt.
- Stored properly.
- Dated when the container is opened.
- Used within a reasonable time (based on available references).
- Visually inspected by the pharmacist when used.

The conditions under which containers of bulk drug substances are opened and the technique of content withdrawal should be strictly controlled. The devices used for withdrawal should be clean to avoid contamination of the remaining contents. The pharmacy

Lot # (Pharmacy)	Name of Chemical	Grade	Date received	Mfg.	Lot # Exp. Date	Quantity received	Remarks	Approval date
UM601	Sodium chloride, cryst	USP	7-7-94	xyz Chem	000726 None	2 x 100lbs	Fiber drums	JAP 7-8-94
UM602	Alcohol 95%	USP	7-8-94	USChem	TI3366 None	1 x 54 Gal.	Metal drum	7-8-94 AR
UM603	Dextrose, Anhydrous	USP	7-10-94	Starch Prod.	MBKX None	5 x 100 lbs.	Bags	PMJ 7-12-94

Figure 14-1. Component inventory record for nonsterile components with manufacturers' certificates of analysis. (Adapted, with permission, from Reference 5.)

may repackage bulk drug substances into smaller, suitable, and properly sealed containers (e.g., shrink-seal or zip-closure plastic bags) to minimize contamination.[3]

Raw materials

When raw materials are received without a certificate of analysis from the manufacturer, they must be quarantined to prevent use until testing is completed. Each lot represents a single batch of raw materials, in one or more containers, represented by a single manufac-turer's control number. Records (Figure 14-2) should be kept of the

- Chemical name
- Grade
- Quantity received
- Date received
- Manufacturer
- Manufacturer's lot number
- Expiration date
- Results of tests for identity and purity

If the raw materials are not graded, an assay report should be obtained from the manufacturer. A decision can then be made about whether the material meets the desired specifications. Assays usually are performed on labile chemicals, such as calcium chloride (anhydrous) and magnesium sulfate, which readily gain or lose moisture. Purity and identification can be tested by various methods. Usually, several chemical and physical tests can identify the material and ascertain its purity. For example, a mixed melting point or optical rotation determination may suffice for purity tests. To identify the drug, a simple chemical color reaction, chemical color change reaction, characteristic odor, taste, or physical appearance may suffice.[5] If the pharmacy cannot perform these tests, the material should be sent to another laboratory.

Components compounded in the pharmacy

Sterile injectable preparations that are compounded in the pharmacy but used as components of other sterile injectables deserve special attention. Lack of quality (e.g., purity, potency, and sterility) of the component solution adversely affects the quality of the resulting preparation. All nonsterile ingredients used to compound sterile component preparations should be inspected; the final preparation also must be tested for sterility, nonpyrogenicity, and potency to ensure that it meets all specifications. An analytical request and results form (Figure 14-3) should be sent to the laboratory along with the test solution. Figure 14-4 illustrates the process used to review analytical results from testing and to approve release of component preparations.

Equipment and Supplies Specifications

The master work sheet should specify all equipment, containers, and supplies needed for compounding. The brand name and model or item number of equipment and supplies should be listed as well as any applicable performance characteristics (e.g., weight limits for scales). Specification of all details, such as lengths and diameters of tubing, ensures that the same items can be reordered if equipment malfunctions or supplies become depleted (Figure 14-5). For complicated equipment setups, a diagram can illustrate the proper sequence of assembly.

The preparation of equipment and supplies also should be part of the master work sheet. For example, a procedure should be established to calibrate or verify the accuracy of automated compounding devices used in aseptic processing.[1] If products are dispensed by weight, the

Pharmacy Lot #	Description	Identification	Solubility	Specific Rotation	Acidity	Color of solution	Heavy metals	Soluble starch	Approval	Analyst date
UM603	passes	passes	passes	passes	passes	passes	0.0005 %	passes	approved	PMJ 7/12/94

Figure 14-2. Raw materials testing record. (Adapted, with permission, from Reference 5.)

PHARMACY - ANALYTICAL REQUEST & RESULTS

Product: _____ Dextrose 50% USP _____ Lot No._____
Testing Bottles Submitted: _____
Anticipated Q.C. Release Date for this Lot: _____
Analyses Requested By:_____ Date of Request: _____

Analyses Requested	Procedure	Production Specification	Laboratory Results					
			Bott.	P/F	Bott.	P/F	Bott.	P/F
pH	2-1-001-85	3.5-6.5						
Specific Gravity	2-1-126-85	1.100 - 1.200						
Dext. Hyd.	2-1-004-82	47.5 - 52.5 g%						
Nitrogen	2-1-006-82							
Acetate	2-1-163-82							
Chloride	2-1-032-82							
Sodium	2-1-013-82							
Potassium	2-1-211-82							
Phosphate	2-1-250-82							
Magnesium	2-1-252-82							
Calcium	2-1-251-82							
Vitamin K_1	2-1-397-82							

Chemistry No. _____ , _____ , _____ By: _____ Checked: _____
Date Received: _____ Date Initiated: _____ Date Completed: _____

Particulate Count	Bottle 2-2-080-	Not >50 p/ml = to 10μm		Particle Description
		Not >5 p/ml = to 25μm		

Sterility (Membrane Filtration)	2-2-113-82	Must Pass	Bottle No.	7 Day Incubation				B &F	
				FTM		SCD			
				+	-	+	-	Pass	Fail	Pass	Fail

Microbiology No. _____ , _____ , _____ By: _____ Checked: _____
Date Received: _____ Date Initiated: _____ Date Completed: _____

Analyses Requested	Procedure	Production Specification	Bottle No.	Basal Temp.	T_1	T2	T3	ΔT	Pass	Fail
USP XX Pyrogens	2-3-001-85	Must Pass								
1.										

Biology No. _____ , _____ , _____ By: _____ Checked: _____
Date Received: _____ Date Initiated: _____ Date Completed: _____

Figure 14-3. Analytical testing request and results form for component solutions.

HOSPITAL PHARMACY

TEST ASSAY OR PROPERTY	METHOD	SPECIFICATIONS	OBSERVATION OR RESULTS 1	2	3
COMPLETE LABEL	Visual	Check for correct formula Cat. # Lot # Exp. date			
INTACT CONTAINER	B/W Bkg Visual	No hairline cracks or Imperfections			
CLARITY	B/W Bkg Visual	No visible particulate Matter			
COLOR	Visual	Clear (No color)			
ODOR	Smell	None			
pH	pH Meter	3.5 - 6.5			
TASTE	Taste	Sweet			
WEIGHT or VOLUME	Volu-metric	1025 - 1060ml			
SPECIFIC GRAVITY	Hydro-meter	1.100 - 1.200			
STRENGTH					
Detrose (Anhydrous)	Chem.	45 (42-46) g%			
PARTICULATE MATTER	Visual	(Yes - No) Inspect Black/White for			
		presence of particular matter			
STORAGE PROCEDURE	Room Temp	Yes - No			

QUALITY CONTROL ANALYTICAL REPORT

RAW MATERIAL — IN-PROCESS — END PRODUCT

NDC # 0264-1128-00

CATALOG # S1280

NO. CONTAINERS

MANUFACTURER LOT NUMBER

NO. CONTAINERS

PRODUCT DEXTROSE 50% USP

MANUFACTURER McGAW

NO. CONTAINERS

STRENGTH

SAMPLE DATE

DATE OF MANUFACTURE

LOT NUMBER

FINAL APPROVAL OF MATERIAL OR PRODUCT FOR USE

	Incomp.	Complete
PHARMACEUTICAL BULK COMPOUNDING MASTER WORKSHEET		
BIOLOGICAL TESTS WORKSHEET		

COMMENTS:

APPROVED: ☐

CONDITIONALLY APPROVED: ☐
EXPLAIN:

REJECTED: ☐
EXPLAIN:

RPh
Analyst — Date

RPh
Released By — Date

Figure 14-4. Form for final approval and release of component solutions.

EQUIPMENT RECORD

1.   Perma-San stainless steel mixing tank and cover (100 gallon)
2.   P-35S 1" stainless steel flush valve
3.   MixMor G-14 stainless steel electric mixer and stand
4.   Stainless steel calibration strip A
5.   Climet 411 printer
6.   Climet CI-4100 particle counter

ASSEMBLY AND POOLING EQUIPMENT (STERILE)

Equipment Code Number

1. Plastic paddle   No. _____   No. _____
2. Beaker 4000 ml   No. _____   No. _____
3. Cylindrical graduate   No. _____   No. _____

FILLING

1.   XX2504700 6-Place manifold   No. _____   No. _____
2.   XX2504705 1/4" NPTM to 3/8' I.D. Hose (6)   No. _____   No. _____
3.   XX6700101 1/4" tee   No. _____   No. _____
4.   XX6700L11 1/4" NPT to tubing adapter (6)   No. _____   No. _____
5.   YY2004040 2" T.C. clamp assembly   No. _____   No. _____
6.   Tubing, latex surgical, 1/4" x 3/32" wall   No. _____   No. _____
7.   XX6700030 1/4" quick release coupling and nipple (7)   No. _____   No. _____
8.   BD needle adapter (6)   No. _____   No. _____
9.   18 gauge 1-1/2" needles   No. _____   No. _____
10. YY1301009 1/4' pipe plug   No. _____   No. _____
11. YY1412229 1/2" T.C. to 1/4" NPT adapter   No. _____   No. _____
12. Pressure tubing 3/8" I.D. PVC   No. _____   No. _____
13. 7549 Masterflex variable speed peristaltic pump   No. _____   No. _____
14. 6408-73 tygon tubing   No. _____   No. _____
15. YY1301015 1/4" Pressure gauge, 0-100 psi   No. _____   No. _____
16. XX6700111 1/4" NPTF Coupling   No. _____   No. _____
17. No. 12122, 0.2 micrometer Gelman Capsule   No. _____   No. _____

Figure 14-5. Equipment record.

---

type of weighing device and the product's specific gravity should be documented.

The pharmacy should ensure that equipment, apparatus, and devices used in compounding operate properly and are within acceptable tolerance limits. Records of equipment calibration, testing, maintenance, and cleaning should be kept on file and be easily retrieved. Routine maintenance checks should be performed as necessary. Before operating the equipment, personnel should receive training and experience. They also should be able to determine whether their equipment is operating properly or malfunctioning.[3]

The master work sheet generally includes requirements for cleaning and disinfecting the compounding area before work is begun.

Sterilization procedures for any equipment heat sterilized by the pharmacy should include review of a biologic indicator to validate that sterilization occurred before use.[3]

All nonsterile equipment (e.g., tubings, filters, and containers) that contacts the sterilized final preparation should be properly cleaned and sterilized before entering the controlled area. The sterilization process should be monitored and documented. Equipment that does not contact the finished preparation should be properly cleaned, rinsed, and disinfected. Large equipment (e.g., tanks, carts, and tables) kept in the controlled area or cleanroom should be made of a material, such as stainless steel, that can be easily cleaned and disinfected.[1]

Requirements for packaging of compounded preparations (e.g., types of containers and methods of closure) should be included in the master work sheet. The final container for the sterile preparation should maintain its integrity (i.e., sterility, identity, strength, quality, and purity) throughout the shelf life.[6] Presterilized containers from licensed manufacturers should be used when possible. In an aseptic filling operation, the container should be sterile at the time of the operation; if nonsterile containers are used, methods for sterilization should be established.[1]

Compounding Procedure Checks

Procedures should be written clearly and be easily understood so that personnel who follow the master work sheet can compound the preparation uniformly. The order of addition of ingredients also should be specified if a certain sequence is required (e.g., calcium and phosphate or amino acids, dextrose, and lipids). A step-by-step procedure should be developed for all compounding activities, including in process tests (e.g., pH checks).

Conditions suitable for compounding each preparation should be documented. For example, Risk Level 3/high risk preparations must be prepared in an ISO Class 5 (Class 100) certified laminar-airflow hood within an ISO Class 7 (Class 10,000) cleanroom according to the ASHP Guideline, ISO Class 8 (Class 100,000) cleanroom according to USP Chapter <797>, or in a properly maintained and monitored ISO 5 (Class 100) cleanroom.[1,3] Other required operating conditions, such as cleaning and disinfection of work surfaces, also should be included.

Compounding Directions

Compounding procedures should be checked and double-checked. Technicians should be adequately supervised by a licensed pharmacist in the compounding area. The pharmacist should check that correct ingredients are selected and that correct volumes or weights are added. Finally, the pharmacist must verify that the volume of the final container is correct and check the labeled preparation.

Data entered into an automated compounding device should be verified by a pharmacist before compounding is begun, and checks should verify the accuracy of ingredients delivered. These checks may include weighing (Figure 14-6) and visually inspecting the final preparation. The expected weight, based on the specific gravities of the ingredients and their respective volumes, can be documented on the batch record, dated, and initialed by a pharmacist. Once compounding is completed, each final preparation can be weighed and compared with the expected weight. The product's actual weight should fall within an established threshold for variance.[7]

To verify a preparation visually, the beginning level of each bulk container should be marked before the start of automated mixing. Then the container should be checked after completion of the mixing to determine whether the final volumes are reasonable compared to expected volumes. The operator should periodically observe the automated compounding device during mixing to ensure its proper operation.[8]

Other quality controls may be needed when multiple sterile ingredients are combined into a single sterile or nonsterile reservoir for subdivision into multiple units. Associated calculations should be verified by a second pharmacist and documented.[1] Methods of sterilization and testing of preparations for sterility are discussed in Chapters 13 and 21, respectively. If there are doubts about whether a preparation has been properly prepared or sterilized, it should not be used.

Sample Label

A sample label should be part of the master work sheet. Standardized label text should be developed for each commonly batch compounded preparation to ensure consistency among batches. If preparations are compounded in advance, stored, and then dis-

COMPOUNDED BY: __SE__

PHARMACIST: __Coronado__

500.00 ml X ‾‾‾ O.F. X __1.07__ S.G. = __535__ Grams

UNIT#	WEIGHT	UNIT#	WEIGHT	UNIT#	WEIGHT	UNIT#	WEIGHT	UNIT#	WEIGHT
1	535	9	536	17		25		33	
2	540	10	535	18		26		34	
3	539	11	540	19		27		35	
4	538	12	539	20		28		36	
5	537	13	538	21		29		37	
6	536	14	537	22		30		38	
7	535	15		23		31		39	
8	540	16		24		32		40	

Figure 14-6. Weight record. (Reproduced, with permission, from PharmaThera, Memphis, TN.)

pensed to individual patients, both a preparation label and a final patient-specific label are required.

When the patient-specific label is affixed, the original preparation lot number and assigned expiration date must still be visible. The issuing and use as well as destruction of any unused or damaged preprinted labels should be documented. Labeling of compounded preparations are discussed further in Chapter 9.

Inprocess Testing

Inprocess testing verifies that the compounding environment and the actual preparation meet established criteria. No sterile preparations should be compounded in a controlled area that fails to meet these criteria. Environmental checks might include:

- Counting of airborne particles with a calibrated particle counter
- Monitoring of the positive pressure of the compounding room relative to other areas
- Microbial sampling of the air and surfaces
- Temperature and humidity monitoring

This monitoring may be performed routinely (e.g., weekly) or before or during compounding, depending on the risk level of the preparation. Techniques for environmental monitoring are discussed in Chapter 18.

When the environment does not meet established criteria, the compounding of sterile preparations should immediately cease and corrective action should be taken. The compounding of Risk Level 3/high risk sterile preparations is especially critical. Steps taken to correct the problem and their results should be documented.

In process testing may be as simple as visual inspections for physical properties (e.g., color, smell, and clarity) or as complex as detailed chemical analyses for content. Checks for pH can easily be performed with a small, hand-held meter. This meter monitors the adjustment of product pH before and after subsequent additions of acid or base (e.g., acetic acid or sodium bicarbonate). Refractive index measurements may help to verify the addition of certain ingredients.[9] For example, these measurements can approximate the concentration of dextrose in batch-compounded parenteral nutrition solutions. Similarly, specific gravity measurements can check the dextrose content of parenteral nutrition solutions.[10]

Testing and Quarantine Requirements for Final Compounded Preparations

The master work sheet should list the appropriate checks and tests to ensure that batch compounded sterile preparations are free from defects and meet all quality specifications. A sterile preparations should not be released until all quality specifications have been reviewed and all release requirements are met.[3] For Risk Level 3/high risk preparations, tests should include visual inspection as well as checks for compounding accuracy and formulation integrity, including sterility, pyrogenicity, and potency.

Visual inspection

As a condition of release, each compounded unit should be inspected immediately after compounding against lighted white and black backgrounds for visible particulates or other foreign matter. The final preparation should also be inspected for proper labeling, container leaks and integrity, and solution cloudiness, color, and volume (Figure 14-7). Defective preparations should immediately be discarded or marked and segregated to prevent their administration. When preparations are not

distributed promptly after compounding, a predistribution inspection should be conducted because defects (e.g., precipitation, cloudiness, and leakage) may develop.[3]

Compounding accuracy

A pharmacist should verify that the preparation was compounded accurately with the correct ingredients, quantities, containers, and reservoirs. The additive containers and the syringes used to measure additives should be quarantined with the final preparations for a final check. Syringe plungers should be drawn back to the volume mark used for each additive if the additive volume was not checked before the addition.

Automated pump settings should be verified just before or just after pumping and mixing. The volumes of each pumped ingredient should be checked to establish that the automated pump is within the accuracy limits set by the manufacturer. All compounded units used should be accounted for according to

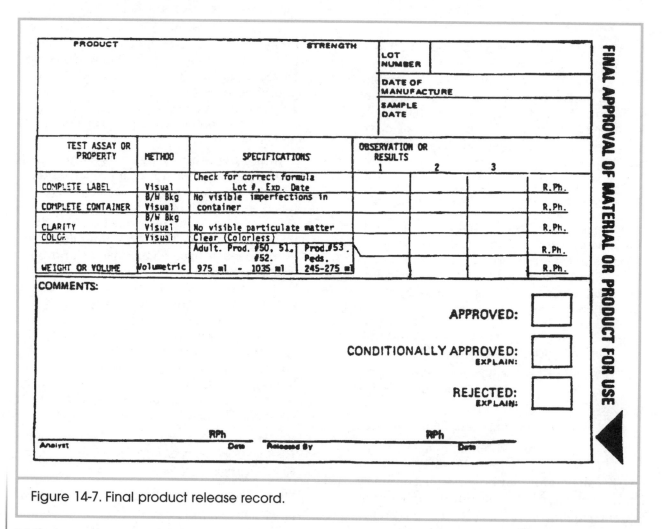

Figure 14-7. Final product release record.

written procedures.[3] Other methods (e.g., observation during compounding, calculation checks, and documented records) also may be used for verification.[1]

Formulation integrity

Formulations involving nonsterile ingredients require additional evaluations to ensure that the final preparations meets desired specifications for potency, purity, identity, and quality. Quality-control tests demonstrate the unique properties of parenteral dosage forms (e.g., sterility and freedom from pyrogens and visible particulate contamination). (Figure 14-8.)

Sterility tests evaluate the preparation for contamination with microbiological impurities. Sterility tests should be performed on Risk Level 3/high risk preparations after sterilization. This test, including the sampling scheme, should be conducted according to a USP method. The USP methods estimate the probable not actual sterility of numerous preparations. After a few batch samples are tested for sterility, they are assumed to be representative of every article from the batch. These samples can be inadvertently contaminated during the testing procedure. Despite these limitations, some final testing must be performed to protect consumers from contaminated preparations. Although the sterility of every preparation is not guaranteed, the sterility test indicates that a representative sample of a lot or batch is uncontaminated. Final testing also checks the sterility of preparations sterilized in the pharmacy, such as those compounded by a filtration process.[11]

The capability of the preparation to form a gel in the presence of limulus amoebocyte lysate is used to test for pyrogens. The prevention of pyrogens is preferred over their removal in parenteral products. Pyrogen testing should be performed on all preparations compounded from nonsterile drug components or with nonsterile equipment.[11] The limulus amoebocyte lysate test is convenient and offers rapid results (generally within 1 hr). The preparation should not be released until it has been determined that the specified endotoxin limit has not been exceeded. Pyrogen testing is not required for ophthalmic or topical solutions.[3]

Clarity tests check for visible particulate contamination, and particulate analytical tests quantify the number and size of the particulates. Package integrity tests are performed, for glass-sealed ampuls and other parenteral packaging systems, to check for microbiological contamination.[10]

Sterility and pyrogen testing typically requires quarantine of final preparations until the results are available. If preparations compounded from nonsterile components must be dispensed before final testing is completed, a procedure must allow for their immediate recall.[1] Evaluation of final products and procedures for quarantine are discussed further in Chapter 21.

Batch Preparation Records

The master work sheet is the recipe for compounding of multiple, identical batches of a given preparation. The batch record, however, documents the compounding of a *single* batch preparation. Typically, master work sheets are only needed for commonly compounded batches or for high-risk preparations. However, the batch record may be helpful for compounding directions and documentation of any preparation compounded as a batch.

Each time a preparation is compounded, the batch record documents its preparation, control, and distribution. To save time, batch records can be standardized, computerized, and reprinted whenever a preparation is compounded. When compounding is begun, the batch record is filled out with the following items:

- Date
- Number of units compounded
- Component quantities
- Lot numbers and expiration dates of components
- Initials of personnel who check each step of the process
- Results of inprocess and final evaluations
- Lot number assigned to the batch
- Beyond-use dating assigned to the batch
- Names of personnel directly involved in compounding

A batch record offers several advantages. It helps to ensure that all subsequent refills are compounded in exactly the same manner, using the same brands of ingredients and the same diluents. The batch record provides a clear list for gathering the necessary drugs,

PHARMACY - ANALYTICAL REQUEST & RESULTS

Product: _____ TROPHAMINE 2% w DEXTROSE 15% 1000 ML _____ Lot No. __57__

Testing Bottles Submitted: _#3, 5, 6, 10, 20, 30, 40, 50, 60, 70, 80, 90, 96, & 97_____

Anticipated Q.C. Release Date for this Lot: _____

Analyses Requested By: _____ Date of Request: _____

Analyses Requested	Procedure	Production Specification	Laboratory Results					
			Bott.	P/F	Bott.	P/F	Bott.	P/F
pH	2-1-001-85	5.0-7.0						
Specific Gravity	2-1-126-85	1.0 - 1.2						
Dext. Hyd.	2-1-004-82	13.3 - 16.5 gm%						
Nitrogen	2-1-006-82	2.79 - 3.41 g/L						
Acetate	2-1-163-82	17.4 - 21.4 mEq/L						
Chloride	2-1-032-82	18 - 22 mEq/L						
Sodium	2-1-013-82	4.5 - 5.5 mEq/L						
Potassium	2-1-211-82	21 - 27 mEq/L						
Phosphate	2-1-250-82	5.4 - 6.6 mEq/L						
Magnesium	2-1-252-82	4.5 - 5.5 mEq/L						
Calcium	2-1-251-82	4.1 - 5.1 mEq/L						
Vitamin K_1	2-1-397-82	1.0 mg/L Yes-No						

Chemistry No. _____ , _____ , _____ By: _____ Checked: _____

Date Received: _____ Date Initiated: _____ Date Completed: _____

Particulate Count	Bottle # 6 2-2-080-85	Not >50 p/ml = to 10μm				
		Not >5 p/ml = to 25μm				

Sterility (Membrane Filtration)	2-2-302-85	Bottle No.		7 Day Incubation		B &F	
		10, 20, 30, 40, 50, 60, 70, 80, 90, & 97		Pass	Fail	Pass	Fail

Microbiology No. _____ , _____ , _____ By: _____ Checked: _____

Date Received: _____ Date Initiated: _____ Date Completed: _____

Analyses Requested	Procedure	Bottle No.	Basal Temp.	T_1	T2	T3	Δ T	Pass	Fail
USP PYROGEN	2-3-001-85	# 5							
USP PYROGEN	2-3-001-85	# 96							

Biology No. _____ , _____ , _____ By: _____ Checked: _____

Date Received: _____ Date Initiated: _____ Date Completed: _____

Figure 14-8. Analytical testing request and results form for finished product.

solutions, and supplies from storage areas. It provides precise directions for compounding, which may be particularly helpful for technicians. Errors also can be minimized by using the documented system of checks. A record of lot numbers and expiration dates of components can help in the event of a product recall.

For low-risk preparations, completion of a batch record may not be time consuming. Some pharmacy software programs automatically generate simple batch records along with preparation labels (Figure 14-9). These records typically document the component, strength, and volume to be added for each ingredient. To save cost and time, one extra label can be generated to document the exact components, strengths, and volumes used for compounding. This batch record can then be attached to the prescription or medication order to document the compounding process.

For high-risk preparations, a more thorough batch record is required (Figure 14-10). Because these preparations may be stored or administered over prolonged periods or given to multiple patients, records should be maintained of lot numbers and beyond-use dates. These records are invaluable if a component is recalled, if the preparation fails a final test (e.g., sterility or pyrogen), or if the sterility or potency of the preparation is questioned.

Preparations compounded for multiple patients may be given a lot number so they can be identified and retrieved if there are defects. Simple strategies can be devised for assigning a lot number. For example, a sequential number may be assigned to each batch of a particular preparation. Alternatively, numbers representing the month, date, year, and batch prepared in a day can be used (e.g., 101203-6 for the sixth batch prepared on October 12, 2003). A batch log is useful to track preparations easily by lot number and to avoid the assignment of the same sequential number to two preparations compounded at approximately the same time. If there are separate compounding areas, an identifying letter can be used with the lot number to determine the compounding area.

To assign responsibility for the process and the preparation, the involvement of all personnel must be documented. For short or uncomplicated procedures (e.g., combination of two solutions), the signatures should appear at the end of the document. By signing, these individuals attest that all information is accurate and that they are responsible for the preparation. For preparations requiring several components or several compounding steps, each step must bear the signature or initials of the persons responsible. A pharmacist must still take responsibility for the finished preparation.

Criteria for the release and use of the preparation must be established in advance and adhered to from batch to batch. Release data may include laboratory analysis, physical and visual inspection, and results of other parameters (e.g., environmental testing, proper labeling, accurate weight or volume, and container/closure integrity). The finished preparation is then compared to established specifications. If the preparation meets these criteria, it is released for use. If the criteria are not strictly met, the preparation may be conditionally released, pending results of further investigation. This occurrence is usually rare and the decision for conditional release should be made only after careful analysis.

If the preparation fails any major specification, it must be rejected. Rejected preparations may be reprocessed, depending on the reason for failure or destroyed. A pharmacist who is trained and knowledgeable in compounding sterile preparations and analysis must be responsible for the product's release. Two phar-

```
 5/15/95  Location:D-416      Volume:1257ml IV#:  1
      * * *  S O L U T I O N   F O R M U L A  * * *
 __ Additive _____ ml __    Additive _____ ml __
  Aminosyn II 10% 600.00       MgSO4 50% .....    2.40
  Dextrose 70% .. 428.57       M.T.E.-5 ......    3.60
  NaCl 2.5mEq ...  24.00       M.V.I.-12 .....   12.00
  KCl 2mEq ......  24.00       Albumin 25% ... 120.00
  K Phosphate 3mM  8.00        Selepen .......    1.50
  Ca Gluconate ..  25.81       Ranitidine inj    7.20


      5/15/95  Location:D-416        Volume:1257ml IV#:  1

  Ion  Conc. delivered     Ion  Conc. delivered
  Na    69.69 mEq/L        Zn     2.86  mg/L
  K     66.19 mEq/L        Cu     1.15  mg/L
  Ca     9.55 mEq/L        Mn     0.29  mg/L
  Mg     7.64 mEq/L        Cr    11.46  mcg/L
  PO4   19.09 mM/L         Se   105.01  mcg/L
  Ace   34.37 mEq/L        I      0.00  mcg/L
  Cl    85.92 mEq/L
```

Figure 14-9. Batch preparation record for a Risk Level 1 parenteral nutrition solution. (Reproduced, with permission, from PharmaThera, Memphis, TN.)

PRX525-2   COMPOUNDING RECORD CHECK AND LOT NUMBER RECORD   05/15/95   10:19

Patient:
 Nbr:
Rx Nbr: Hood Nbr:
Physician: F.G. List-IC: 999910-51
Date Compounded: A96700 Approximate Container Volume: 1350   ml
Patient Order is for containers   100 through 128
Total Number of Units   29

Initial Master Approved   R.Ph.   sign/date
Final Product Approval   R.Ph.   sign/date

Pharmacist's initials each drug. This check is for containers:

Drug Item	Order Qty	List-Size Cd	Lot Number Rcrd Multi Lots	Original Drug Conc	Amount per Container	Final Conc Per Cont
1. TRAVASOL 10% 1000ML	17	629-04	exp.	10.00%	552.00 ml	4.09%
2. DEXTROSE 70% 1000ML	21	1519-05	exp.	70.00%	699.00 ml	36.26%
3. SODIUM CHLORIDE 2.5MEQ/ML 250ML	2	4219-02	exp.	2.5 meg/ml	12.00 ml	30.00MEG
4. SODIUM ACETATE 2MEQ/ML 100ML	5	3299-06	exp.	2.0 meg/ml	15.00 ml	30.00MEG
5. POTASSIUM CHLORIDE 2MEQ/ML 250ML	1	1513-02	exp.	2.0 meg/ml	5.00 ml	10.00MEG
6. CALCIUM GLUCONATE 10% 4.65MEQ/10ML 100ML	4	6522-00	exp.	0.46 meg/ml	10.86 ml	5.00MEG
7. MAGNESIUM SULFATE 50% 4.06MEQ/ML 50ML	5	2168-03	exp.	4.1 meg/ml	7.38 ml	30.00MEG
8. MULTI-TRACE (MTE-4) 10ML SDV	9	8100-30	exp.		3.00 ml	3.00ml
9. SELEPEN 40MCG/ML 10ML	3	8820-30	exp.	40.0 mcg/ml	1.00 ml	40.00mcg
10. STERILE WATER FOR INJ 2000ML	2	7118-07	exp.		98.00 ml	98.00 ml
11. EMPTY IV BAG 2000ML		113610-25				1.35
12.						
13.						
14.						
15.						

*Lot Nbr - Record Responsibility

Check not required when R.Ph. compounding

1) Tech. or R.Ph. responsible for compounding.......... sign _____ (Signature/Date)

2) Second Tech. or R.Ph. responsible for compounding........ _____ (Signature/Date)

Pharmacists Performing Check: _____ (Signature/Date)

Figure 14-10. Batch preparation record for a high-risk product. (Reproduced, with permission, from PharmaThera, Memphis, TN.)

macists probably should review all results. Regardless of the outcome, the pharmacists must document their decision in the batch record and sign the release document (Figure 14-11).

As in the master work sheet, batch compounding records may contain the following:

- A component test record for nonsterile ingredients, with manufacturers' certificates of analysis to document their acceptability (see Figure 14-1).

- A raw materials testing record (see Figure 14-2).

- An analytical request and results form for testing components of sterile solutions compounded in the pharmacy (see Figure 14-3).

- A final approval and release form for components of sterile solutions compounded in the pharmacy (see Figure 14-4).

- An equipment form to record the supplies used for compounding and, if necessary, the checks of calibration, filter integrity, etc. (see Figure 14-5).

- Records of component lot numbers and expiration dates as well as quantities used (see Figure 14-10).

- Inprocess test records, including the weight of the final preparation (Figure 14-6) and various other tests.

- A final release form for the preparation, including results of tests and release from quarantine (see Figure 14-11).

Finally, a sample label for each lot number is affixed to the batch record, and the batch is visually checked for container integrity, clarity, color, and weight or volume before any preparation is released (see Figure 14-7). A separate document is not necessary for each type of record. One form usually can be used for components, equipment, and results of tests (see Figure 14-12). Then, the label is affixed to the back of the form.

Summary

Batch compounding of multiple sterile preparations, if done correctly, can result in cost savings in labor, drugs, and materials. This requires strict adherence to procedure. Any failure in the process of compounding can lead to waste and/or pose a threat to patient safety.

Master work sheets and batch compounding records can establish a uniform approach to the compounding process. The work sheet provides exact directions on the standard compounding of the batch preparation. The batch record then records the completion of these tasks and identifies that each step has been followed.

References

1. American Society of Hospital Pharmacists. ASHP Guidelines on quality assurance for pharmacy-prepared sterile products. *Am J Hosp Pharm.* 2000;57:1150–69.
2. Turco S. *Sterile Dosage Forms: Their Preparation and Clinical Application.* 3rd ed. Philadelphia, PA: Lea & Febiger; 1994.
3. Pharmaceutical compounding—sterile preparations. In: United States pharmacopeia, 27th rev/national formulary, 22nd ed., first supplement. Rockville, MD: United States Pharmacopeial Convention; 2004. Available at: www.uspnf.com. Accessed on April 1, 2004.
4. U.S. Food and Drug Administration MedWatch. Available at: http://www.fda.gov/medwatch/. Accessed on February 22, 2004.
5. Patel JA. Quality control and standards. In: Brown TR, Smith MC, eds. *Handbook of Institutional Pharmacy Practice,* 2nd ed. Baltimore, MD: Williams & Wilkins; 1986:402–11.
6. Nedich RL. Selection of containers and closure systems for injectable products. *Am J Hosp Pharm.* 1983;40:1924–7.
7. Murphy C. Ensuring accuracy in the use of automatic compounders. *Am J Hosp Pharm.* 1993;50:60. Letter.
8. Brushwood DB. Hospital liable for defect in cardioplegia solution. *Am J Hosp Pharm.* 1992;49:1174–6.
9. Bardas SL, Ferraresi VF, Lieberman SF. Refractometric screening of controlled substances used in operating rooms. *Am J Hosp Pharm.* 1992; 49:2779–81.
10. Silverberg JM, Webb B, Pawlak R. Specific gravity-based determination of dextrose content of total parenteral nutrient solutions for neonates. *Am J Hosp Pharm.* 1993; 50:2090–1.
11. Akers MJ. *Parenteral Quality Control.* New York, NY: Marcel Dekker; 1985.

TPN QC SUMMARY/ RELEASE

TPN: 4.25% Amino Acids / 20% Dextrose   Date:_____

Formula No. : _____HP20 1L_____   Lot No. : _____

BACTERIOLOGY

Sterility:_____ Pass _____ Fail
Lab Test No. _____

Pyrogen:_____ Pass _____ Fail
Lab Test No. _____

STERILITY RETEST

Reason for Retest:_____
Number of Bags Sent:_____
Date Samples Sent:_____

RESULTS: _____ Pass _____ Fail
Lab Test No. _____

INGREDIENT	Labeled Content	Test Result	Satisfactory	Discrepant
Amino Acid	4.25 %			
Dextrose	20.00 %			
Sodium	35.00 mEq/L			
potassium	30.00 mEq/L			
magnesium	10.00 mEq/L			
chloride	35.00 mEq/L			
acetate	64.60 mEq/L			
calcium	5.00 mEq/L			
phosphorous	10.00 mM/L			
copper	1.00 mg/L			
zinc	2.00 mg/L			
selenium	40.00 μg/L	N/A		

PRODUCT RELEASE

Pharmacist: _____

Date:_____

PRODUCT REJECTED

Reason: _____
Date: _____
Discarded Date:_____
Pharmacist: _____

Figure 14-11. Final product quality-control summary/release.

CARDIOPLEGIA SOLUTION, TYPE "C"
LOG SHEET

Date:_____

Quantity of bags to be made, Type "C" _____

Prepared by: _____   Checked by: _____
          (print name)   (print name)

Assigned Lot # _____   Expiration Date: _____

SOLUTIONS USED:	MFG:	VOLUME:	LOT#	EXPIRATION
Sterile Water for Inj.	(Baxter)	2000 ml		_____
Anticoagulant CPD Soln.	(Abbott)	500 ml		_____
Tham 0.3 Molar Soln.	(Abbott)	500 ml		_____
Potassium Chloride 2mEq/ml	(_____)	200 ml		_____
Dextrose 50% in Water	(_____)	50 ml		_____
Glutamate-Aspartate Sol.	(UIH)	30 ml		_____
Viaflex Automix Bag	(Baxter)	1000 ml		_____

PHASE I

New Transfer Set Used?   YES   /   NO   : _____ (R.Ph. Initials)

Automix Calibrated?   YES   /   NO   : _____ (R.Ph. Initials)

Automix Set-up Checked
and Verified for Base
Solution Compounding?   YES   /   NO   : _____ (R.Ph. Initials)

PHASE II

Additive Set-up Checked
and Verified?   YES   /   NO   : _____ (R.Ph. Initials)

Compounding Process Completed: _____ (R.Ph. Signature)

END PRODUCT TESTING

End Product Testing Done? YES   /   NO   : _____ (R.Ph. Initials)

Microbial Testing Results? POS.   /   NEG. : _____ (R.Ph. Initials)

Potassium Chloride Conc., Type "C" Sample: _____ mEq/ml
                                             (0.034 mEq/ml)

Release Date / Pharmacist: _____ / _____

Figure 14-12. Batch preparation record of components, equipment, and test results.

15 | Pharmacist Education

Philip J. Schneider

Attention to the quality of compounded sterile preparations prompts an assessment of how well pharmacists are educated to perform this function. With the current emphasis on clinical practice, traditional subject matter has been de-emphasized. Therefore, pharmacy schools, professional organizations, and employers must verify that adequate training to compound sterile preparations is offered to their students, pharmacists, and technicians.

This chapter examines the current status of pharmacy school education about compounding sterile preparations.

The technician's role in this area and the current level of technician training are presented in Chapter 16. The need for employers to train and evaluate all employees in compounding sterile preparations is then discussed, followed by a brief description of the importance of this training to pharmacy licensure.

Pharmacy School Education

Professional Perceptions

In 1991, the American Society of Hospital Pharmacists (ASHP, now the American Society of Health-System Pharmacists) held a conference on quality assurance for pharmacy-prepared sterile products.[1] Attendees included representatives from the Food and Drug Administration (FDA), National Association of Boards of Pharmacy (NAPB), and the United States Pharmacopeial Convention (USP), and practitioner-based organizations. Conference proceedings reported several problems related to pharmacist training on this subject[1]:

- Many pharmacists lack education and training on the compounding of sterile preparations.

- Many pharmacists receive little or no formal education and training in pharmacy schools on the compounding of sterile preparations.

- Many pharmacists do not understand applicable quality-assurance principles.

- Mere experience in the compounding of sterile preparations does not impart the knowledge and understanding necessary to ensure their accurate and safe preparation.

- Few pharmacy school faculty members have the knowledge and skill to teach others about this subject area.

- Instructional materials are not readily available.

Several ideas for resolving these problems were identified at the conference:

1. The American Association of Colleges of Pharmacy and the American Council on Pharmaceutical Education (ACPE) should reassess the present curricula of colleges of pharmacy. The compounding of sterile preparations should be a required component.

2. The knowledge and skill of college faculty in compounding sterile preparations should be upgraded, perhaps through videotapes at the teaching site.

Student Perceptions

A study of graduating pharmacy students' evaluated knowledge of aseptic technique to determine if specific factors influenced this knowledge base.[2] Results indicated that:

- Student performance on a test of this knowledge varied widely.

- Students reported limited exposure to compounding sterile preparations as part of their academic programs.

- Only about 19% of the experiential training was in this area.

- Two percent of the students said that they had no exposure to sterile preparations in classes.

- Twenty-seven percent of the students said that they had no exposure in their internships.

- Thirteen percent of the students said that they had no exposure during their externships.

- Eighty-one percent of the students did not take any elective courses in compounding sterile preparations.

Practitioner Perceptions

Another study surveyed hospital externship preceptors and a selected group of home care pharmacists.[3] Its purpose was to address concern about inadequate parenteral medication and IV therapy instruction in the core curriculum in spite of the increased use of these products in both the hospital and ambulatory settings.

According to this study's findings, subjects related to sterile preparations are neglected at many colleges of pharmacy. The topic is often covered in a fragmented fashion, and proper equipment (e.g., cleanrooms and laminar-airflow workbenches) is not available. The current emphasis on therapeutics and clinical practice has occurred at the expense of science and technology, so new pharmacy graduates are inadequately prepared to compound sterile preparations.

Changing the Curriculum

The inadequate exposure to compounding sterile preparations in colleges of pharmacy will not be an easy problem to solve. These institutions make changes slowly and face many curricular issues. Nevertheless, given the attention being devoted by the FDA and the public to problems with sterile preparations compounded in pharmacies, it seems prudent for colleges of pharmacy to revisit their commitment to this area of practice.

A three- or four-credit course with laboratory experience might resolve this problem. Some educators also recommend creating residencies in compounding sterile preparations in strategically located schools with the necessary faculty, facilities, and equipment.[3] The curriculum could emphasize both manufacturing and sterile compounding technologies. Such course work is becoming even more relevant with the increased involvement of compounding community pharmacists and the growth of home infusion practices. At a minimum, the subjects covered in this book should be in the core curriculum for any course on compounding sterile preparations.

Employee Training and Evaluation

Orientation

Because pharmacists are often not well trained in compounding sterile preparations, a new employee must receive proper orientation before being given this responsibility. An orientation consists of two components: (1) providing the employee with information, and (2) measuring baseline performance.

Providing information

Regardless of a staff member's education and training before employment, some information is unique to each institution. Before compounding sterile preparations, a new employee should receive orientation about:

- Dress code and garb requirements.
- Hand-washing techniques, including where and when to wash hands, and personal hygiene.
- Procedures for entering and leaving critical and controlled areas.
- Locations of medications and supplies.
- How orders are recorded and labels are generated.
- Documentation of work, including who made a dose and what was used.
- Types and locations of drug information resources.
- Methods for transmitting medication orders.
- Policies for storing compounded sterile preparations.
- Methods for sending doses to patients.
- Policies for reusing returned doses.
- Special procedures for chemotherapy agents and TPN.
- Quality management procedures, including process validation and environmental monitoring.
- Problem resolution, including spill management.
- Staffing and scheduling, including "safe staffing."

A checklist is recommended for documenting the satisfactory recall of this information. This checklist, with space for the employee's signature and validation by the responsible supervisor, should be placed in the employee's personnel record.

Measuring Performance

Quality improvement requires the ongoing monitoring of an employee's technique (see Chapter 18). Therefore, a baseline evaluation of a new employee's aseptic technique, using process validation, is an important part of the orientation. While sources differ concerning how many process validation samples are needed for a baseline, USP chapter 797 can be considered a standard of practice.[4]

Throughout the process of education, training, and evaluation, it is important to document the attainment of competence for employees who compound sterile preparations.

Continuing Education

To maintain proper quality assurance, pharmacy personnel should regularly receive didactic and experiential training and competency evaluation.[5] Table 15-1 lists recommended continuing education topics about compounding sterile preparations for pharmacists. Although pharmacy managers generally recognize that their staff need training, they often do not understand how adults learn.[6] Six cognitive skill levels are recognized for adult learners and should be incorporated into all education programs about compounding sterile preparations.

Level 1—knowledge

Knowledge includes the recall of ideas or material about compounding sterile preparations. Although knowledge does not necessarily connote understanding, even recall is impossible without adequate training. A training course should introduce pharmacy personnel to basic and important information. Many topics for such a training course are listed in Table 15-1. The reading of this book constitutes the transmission of knowledge of facts about compounding sterile preparations. Other texts are available as training resources[7,8] and the policies and procedures for compounding sterile preparations should also be included.

Level 2—comprehension

Comprehension of a subject the mental grasping of ideas, facts, and concepts is manifested by a person's ability to communicate via translation, interpretation, and extrapolation. Comprehension can be enhanced by examples, multimedia (e.g., videos), and quizzes to illustrate key points.

Level 3—application

Application is the ability to use and comprehend knowledge in specific and concrete ways. For example, the application of aseptic technique requires that an individual choose, orga-

Table 15-1.

Pharmacist Continuing Education Topics for Compounding Sterile Preparations

- Aseptic technique
- Critical area contamination factors
- Environmental monitoring
- Facilities
- Equipment and supplies
- Sterile product calculations and terminology
- Sterile compounding documentation
- Quality-assurance procedures
- Proper gowning and gloving techniques
- General conduct in controlled area
- Good manufacturing practices
- Environmental quality control
- Component and testing of final preparations
- Sterilization techniques

nize, restructure, develop, and generalize facts and concepts. Since adult learners must apply what they learn to retain the information, experiential training is recommended. At first, such practice should be observed by a pharmacist validated in the processes being taught.

Level 4—analysis

The ability to break down systems into parts so that the organization of ideas becomes clear is termed analysis. For instance, a well-trained person can use analysis to identify ways to eliminate sources of contamination or to create more efficient compounding processes. For quality and performance improvement, advanced learners must contribute ideas or analyses from their experience and understanding of compounding sterile preparations.

Level 5—synthesis

Synthesis is the creation of a new system or procedure. For example, designing a new sterile compounding area based on previous analysis would show synthesis. Therefore, an expert is required to create effective training aids for teaching new learners.

Level 6—evaluation

Evaluation consists of judging (1) the value of materials and methods for achieving a goal or (2) the appropriateness of others' work. Experts evaluate performance against internal standards (e.g., environmental contamination) or external evidence (e.g., nosocomial infection rates). Evaluation of another person's technique requires an expert in the subject matter.

Adult learners are oriented to goals that will help them perform; they are primarily self-directed in learning new skills. Trainers should consider using ASHP's goals and objectives that pertain to sterile compounding for residencies in pharmacy practice and home care pharmacy practice.[11,12]

Here is an example of a learning goal and the associated objectives.[12]

> **Goal:** Prepare and dispense medications using appropriate techniques and following the home care pharmacy's policies and procedures.
>
> *Objective 1:* (Application) Follow the home care pharmacy's policies and procedures to maintain the accuracy of the patient profile.
>
> *Objective 2:* (Mechanism) Prepare IV admixtures using aseptic technique.
>
> *Objective 3:* (Mechanism) Prepare chemotherapeutic agents observing rules for safe handling of cytotoxic or hazardous agents.
>
> *Objective 4:* (Evaluation) Appraise admixture solutions for appropriate concentrations, rates, compatibilities, stability, storage, and freedom from defects (e.g., leaking and particulates).
>
> *Objective 5:* (Evaluation) Determine situations when it is appropriate to compound preparations extemporaneously.
>
> *Objective 6:* (Synthesis) Formulate a strategy for extemporaneously compounding drugs to produce the desired preparation.
>
> *Objective 7:* (Application) Label drug products in accordance with the home care pharmacy's policies and procedures.
>
> *Objective 8:* (Comprehension) Discuss standards of practice for the compounding of drug preparations (ASHP and USP guidelines for compounding of sterile preparations).
>
> *Objective 9:* (Application) Follow the home care pharmacy's quality-control standards in the compounding of sterile drug preparations.

An organized training program for compounding sterile preparations uses learning objectives such as these for evaluating the competence of pharmacy personnel. The trainer also should provide new learning opportunities through increasingly complex levels of cognitive skills. Furthermore, training must be combined with implementation of improved methods and reinforcement of positive results (e.g., posting team scores on process validation).[6] Enhancements to methods should be recognized and rewarded.

Continuing Education Resources

ASHP has the following recourses to assist pharmacists in developing, updating or validating their knowledge of the principles of compounding sterile preparations:

- Quality Assurance for Pharmacy-Prepared Sterile Products Videotape
- Quality Assurance for Pharmacy-Prepared Sterile Products Workbook
- Sterile Product Preparations Multimedia Learning Tool CD ROM
- Safe Handling of Cytotoxic and Hazardous Drugs Videotape

ASHP's video tape and workbook includes continuing education credit testing.[9] ACPE maintains a continually updated data base, the "Pharmacists' Learning Assistance Network (PLAN)," of all continuing education programs offered by ACPE-approved providers.[10]

State Board Examination for Pharmacists

Twice a year, NABP administers a nationwide examination (NABPLEX) to pharmacists seeking licensure in 49 states plus Puerto Rico. (California has its own examination.) NABPLEX covers five areas of competency, including "Compounding and Calculation Involved in Dispensing of Prescriptions and Medication Orders." This area has a subcompetency on aseptic technique.[13]

As part of their practical examinations, some State Boards require the compounding of sterile preparations. Compounding technique and accuracy may be evaluated via direct observation by an examiner and quantitative product analysis, respectively. Candidates should review the principles of compounding sterile preparations before taking their State Pharmacy Board examinations.

Although 48 state boards require continuing education for pharmacist relicensure, none specifies that sterile compounding must be part of that education.[14]

Summary

Pharmacists do not always receive the education and training required to compound sterile preparations. Colleges of pharmacy should recognize the regulatory and public scrutiny being placed on the profession and its responsibility to compound sterile preparations competently. Regardless of the setting, pharmacy programs should orient and train staff who are responsible for compounding sterile preparations and verify their skill levels initially and regularly.

References

1. ASHP invitational conference on quality assurance for pharmacy prepared sterile products. *Am J Hosp Pharm.* 1991;48:2391–7.
2. Brown RE, Birdwell SW, Schneider PJ, et al. *Assessing factors affecting graduating pharmacy students' scores on a standardized aseptic technique test* [master's thesis]. Columbus, OH: Ohio State University, College of Pharmacy; 1993.
3. Allen LV, Bloss CS, Brazeau GA, et al. Educational issues related to the science and technology of sterile products: academic and industrial perspectives. *Am J Pharm Educ.* 1993; 57:257–65.
4. Pharmaceutical Compounding – Sterile Preparation. United States pharmacopeia, 27th rev/national formulary, 22nd ed. Rockville, MD: United States Pharmacopeial Convention; 2004:2350–70.
5. American Society of Hospital Pharmacists. ASHP guideline on quality assurance for pharmacy-prepared sterile products. *Am J Health-Syst Pharm.* 2000;57:1150–69.
6. Fitch HD. Workplace training must recognize how people learn. *CleanRooms.* 1994; 8:602.
7. Hunt ML. *Training Manual for Intravenous Admixture Personnel.* 4th ed. Chicago, IL: Pluribus Press; 1989.
8. Turco S. *Sterile Dosage Forms: Their Preparation and Clinical Application.* 4th ed. Philadelphia, PA:Lea & Febiger; 1994.
9. Quality assurance of pharmacy-prepared sterile products. Bethesda, MD: American Society of Hospital Pharmacists; 1994. Videotape and workbook.
10. Accreditation Council for Pharmacy Education (ACPRE) website. http://www.acpe-accredit.org/frameset_Plan.htm. Accessed February 22, 2004.
11. American Society of Health-System Pharmacists (ASHP) website. http://www.ashp.org/rtp/Word/Final%20Pharmacy%20Practice%20G&Os%20-%20March%207,%202001.doc. Accessed February 22, 2004.
12. American Society of Health-System Pharmacists (ASHP) website. Home care pharmacy practice. http://www.ashp.org/rtp/Word/HomeCarePharmacyPractice G&Os-2001. Accessed February 22, 2004.
13. National Association of Boards of Pharmacy (NABP) website. http://www.nabp.net/ftpfiles/bulletins/NAPLEX_MPJE2003_Bulletin.pdf. Accessed February 22, 2004.
14. *NABP 2002-2003 Survey of Pharmacy Law Including all 50 States, D.C. and Puerto Rico.* Park Ridge, IL: National Association of Boards of Pharmacy; 2003.

16 | Pharmacy Technician Education, Certification, Training, Evaluation, and Regulation

E. Clyde Buchanan

In 1991, the American Society of Hospital Pharmacists (ASHP, now the American Society of Health-System Pharmacists) held a conference on quality assurance for pharmacy-prepared sterile preparations.[1] Attendees included representatives from the Food and Drug Administration (FDA), National Association of Boards of Pharmacy (NABP), and the United States Pharmacopeial Convention (USP) as well as practitioner-based organizations. Conference proceedings noted several apparent problems related to pharmacy technician training on this subject[1]:

- Many pharmacy technicians lack education and training on the preparation of sterile preparations.

- Many pharmacy technicians do not understand applicable quality-assurance principles.

- Mere experience in the preparation of sterile preparations does not impart the knowledge and understanding necessary to ensure their accurate and safe preparation.

Advances in Technician Education, Certification, Training, and Regulation

Since 1991, there have been many advances in teaching and evaluating pharmacy technicians, including improved education and training in sterile preparations[2]:

- 1991 The Pharmacy Technician Educators Council (PTEC) was formed.

- 1994 The Scope of Pharmacy Practice Project was completed, including a task analysis of what technicians do.[3]

- 1995 ASHP, the American Pharmaceutical Association (now the American Pharmacists Association—APhA), the Illinois Council of Health-System Pharmacists and the Michigan Pharmacists Association created the Pharmacy Technician Certification Board (PTCB) as an independent body to develop and administer national voluntary pharmacy technician certification examinations.

- 1996 ASHP and APhA prepared a White Paper on pharmacy technicians,[4] urging planning for uniform national standards for pharmacy technician training.

- 1997 ASHP, APhA, the American Association of Colleges of Pharmacy (AACP), the American Association of Pharmacy Technicians (AAPT) and PTEC collaborated to create the *Model Curriculum for Pharmacy Technician Training.*

- 2000 The PTCB conducted an updated task analysis of what pharmacy technicians do.

- 2001 The second edition of the *Model Curriculum for Pharmacy Technician Training* was published.[5]

- 2002 The PTCB and the National Association of Boards of Pharmacy (NABP) joined forces on the national certification program for pharmacy technicians.[6]

- 2002 The *White paper on Pharmacy Technicians 2002: Needed Changes Can No Longer Wait* was published.[7]

Technician Involvement in Sterile Preparations

Pharmacy technicians are actively involved in all aspects of pharmaceutical care. The Scope of Pharmacy Practice Project[3] found that 26% of technicians' time is spent in collecting, organizing, and evaluating information. The second most time-consuming functions (total of 21%) involve preparing, dispensing, distributing, and administering medications. A smaller survey identified what percentages of hospital pharmacy technicians prepare certain sterile dosage forms (Table 16-1).[8]

The second edition of the *Model Curriculum*[5] has 35 stated goals. Many of these goals have measurable objectives (what the trainee must do) and three sets of goals and objectives have particular relevance to training pharmacy technicians to prepare sterile medications (Table 16-2).

Technician Education

Technician Educators

The Pharmacy Technician Educators Council (PTEC) was organized in 1991 with a mission "to assist the profession of pharmacy in preparing quality well-trained technical personnel through education and practical training."[9] PTEC says that informal, on-the-job training is still the most common education for phar-

Table 16-1.

Percentage of Pharmacy Technicians Who Participate in Sterile Compounding by Preparation Type [8]

Sterile Dosage Form	Pharmacy Technician Participation in Extemporaneous Compounding Percentage
Unit dose injections	60
Large volume parenteral admixtures	81
TPNs	57
IV piggybacks	85
Chemotherapy agents	31
Narcotic infusions	38

macy technicians. For a variety of reasons, many employers are looking for technicians with relevant training and experience that fits their pharmacy.

Formalized pharmacy technician education was first offered by the armed forces, but is now offered by many teaching hospitals and community colleges. PTEC members serve as faculty for some of these programs.

Educational Programs

Most formal programs include didactic and practical training in areas such as medical and pharmaceutical terminology, pharmacology, pharmaceutical dosage forms, pharmacy laws and record-keeping, pharmaceutical calculations, and non-sterile and sterile compounding and dispensing of medications. PTEC is recommending that, within 5 years, all technician training programs evolve into at least 9 months and/or 45 quarter credit programs, and that within 10 years, all technician training programs evolve into 2-year associate degree programs.[9] Graduates of educational programs may receive a certificate, a diploma or an associate degree—depending on the length, nature, and site of the program.

Accreditation of Pharmacy Technician Educational Programs

Since 1983, ASHP has encouraged the formal

education of pharmacy technicians, either in hospitals or academic settings, by means of accrediting these educational programs. Accreditation is the process of granting recognition or vouching for conformance with a standard and usually is conferred on a specific institution.

To be accredited, pharmacy technician educational programs must be surveyed according to ASHP regulations[10] and meet the accreditation standard.[11] This standard states a goal that technicians should know how to prepare medications for distribution (including sterile preparations) and makes specific reference to use of the most recent edition of the *Model curriculum.*[5] By 2003, ASHP's Commission on Credentialing had accredited 97 pharmacy technician training programs in 24 states. ASHP accreditation is the only established mechanism for ensuring a minimum quality of pharmacy technician education.

Technician Certification

The Pharmacy Technician Certification Board (PTCB) offers a voluntary, national pharmacy technician certification examination. These exams certify the competence of persons who demonstrate the knowledge required to practice as a pharmacy technician. The goal of these exams is to enable pharmacy technicians to work more effectively with pharmacists to offer safe and effective patient care. The National Pharmacy Technician Certification Examination is offered in all 50 states. PTCB requires renewal of certification every 2 years. A total of 20 hours in pharmacy-related topics is required within the 2-year period. At least one hour in the area of pharmacy law is required. A maximum of 10 hours may be carried out in practice sites (in-service training) under the supervision of pharmacists for whom the certified technicians work.[12]

Often technicians who were trained on the job choose to establish their credibility as a competent pharmacy technician by taking the PTCB certification exam. Many employers prefer to hire formally educated and/or examination-certified pharmacy technicians. Since the exam's inception in 1995, PTCB has certified almost 165,000 pharmacy technicians.[12] A 1998 PTCB pharmacy technician task analysis found that 73% of certified pharmacy technicians who work in hospitals prepare IV admixtures.[13]

Table 16-2.

Pharmacy Technician Training Goals and Objectives Related to Sterile Preparations

Goal 3: Prepare Medications For Distribution

Objective 3.4 Knowledge of a site's storage system to efficiently secure all the prescribed medications or devices from inventory.

Objective 3.5 Accurately count or measure finished dosage forms as specified by the prescription/medication order.

Objective 3.6 Collect the correct ingredients for sterile preparations that require compounding.

Objective 3.7 Accurately determine the correct amounts of ingredients for a compounded preparation.

Objective 3.8 Compound sterile preparations using appropriate techniques, equipment, and devices.

Objective 3.10 Compound cytotoxic and other hazardous medication preparations using appropriate technique.

Objective 3.11 Follow safety policies and procedures in the preparation of all medications.

Objective 3.12 Follow safety policies and procedures in the disposal of all hazardous and non-hazardous wastes generated during medication preparation.

Objective 3.13 Package the preparation in the appropriate type and size of container using a manual process or automated system.

Objective 3.14 Follow an established manual procedure or electronic procedure to generate accurate and complete preparation labels.

Objective 3.15 Affix the appropriate primary and auxiliary labels to containers.

Objective 3.19 Follow the manufacturer's recommendation and/or the pharmacy's guidelines for storage of all medications prior to distribution.

Goal 5: Distribute Medications

Objective 5.1 Efficiently deliver the correct medication, equipment, device or supplies to the correct patient or patient's representative.

Objective 5.2 Follow established policies and procedures to record the distribution of prescription medications.

Goal 12: Maintain Pharmacy Equipment And Facilities

Objective 12.1 Follow policies and procedures for sanitation management, hazardous waste handling (e.g., needles) and infection control (e.g., protective clothing).

Objective 12.2 Clean laminar flow biological safety cabinets using approved technique.

Objective 12.3 Maintain a clean and neat work environment.

Objective 12.4 Given a weighing or counting device, fluid compounder, or syringe pump used at a specific site, accurately calibrate the device, compounder, or pump.

Objective 12.5 Follow manufacturer's guidelines in trouble-shooting, maintaining, and repairing electronic devices used by the pharmacy in the preparation and dispensing of medications.

PTCB's validated (psychometrically sound and legally defensible) examination focuses on three broad functions[14]:

- Assisting the pharmacist in serving patients—64% of the exam.

- Medication distribution and inventory control systems—25%.

- Participating in the administration and management of pharmacy practice—11%.

The medication distribution and inventory control part of the exam includes questions about:

- Calibrating equipment needed to compound medications.
- Compounding.
- Preparing IV admixtures.
- Dispensing documentation.

The topics covered in this national technician certification examination further emphasize the need for a formalized approach to training in sterile preparation of medications.

Technician Employee Competency and Evaluation

While it is easier to train new employees for their job if they already have formal education, certification and experience, new employees must be oriented to a new work environment and their training must continue as pharmacy policies and procedures change. Pharmacy employers are obligated to have competent employees, especially when their work involves patient care.

Orientation

Because pharmacy technicians often are not well trained in sterile preparation of medications, a new employee must receive proper orientation before being given this responsibility. An orientation consists of two parts: (1) providing the employee with information, and (2) measuring baseline performance.

Providing information

Before compounding preparing sterile preparations, a new employee should receive orientation on

- Dress code and garb requirements.
- Hand washing techniques, including where and when to wash hands, and personal hygiene.
- Procedures for entering and leaving critical and controlled areas.
- Locations of medications and supplies.
- How orders are recorded and labels are generated.

- Documentation of work, including who made a dose and what was used.
- Types and locations of drug information resources.
- Methods for transmitting medication orders.
- Policies for storing compounded sterile preparations.
- Methods for sending doses to patients.
- Policies for reusing returned doses.
- Special procedures for chemotherapy agents and TPN.
- Quality management procedures, including process validation and environmental monitoring.
- Problem resolution, including spill management.
- Staffing and scheduling, including "safe staffing."

A checklist is recommended for documenting the satisfactory recall of this information. This checklist, with space for the employee's signature and validation by the responsible supervisor, should be placed in the employee's personnel record.

In addition to this text, ASHP publishes other valuable teaching aids for employee orientation:

1. Kastango ES. *Sterile Product Preparation: A Multimedia Tool.* This is a network-based learning program that provides a thorough way to train technicians and pharmacists. The program contains two modules, the first focusing on initial training of pharmacists and technicians; the second, focusing on the supervisor's responsibility in assuring quality within the sterile preparation process. Media include self-assessment exams, photos, video clips, a virtual clean room tour and other teaching aids. 2002; Product code P638P.

2. Anon. *Safe Handling of Cytotoxic and Hazardous Drugs.* This is a videotape and study guide. It demonstrates recommended procedures for preparing, administering, and cleaning up spills of these substances. Order Code PL40.

Measuring baseline performance

Quality management requires the ongoing monitoring of an employee's technique. Therefore, a baseline evaluation of a new employee's aseptic technique, using process validation, is an important part of the orientation (see Chapter 20).[15]

Technician Competency and Evaluation

Regarding assessing, maintaining, and improving staff competence, the Joint Commission on Accreditation of Healthcare Organizations (JCAHO), has a human resource standard requiring ongoing, periodic competence assessment that evaluates staff members' continuing abilities to perform throughout their association with the hospital.[16] Thus pharmacy technicians must maintain their competence in compounding sterile preparations if they continue to have these responsibilities.

To help fulfill the identified need for technician training in sterile preparations, ASHP published outcome competencies and training guidelines for institutional technician programs.[17]

According to this 1982 bulletin, technicians should be able to:

1. List five possibilities for contamination of an injectable solution during its preparation as well as a precaution that would prevent each possibility.

2. Demonstrate proper technique for using a syringe and needle for aseptic withdrawal of the contents of a rubber-capped vial and a glass ampul.

3. Demonstrate proper technique for aseptic reconstitution of an antibiotic injection.

4. Describe when hand washing is required and demonstrate proper technique.

5. Demonstrate correct techniques and procedures for preparing at least three parenteral admixtures, including the label and control records.

6. Identify major components of a laminar-airflow hood and state their functions.

7. Define and describe (1) microbial growth and transmission; (2) origin, pharmacologic effect, and prevention of pyrogens; (3) sterility; (4) heat sterilization; and (5) cold sterilization.

8. Designate, from a list of 10 sterile preparations, those that may be safely heat treated.

9. Demonstrate proper technique for visual inspection of parenteral solutions.

Since 1982, many competencies have been added through the evolution of model training programs for pharmacy technicians. While too detailed to list in this manual, the second edition of the *Model Curriculum*[5] now covers outcome competencies such as:

- Compounding cytotoxic and other hazardous medication products using appropriate technique. (*Model Curriculum* Objective 3.10)

- Given a weighing or counting device, fluid compounder or syringe pump used at a specific site, accurately calibrating the device, compounder or pump. (*Model Curriculum* Objective 12.4)

Depending on the pharmacy site, pharmacy managers may need to develop additional competencies concerning:

- Working in cleanroom environments (Chapter 5).

- Working in isolator environments (Chapter 4).

- Preparing sterile medications for patients who are sensitive to latex (Chapter 19).

Technician Continuing Education

To maintain proper quality assurance, pharmacy personnel should regularly receive didactic and experiential training and competency evaluation.[18] Table 16-3 lists recommended continuing education topics on sterile preparation for technicians.

Although pharmacy managers generally recognize that their staffs need training, they may not understand how adults learn.[19] Six cognitive skill levels are recognized for adult learners and should be incorporated into all training programs on sterile preparations.

Level 1—Knowledge

Knowledge includes the recall of ideas or material about sterile compounding. Although knowledge does not necessarily connote understanding, even recall is impossible without adequate training. A training course should introduce pharmacy personnel to basic and important information.

Table 16-3.

Examples of Technician Continuing Education Topics for Sterile Preparations

1. Parenteral routes of administration (rationale, precautions, and problems; routes; and methods)
2. Equipment and systems used in parenteral administration (needles and syringes, administration sets, fluid containers, pumps, etc.)
3. Equipment used to prepare parenteral admixtures (laminar-airflow workbenches, filters, pumps, etc.)
4. Aseptic compounding techniques specific to fluid system used (prefilling IV admixtures, preparing syringes, preparing ophthalmic solutions, etc.)
5. Labeling and record keeping (bottle labels, fluid orders and profiles, compounding records, etc.)
6. Incompatibilities (visual and chemical incompatibilities, pH and concentration effects, reference sources, etc.)
7. Quality control (particulate matter inspection and monitoring of contamination)

Level 2—Comprehension

Comprehension of a subject—the mental grasping of ideas, facts, and concepts—is manifested by a person's ability to communicate via translation, interpretation, and extrapolation. Comprehension can be enhanced by examples, multimedia (e.g., videos), and quizzes to illustrate key points.

Level 3—Application

Application is the ability to use and comprehend knowledge in specific and concrete ways. For example, the application of aseptic technique requires that an individual choose, organize, restructure, develop, and generalize facts and concepts.

Since adult learners must apply what they learn to retain the information, experiential training is recommended. At first, such practice should be observed by a pharmacist or

technician validated in the processes being taught (Chapter 20).

Level 4—Analysis

The ability to break down systems into parts so that the organization of ideas becomes clear is termed analysis. For instance, a well-trained person can use analysis to identify ways to eliminate sources of contamination or to create more efficient processes. For quality and performance improvement, advanced learners must contribute ideas or analyses from their experience and understanding of sterile compounding.

Level 5—Synthesis

Synthesis is the creation of a new system or procedure. For example, creating a new sterile compounding formula based on analysis of the literature would show synthesis. Synthesis could also be creating effective training aids.

Level 6—Evaluation

Evaluation consists of judging (1) the value of materials and methods for achieving a goal or (2) the appropriateness of others' work. Experts evaluate performance against internal standards (e.g., environmental contamination) or external evidence (e.g., benchmarked nosocomial infection rates). Evaluation of another person's technique requires an expert in the subject matter.

Adult learners are oriented to goals that will help them perform; they are primarily self-directed in learning new skills. Trainers should consider using the *Model Curriculum*'s goals and objectives that pertain to sterile preparations.[5]

Here is an example of a learning goal and the associated objectives.

Goal: Prepare and dispense medications using appropriate techniques and following the home care pharmacy's policies and procedures.

Objective 1: (Application) Follow the home care pharmacy's policies and procedures to maintain the accuracy of the patient profile.

Objective 2: (Mechanism) Prepare IV admixtures using aseptic technique.

Objective 3: (Mechanism) Prepare chemo-therapeutic agents observing rules for safe handling of cytotoxic or hazardous agents.

Objective 4: (Evaluation) Appraise admixture solutions for appropriate concentrations, rates, compatibilities, stability, storage, and freedom from defects (e.g., leaking and particulates).

Objective 5: (Evaluation) Determine situations when it is appropriate to compound preparations extemporaneously.

Objective 6: (Synthesis) Formulate a strategy for extemporaneously compounding drugs to produce the desired end preparation.

Objective 7: (Application) Label drug preparations in accordance with the home care pharmacy's policies and procedures.

Objective 8: (Comprehension) Discuss standards of practice for compounding drug preparations (ASHP and USP standards for preparation of sterile preparations).

Objective 9: (Application) Follow the home care pharmacy's quality-control standards in the compounding of sterile preparations.

An organized sterile preparation training program uses learning objectives such as these for evaluating the competence of pharmacy technicians. O'Neal et al. found that only 81.4% of hospital pharmacies evaluate the aseptic technique of each person preparing sterile medications at least annually.[20] Morris et al. found that only 78% of pharmacy personnel are assessed for their sterile compounding skill after they are first trained. Indeed, only 34% are ever given written tests and 26% ever show that they are capable of compounding sterile preparations by preparing sterile media fills (Table 16-4).[20] There is still much to be done in training technicians to compound sterile preparations more than 12 years after the 1991 ASHP-led conference pointed out this problem.[1]

The trainer also should provide new learning opportunities through increasingly complex levels of cognitive skills. Furthermore, training must be combined with implementation of improved methods and reinforcement of positive results (e.g., posting team scores on process validation).[19] Enhancements to methods should be recognized and rewarded.

Table 16-4.

Personnel Education, Training and Evaluation[21]

Item	Weighted % (n = 182)
Staff who receive training	
● Pharmacists	95.9
● Technicians	89.0
● Nurses	50.2
Methods used to train staff	
● On-the-job training	96.1
● Lectures and videotapes	77.8
● Supervised laboratory exercises	48.6
Areas covered in training	
● I.V. compounding	95.6
● Labeling and record keeping	87.7
● Quality assurance procedures	74.1
Assessment of compounding skills after training	77.8
Methods used to assess compounding skills	
● Direct observation of technique	91.9
● Written tests for knowledge	33.5
● Aseptic technique validation (media fills)	25.7
Follow-up assessment of compounding skills	71.6
Methods used to assess compounding skills	
● Direct observation of technique	89.8
● Written tests for knowledge	38.5
● Aseptic technique validation (media fills)	29.8

Adopted from Morris AM, Schneider PJ, Pederson CA, et al. National survey of quality assurance activities for pharmacy-compounded sterile preparations. *Am J Health-Syst Pharm.* 2003;25:67–76.

Technician Regulation

The practice of pharmacy is regulated at the state level where state legislatures pass laws or statutes and state agencies such as boards of pharmacy promulgate rules and regulations to enable the laws and regulations to be followed. Most state boards of pharmacy are responsible for maintaining and updating rules and regulations for their states pharmacy practice act—a set of laws that govern the practice of pharmacy within a state. State boards of pharmacy may register or license pharmacy practitioners (pharmacists and pharmacy technicians). The process of registering is simply a listing of the practitioner and the licensed pharmacy where the practitioner works. A pharmacy technician may not have to be certified to be registered in a state; it depends on state laws, rules and regulations. Licensing implies that the practitioner has passed an examination recognized by the respective board of pharmacy.

By 2002, nearly every state recognized the position of pharmacy technician and permitted pharmacy technicians to assist pharmacists; 32 states licensed or registered pharmacy technicians; 27 states have mandatory training requirements for technicians; 5 states (LA, MT, TX, UT, and WY) require technician examination and 9 states have continuing education (CE) requirements for technicians.[20] Wyoming recognizes the PTCB certification exam as one way for a technician to become licensed. Kentucky gives certified technicians (C.Ph.T.) additional responsibilities. Virginia and Georgia allow an increased technician to pharmacist ratio for C.Ph.T's. Arkansas allows the PTCB examination in lieu of technician CE for renewal of technician licensure.[13]

In 2002, the National Association of Boards of Pharmacy (NABP) joined with the PTCB to encourage acceptance of the PTCB certification program as a recognized assessment tool for pharmacy technicians. In addition, NABP will incorporate the use of the PTCB certification program into its Model State Pharmacy Act and Model Rules.[6]

Summary

Pharmacy technicians do not always receive the education and training required to competently compound sterile preparations. Technician education programs and pharmacies should recognize the regulatory and public scrutiny being placed on the profession of pharmacy and technicians responsibility to compound and dispense sterile preparations competently.

References

1. ASHP invitational conference on quality assurance for pharmacy prepared sterile products. *Am J Hosp Pharm.* 1991; 48:2391–7.
2. Anon: Sesquicentennial Stepping Stone Summits—Summit Two: Pharmacy Technicians. *J Am Pharm Assoc.* 2003;43:84–92.
3. Anon. Summary of the final report of the Scope of Pharmacy Practice project. *Am J Hosp Pharm.* 1994;51:2179–82.
4. ASHP. White paper on pharmacy technicians. *Am J Health-Syst Pharm.* 1996; 53:1793–6.
5. *Model Curriculum for Pharmacy Technician Training.* 2nd ed. Bethesda, MD: American Society of Health-System Pharmacists. 2001. Available at: www.ashp.org/technician/model_curriculum. Accessed January 28, 2004.
6. Anon. The Pharmacy Technician Certification Board (PTCB) and the National Association of Boards of Pharmacy to join together on national certification for pharmacy technicians. 2002. Available at: www.ptcb.org. Accessed February 20, 2003.
7. Anon. White paper on pharmacy technicians 2002: Needed changes can no longer wait. *Am J Health-Syst Pharm.* 2003;60:37–51.
8. Anderson RJ. Pharmacy technician survey in the state of Georgia. *Ga J Hosp Pharm.* 1993;7(summer):179.
9. Anon. PTEC Mission Statement. Available at: www.rxptec.org. Accessed January 28, 2004.
10. American Society of Health-System Pharmacists Commission on Credentialing. ASHP regulations on accreditation of pharmacy technician training programs. Available at: http://www.ashp.org/technician/Reg-Final-AccTechProg.PDF. Accessed January 28, 2004.
11. American Society of Hospital Pharmacists. ASHP accreditation standard for pharmacy technician training programs.

Available at: www.ashp.org/technician/ finaldraftAugust2002.pdf. Accessed February 24, 2003.

12. Anon. PTCB statistics. Available at: www.ptcb.org Accessed January 28, 2004.

13. Muenzen PM, Greenberg S, Murer MM. PTCB task analysis identifies role of certified pharmacy technicians in pharmaceutical care. *J Am Pharm Assoc.* 1999 (Nov/Dec);39:857–64.

14. Murer MM. Pharmacy technicians 2002 summit on pharmacy technicians. Available at: www.ptcb.org. Accessed February 26, 2003.

15. Pharmaceutical compounding—sterile preparations. In: United States pharmacopeia, 27th ed./national formulary, 22nd rev. Rockville, MD: United States Pharmacopeial Convention. Available at: http://www.uspnf.com. Accessed on April 1, 2004.

16. Anon. *2002 Comprehensive Accreditation Manual for Hospitals, Automated.* Joint Commission on Accreditation of Healthcare Organizations. Available at: www. jcrinc.com/publications. Updated November 2002.

17. American Society of Hospital Pharmacists. ASHP technical assistance bulletin on outcome competencies and training guidelines for institutional pharmacy technician training programs. *Am J Hosp Pharm.* 1982;39:317–20.

18. American Society of Hospital Pharmacists. ASHP Guidelines on quality assurance for pharmacy-prepared sterile products. *Am J Health-Syst Pharm.* 2000; 57:1150–69.

19. Fitch HD. Workplace training must recognize how people learn. *CleanRooms.* 1994; 8:602.

20. O'Neal BC, Schneider PJ, Pedersen CA, et al. Compliance with safe practices for preparing parenteral nutrition formulations. *Am J Health-Syst Pharm.* 2002; 59:264–9.

21. Morris AM, Schneider PJ, Pederson CA, et al. National survey of quality assurance activities for pharmacy-compounded sterile preparations. *Am J Health-Syst Pharm.* 2003; 25:67–76.

17 | Sterile Preparation Facilities and Equipment

E. Clyde Buchanan

Cleanroom Description

Recently published professional guidelines (see Chapter 1 and Appendices) should persuade pharmacists to evaluate their existing sterile compounding facilities. These guidelines specify that sterile preparations be compounded in an area separate from other pharmacy activities. The American Society of Health-System Pharmacists (ASHP) calls this space the "controlled area,"[1] and the United States Pharmacopeial Convention (USP) calls it the "buffer room."[2] In both common and international parlance, it is called a "cleanroom."

Both ASHP and USP discuss the concepts of anterooms and cleanrooms. ASHP recommends an anteroom for Risk Level 2 preparations and requires an anteroom for Risk Level 3 preparations. USP requires an "ante area" for low and medium risk level preparations and requires an anteroom for high-risk level preparations. ASHP specifies a Class 10,000 cleanroom for Risk Levels 2 and 3; while USP requires Class 100,000 for its low, medium, and high risk cleanrooms. (Table 17-1.)

Air Cleanliness

To interpret ASHP and USP guidelines, pharmacists must understand cleanroom classifications. For nearly 40 years, U.S. Federal Standard 209 (FS 209) defined air cleanliness in contamination control,[3] but FS 209 has been dropped by the U.S. General Services Administration[4] in favor of the internationally-accepted definitions for cleanrooms and clean zones promulgated by the International Organization of Standardization (ISO).[5] (Table 17-2.) Since FS209e classifications are still commonly used in the literature, this chapter cross-references both ISO and FS209e nomenclatures.

Regulatory Requirements for Facilities

In addition to the ASHP and USP standards for air cleanliness, two regulatory organizations have requirements for sterile preparation facilities. The Food and Drug Administration (FDA) requires pharmacists to use good manufacturing practices,[6] including a facility of suitable size, construction, and location to

Table 17-1.

Facilities and Equipment Requirements by Risk Level

ASHP Guidelines	USP Monograph <797>
Risk Level 1	**Low Risk**
• Controlled area separate from other operations.	• Appropriate solid surfaces.
• Clean, well-lighted and of sufficient size.	• Limited (but necessary) furniture, fixtures etc.
• Class 100 environment (laminar or horizontal air-flow workbench or barrier/isolator).	• Anteroom area (diagram shows ante area either demarked or physically separate from buffer zone).
	• Buffer zone (cleanroom) of ISO Class 8 (Class 100,000).
Risk Level 2	**Medium Risk**
In addition to Risk Level 1 requirements,	Same as low-risk level.
• Controlled area must meet Class 10,000 standards.	
• Anteroom is desirable.	
Risk Level 3	**High Risk**
In addition to Risk Level 2 requirements,	Same as low-risk level.
• Anteroom should be Class 100,000	• Diagram shows anteroom, physically separate from buffer room.

Table 17-2.

International Organization of Standardization (ISO) Classification of Particilate Matter in Room Air as Limits in Particles 0.5 microns and Larger per Cubic Meter (Current ISO) and Cubic Feet (Former FS 209E)[2]

Class Name		Particle Counts Per	
ISO Class	U.S. FS209E	ISO, m³	FS209E, ft³
3	Class 1	35.2	1
4	Class 10	352	10
5	Class 100	3520	100
6	Class 1000	35,200	1000
7	Class 10,000	352,000	10,000
8	Class 100,000	3,520,000	100,000

Adapted by USP from the Federal Standard 209e, General Services Administration, Washington, DC 20407 (September 11, 1992) and ISO 14644-1:1999 Cleanrooms and associated controlled environments—part 1: Classification of air cleanliness.

facilitate cleaning, maintenance, and proper operations. Second, the Joint Commission on Accreditation of Healthcare Organizations (JCAHO) standards for hospitals simply state:

Whenever medications are prepared, staff uses appropriate techniques to avoid contamination during medication preparation, which include but are not limited to:

● Using clean or sterile technique as appropriate,

● Maintaining clean, uncluttered, and functionally separate areas for product preparation to minimize the possibility of contamination,

● Using a laminar-airflow hood or other class 100 environment while preparing any intravenous (IV) admixture in the pharmacy, any sterile product made from non-sterile ingredients, or any sterile product that will not be used within 24 hours,

● Visually inspecting the integrity of the medications.

Dispensing adheres to law, regulation, licensure, and practice standards, including record keeping."[7]

Darryl Rich of JCAHO added, "The prevailing standard of practice in hospitals in the US includes the use of a laminar-airflow workbench, or other class 100 environment for

preparing sterile preparations, but the Joint Commission makes no environmental requirements beyond that. The JCAHO standards for home care and ambulatory organizations also specify the use of a laminar airflow workbench or other class 100 environment for preparing sterile preparations. The standards also require a functionally separate area for sterile preparation to minimize the possibility of particulate and microbial contamination. They further require that traffic flow in the sterile work area be minimized and that particulate-generating materials (e.g., boxes) not be stored within 3 feet of the sterile work area. . . JCAHO would expect you to comply with FDA and OSHA requirements."[8] Rich also said, "Because USP Chapter 797 is considered law and regulation enforceable by FDA, JCAHO will expect and survey for compliance with these requirements where ever applicable starting in 2004.[9]

Meeting Current Facility Standards

A 2002 ASHP survey indicated how hospital pharmacy departments conform to ASHP facility guidelines.[10] Of 180 respondents, 1.0% prepared sterile preparations on a clean surface with no laminar-airflow workbench; 18.9% used a workbench in a general dispensing area; 64.5% used a workbench in a limited-access room where air particulate levels are not monitored; 9.2% had a specifically constructed cleanroom where access, and airborne particulate counts were 100,000 or better; 6.3% had a specifically constructed cleanroom where access, and airborne particulate counts were 10,000 or better; 1.8% had a class 100 cleanroom; and 1.4% used a suitable isolator. (The total percentages exceed 100% because some respondents prepared sterile preparations in more than one location.) Fifty-seven percent of survey respondents reported that the highest risk level compounded in their pharmacy was Risk Level 1; 32% reported that Risk Level 2 was their highest risk level compounded, and 11% reported Risk Level 3 as their highest risk level.

In short, almost 20% (1% plus 18.9%) do not meet ASHP facility requirements to compound Risk Level 1 sterile preparations. More than 90% of hospital pharmacies compounded sterile preparations in facilities that do not conform with ASHP or USP requirements to compound Risk Level 2 or 3 sterile preparations. As these percentages illustrate, pharmacy departments need to update their sterile preparation facilities.

Planning the Sterile Preparation Facility

Allen et al. presented a detailed planning process for designing and evaluating a sterile compounding facility.[11] The authors used a strategic functional planning approach. This allowed them to meet hospital goals for efficiency, functionality and a planned future relocation of the sterile compounding center. The functional program development took them through: work flow, work load, equipment, storage, arrangement of work areas, space requirements, floor plan and evaluation of the facility. They were able to improve pharmacist efficiency by 42% and technician efficiency by 29% within a modest-sized facility that met ASHP sterile compounding facility standards extant in 1995. The cost of the equipment and fixtures was $70,000–$75,000.[12]

The functional planning approach includes seven main steps[13]:

1. Developing a master facilities plan.
2. Analyzing existing facilities.
3. Identifying functional needs.
4. Preparing architectural plans.
5. Bidding construction.
6. Building the installation.
7. Evaluating the installation.

Developing a Master Facilities Plan

The first step, developing a master facilities plan, involves identifying and justifying the need for a new facility.

Identifying need

Before updated facilities can be justified, the pharmacy department must determine its specific need based on patient population. Two questions can be asked to determine this need.

What guidelines apply to the patient population? Some state pharmacy laws or regulations (e.g., California, New Jersey, Texas) require that ASHP guidelines be followed. Unless specified otherwise by state law, USP Chapter 797 will hold more legal force.

What are the highest level sterile preparations that will be compounded? Unless there is no chance that Risk Level 3 preparations will ever be compounded, following the ASHP guidelines for Risk Level 3 (or USP High Risk) is the most conservative approach. Many pharmacies prepare some sterile preparations from nonsterile ingredients (Table 17-3).[14]

Justifying need

Pharmacy directors frequently face resistance when justifying the need to improve their facilities. Some commonly asked questions and their corresponding answers follow.

If admixtures are made within a laminar-airflow workbench, why does its location matter? Laminar-airflow workbenches do not eliminate 100% of airborne particles. These workbenches have high-efficiency particulate air (HEPA) filters that remove 99.97% of particles over 0.3 microns when operating properly.[15] A significant increase in airborne contamination outside the workbench significantly increases contamination under the workbench. Workbenches cannot prevent microbial contamination introduced by poor aseptic technique downstream from the HEPA filter (e.g., from air currents pushing room air into the workbench). Table 17-4 shows the effect of increased airborne bacteria on aseptic processing contamination.

If the workbench is already in a separate room, do you really need a cleanroom? A separate room minimizes unnecessary traffic near

Table 17- 3.

Common Nonsterile Ingredients Prepared as Sterile Preparations[13]

- Alum irrigation
- Apomorphine injection
- Brilliant green injection
- Caffeine citrate injection
- Citric acid irrigation
- Cocaine ophthalmic
- Cromolyn sodium ophthalmic
- EDTA irrigation
- Formaldehyde irrigation
- Galactose injection
- Glutamine injection
- Histidine injection
- Methylcellulose ophthalmic
- Phenol injection
- Phosphate buffer
- Renacidin irrigation
- Rose bengal solution
- Talc powder suspension
- Tetracaine adrenalin cocaine (TAC) solution
- Talc powder suspension for injection

Table 17-4.

Effect of Airborne Microorganisms on Vial Contamination[a]

Bacteria per Cubic Foot of Air	Number of Vials Contaminated[b]
0.01	4
2.43	22
5.31	99

[a]Adapted, with permission, from Wythe W, Bailey PV, Tinkler J. An evaluation of the routes of bacterial contamination occurring during aseptic pharmaceutical manufacturing. *J Parenter Sci Technol.* 1982;36:1027.

[b]Approximately 9000 vials filled per condition.

the workbench but not the contamination already in a room. For example:[15]

- A person sitting motionless generates about 100,000 particles/cu ft/min.

- A person sitting down or standing up generates about 2,500,000 particles/cu ft/min.

- A person walking generates about 10,000,000 particles/cu ft/min.

- An open, non-airlocked door can add billions of particles per cubic foot per minute.

The primary functions of a well-designed cleanroom are to remove internally generated contamination and to prevent it from adversely affecting a critical area (i.e., inside workbench environment).[15]

If pharmacy-prepared admixtures have never been implicated in nosocomial infections, why should facilities be upgraded? Pharmacy-prepared sterile preparations are not commonly

implicated because few institutions thoroughly investigate the causes of nosocomial infections. In fact, admixtures in plastic bags prepared under pharmacy laminar-airflow workbenches have shown contamination rates of 0.7-17.7%.[16-18] Even though pharmacists may perform microbial testing on samples of final preparations, such sampling cannot assure sterility of all aseptically filled preparations in a batch.[19] In other words, pharmacists currently have few means of determining whether their preparations are sterile or whether they are causing infections.

Isn't good aseptic technique more important than a cleanroom in preventing microbial contamination? In situations where sterile preparations are contaminated, touch contamination (as evidenced by skin bacteria) is frequently encountered.[20] However, airborne fungi and gram-negative bacteria tend to survive and grow in IV solutions[21] and to be more pathological and difficult to cure. Cleanrooms provide an optimal environment for laminar-airflow workbenches and encourage the practice of aseptic technique.

Since building a cleanroom will be so expensive, why not return the responsibility for admixture preparation to nurses? True, in admixtures prepared just prior to administration, accidentally introduced microbes have less time to grow to pathological levels. But one study showed that 21% of the admixtures were made incorrectly (as to ingredients, dosage, unordered admixture, or incompatibility) on nursing units.[22] Another study showed that 10.9% of the nurse-prepared admixtures in plastic bags were contaminated versus 5.6% for pharmacy-prepared admixtures in plastic bags.[17] Moreover, nurses are less well trained to make admixtures today than when these studies were published. Furthermore, since many sterile preparations are used for 24 hr or more (e.g., TPNs and patient-controlled analgesia syringes), microbes can easily grow to pathological levels at room or body temperatures.[21] There are too many complicated sterile preparations as well as situations where nurses are not involved (ambulatory settings) to remove this activity from the pharmacy.

Finally, is there scientific proof that cleanrooms prevent infections? While definitive studies have not been done, having a controlled cleanroom environment is the only way to know whether sterile preparations are being prepared in a clean place. Creating a cleanroom environment need not be expensive, leaving no excuse for pharmacists not to upgrade their sterile compounding facilities. Physicians, especially surgeons, would expect sterile preparations to be compounded in areas at least as clean as operating rooms.

Analyzing Existing Facilities

Once the need has been justified, the next step is to determine whether a current cleanroom can be updated, whether a new room is needed, or whether a new type of environmental control (e.g., isolator) should be employed. Room size and environment (e.g., temperature, humidity and lighting) as well as cleanliness levels are important considerations.

Size and environment

Table 17-5 can be used to estimate facility size requirements.[23] Allen et al. found that their sterile compounding center required approximately 300 fewer square feet in floor space than the reference for Table 17-5, likely explained by efficiency gains.[11]

For hand washing, a sink with hot and cold running water should be in close proximity but not in the cleanroom itself. Ventilation and room temperature control capabilities should be in accordance with manufacturer and USP preparation labeling requirements. In any enclosed space with heat-producing equipment, the air conditioning must keep personnel comfortable in clean garb. Floors and active work surfaces (i.e., counters and shelves) should be nonporous and washable to enable

regular disinfection.[1] Lighting should ensure that personnel can read packages easily (e.g., syringe gauges and drug labels) and visualize contaminants (e.g., glass fragments in ampuls and rubber cores in vials).[24]

Room cleanliness

Forty-three percent of hospital pharmacies compound ASHP Risk Level 2 and 3 preparations: long expiration dated preparations, batch-prefilled syringes without preservatives, batch-reconstituted antibiotics, and a few preparations from nonsterile components.[10] To handle all eventualities, an ISO Class 7 (FS209 Class 10,000) cleanroom is recommended. This environment requires a positive-pressure differential, relative to adjacent less clean areas, of at least 0.05 inches of water. According to ASHP, the anteroom to an ISO Class 7 environment should meet ISO Class 8 specifications. ISO Classes 7 and 8 conditions simply mean that the areas are routinely monitored to ascertain that there are no more than 10,000 or 100,000 airborne particles greater than 0.5 micron/cu ft of air, respectively. (Table 17-2.)

Identifying Functional Needs

The key point in functional programming is to identify every specific function along with the required methods and systems to be performed in the facility. After existing facilities have been analyzed, one primary decision has to be made: Should a custom-built cleanroom be planned or should a modular cleanroom be purchased? Or can an existing room be remodeled or procedures be implemented to

Table 17-5.

Estimated Size Requirements for IV Admixture Center[22]

Workload, Orders/Day	Floor Space, Sq Ft[a]
100	540
200	637
300	723
400	959
500	1118

[a] Floorspace covers equipment, inventory,

create a facility that meets cleanroom air quality standards?

Cleanrooms and anterooms

The cleanliness of surrounding air, in conjunction with an operator's aseptic expertise, is critical to maintaining ISO Class 5 (FS209 Class 100) conditions in a laminar-airflow workbench.[2] A high-cleanliness anteroom reduces the number of particles in the cleanroom. Appropriate activities for the anteroom include but are not limited to hand washing, gowning and gloving, removal of packaging, and cleaning and disinfecting of hard-surface containers and supplies before they are placed in the cleanroom.[1] (See Chapter 11.)

USP provides further guidance for cleanroom floor planning.[2] Figure 17-1, modified from a USP plan, shows the important parts and spatial relationship of a cleanroom (buffer room) to an ante area suitable for low and medium risk sterile compounding. Figure 17-2 represents USP's floor plan for high-risk sterile compounding facility. Appropriate air-conditioning and humidity controls should be in place for the buffer room.[2]

Cleanroom ceilings, walls, floors, fixtures, shelves, counters, and cabinets should be resistant to sanitizing agents.[2] Furthermore, junctures of ceilings to walls should be covered or caulked to avoid cracks and crevices where dirt can accumulate.[2] If ceilings consist of inlaid panels, they should be impregnated with a polymer to render them impervious and hydrophobic; they also should be caulked with an elastic sealant around the perimeter and clamped to the support frame. The HEPA filter in the ceiling air supply should be placed to avoid creating air currents inside the laminar-airflow workbench. Prefilters on the heating, ventilation, and air conditioning (HVAC) air blower should be changeable from outside the cleanroom.[25]

Walls may be of hard panels locked together and sealed or of epoxy-coated gypsum board[2]

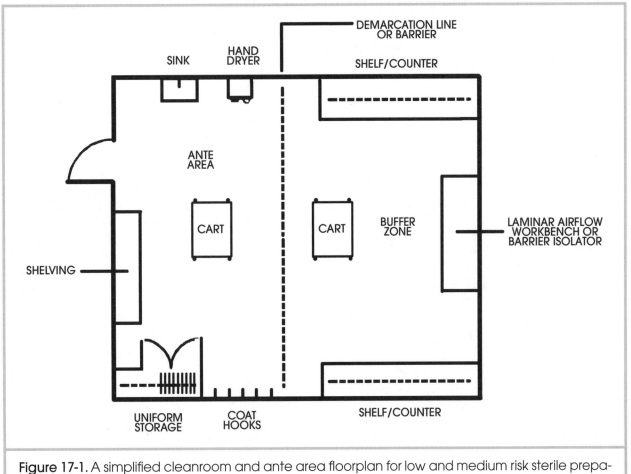

Figure 17-1. A simplified cleanroom and ante area floorplan for low and medium risk sterile preparation. (Adapted, with permission, from Reference 2.)

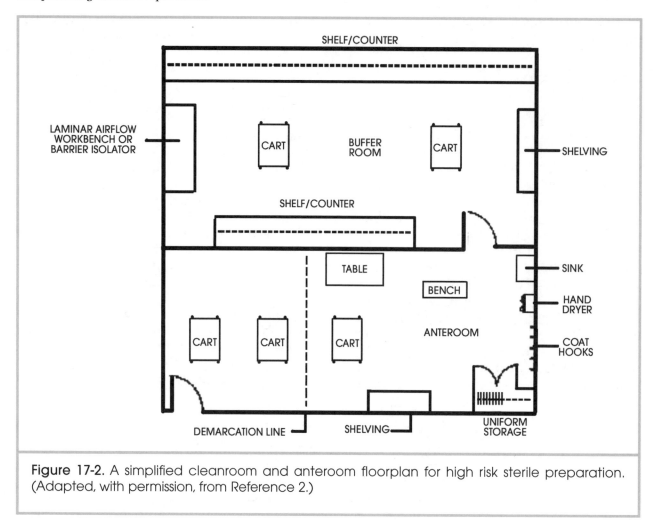

Figure 17-2. A simplified cleanroom and anteroom floorplan for high risk sterile preparation. (Adapted, with permission, from Reference 2.)

or of soft-wall plastic. Flooring should be a continuous, noncracking material that is mechanically and chemically robust.[26] Preferably, floors should be overlaid with wide sheet vinyl flooring with heat-welded seams and coving to the sidewall.[2] Dust-collecting overhangs (e.g., ceiling pipes) and ledges (e.g., windowsills) should be avoided.[2] The exterior lens surface of ceiling lights should be smooth, mounted flush, and sealed. Any other penetrations through the ceiling or walls also should be sealed.[2] The cleanroom should contain no sinks or floor drains.[2]

Access to the cleanroom should be via the anteroom door for personnel and an airlock pass through for most supplies. As supplies are moved from the anteroom into the cleanroom and then into the laminar-airflow workbench, a series of cleaning steps should be followed (see Chapter 11). A sink with air hand dryer or disposable non-shedding towels should be near the cleanroom entrance but

not inside the cleanroom.[2] Faucet handles should be designed so that they can be shut off with the elbows or feet.[2] Near the cleanroom doorway, a movable bench can provide a barrier and place for personnel to don shoe covers just before entering.[2] In the anteroom, a storage area for clean gowning supplies should be conveniently located.[2] The cleanroom door should remain automatically closed; personnel should be able to open it with elbow hooks or other means without using their clean hands.[2]

Modular cleanrooms

Modular cleanrooms (as opposed to custom built) have several advantages:

1. Modular cleanrooms can be customized to specific needs of the institution.

2. No sanding, spackling, or painting of walls are necessary, leaving a cleaner environment.

3. Modularity allows future change if you anticipate changes in aseptic processes or volume, or relocation to another site.

4. Modular cleanrooms cost less and are more rapidly installed.

5. Modular systems use standard components that are often available from different suppliers.

6. Shipping costs for aluminum and vinyl components are less costly than steel and unassembled components.

7. Installion costs are less because the vendor will do most of the installation, with the exception of electrical, water and HVAC hook-ups.

For low-volume operations, soft-wall cleanrooms are available at a lower cost than modular hard-wall installations. The pharmacy at Memorial Hospital in Carthage, IL, had a soft-wall cleanroom (Figure 17-3) installed for under $20,000 that satisfied a JCAHO home care survey. Some facts about this cleanroom include[27]:

- Setup of tubular frame and vinyl plastic panels took 10-12 hr for two company personnel.

- Dimensions are 8 ft by 16 ft, with an 8-ft ceiling height.

- Three "movable" walls are connected to one rigid wall. The rigid wall contains electrical and plumbing fixtures. It is made of aluminum stud supporting fire-rated dry wall and is painted with epoxy paint to provide durability and prevent particle shedding.

- Soft walls are made of 16-mil, replaceable, clear vinyl panels attached to a strong tubular frame.

- The cleanroom door is the same vinyl-on-tubular frame construction.

- The pass-through chamber is 16 inches by 16 inches.

- Two 2-ft by 4-ft HEPA filters are suspended in the cleanroom ceiling. Air from the pharmacy proper is blown through two standard fiberglass filters before passing through the HEPA filters into the cleanroom.

- Louvered dampers in the door and below the pass-through chamber permit airflow out of the positive-pressure room. They can be closed if power is lost to the blower.

- Ceiling tiles are vinyl-coated gypsum panels.

- Vinyl panels are easy to clean with detergent and water and can be replaced inexpensively if torn.

- A "hands free" faucet and hand dryer are just outside the cleanroom.

- The airborne particle count in the cleanroom is about 65 of 0.5 microns or larger per cubic foot, easily qualifying the environment as ISO Class 7 or even ISO Class 5. Particle counts inside the laminar-airflow workbench average 5–10 of 0.5 microns or larger.

Compared to soft-wall cleanrooms, hard-wall modular cleanrooms with rigid panels attached to a frame offer more stability and better seals to maintain cleanroom integrity.[28] Hard-wall cleanrooms are also easier to keep clean and are more durable.

Remodeling existing space

Kuster and Snyder gave reasons for renovating their pharmacy to create an ISO Class 7 cleanroom.[29] They prepared various sterile preparations, including Risk Level 3 preparations such as glycerin and phenol injection and sterile talc injection. To lessen the chance of error due to interruptions, they placed no phone in their cleanroom and included only a foot-activated intercom for outside communi-

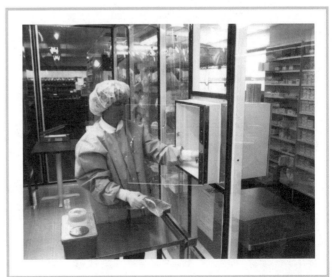

Figure 17-3. Pharmacist in a soft-wall cleanroom at Memorial Hospital, a 67-bed hospital in Carthage, IL.

cations. Figure 17-4 shows a general floor plan of their pharmacy and cleanroom.

Samuelson and Clark described the planning for an ISO Class 7 cleanroom with an ISO Class 8 anteroom at the University of Illinois Hospital.[30] They decided to convert an existing 32-ft by 22-ft sterile preparations room 40% into a cleanroom and 60% into an anteroom by constructing a wall across it. (A detail of the elevation of the cleanroom side of the wall is shown in Figure 17-5.) The large anteroom was needed for stock storage and reference materials. The larger pass-through window is used for supplies going into the cleanroom, and the smaller window is for completed preparations going back to the anteroom where a pharmacist checks them. The glass panel around the windows preserves a sense of openness and allows the pharmacist to monitor activities in the cleanroom. Since the existing walls and floor were seamless, they could be sealed with a polymer coating. However, ventilation had to be changed to incorporate HEPA filtration of the air supply in conjunction with a new 2-in ceiling grid system. The cost of the University of Illinois renovation was about $60,000–$70,000.[31]

In a 321-bed community hospital, Schumock et al. described their remodeling project to create a Class 10,000 cleanroom.[32] The authors planned and implemented a 361 square foot facility that paid for itself ($39,486 in 1996 dollars) in less than 2 years via the batch production of selected unit-of-use syringes not available commercially, i.e., savings were from reduced waste and extended expiration dating.

Minimal facility change

New procedures can also minimize airborne particulate matter. Lau et al.[33] described procedural changes in their large (six workbench) centralized admixture room that produced an ISO Class 7 environment from what had been ISO Class 8. Some of their changes were limiting personnel traffic, having personnel wear sterile garb, and removing cardboard containers outside the room.

Moreover, Chandler et al.[34] found that their large (four workbench) sterile preparation room met ISO Class 8 standards without modifications to either the room or procedures. Therefore, pharmacists should test the air quality in their sterile compounding room before embarking on expensive facility changes.

Preparing Specifications for a New Facility

After testing their sterile compounding environment, many pharmacists will decide to improve the air quality. Pharmacists should prepare plans with a hospital designer or architect. For the hospital architect unfamiliar with cleanroom design, ISO Standard 14644-4 specifies the requirements for the design and construction of cleanroom facilities.[35] This standard is intended for use by purchasers, suppliers and designers of cleanroom installations and provides a checklist of important parameters of performance. Construction guidance is provided, including requirements for start-up and qualification.

The pharmacist has the following roles in functional planning[13]:

- Identify functions to be performed in the cleanroom and anteroom.

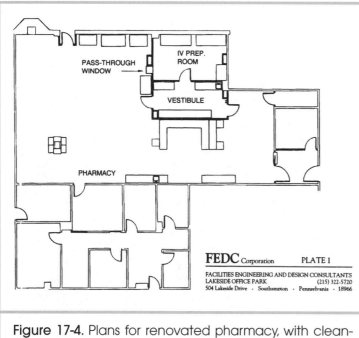

Figure 17-4. Plans for renovated pharmacy, with cleanroom and anteroom, at Lehigh Valley Hospital, an 800-bed nonprofit community teaching hospital in Allentown, PA. (Reproduced, with permission, from Reference 29.)

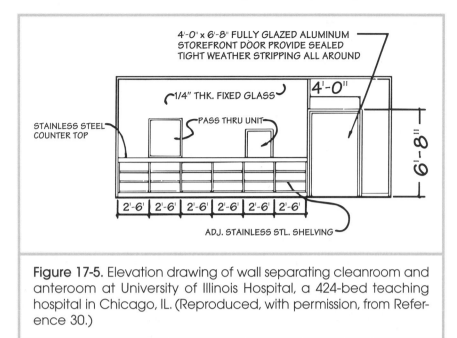

Figure 17-5. Elevation drawing of wall separating cleanroom and anteroom at University of Illinois Hospital, a 424-bed teaching hospital in Chicago, IL. (Reproduced, with permission, from Reference 30.)

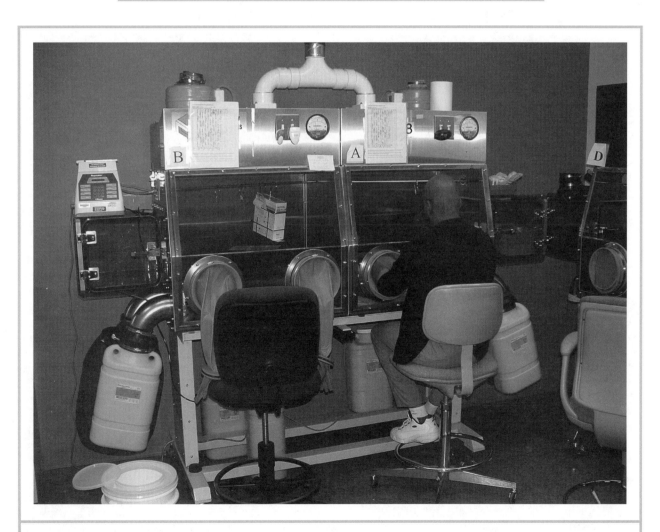

Figure 17-6. Pharmacy technician preparing chemotherapy in an insolator, Winship Cancer Institute at Emory University.

- Determine workflow in the cleanroom and anteroom.

- Identify work areas to be remodeled.

- Decide how to handle workload during the renovation process.

- Specify requirements for the cleanroom and anteroom:

  - Workload (e.g., average and maximum daily numbers of parenteral nutrition solutions, batches of syringes, chemotherapy compounding, peritoneal dialysates, stat admixtures).

  - Equipment types and numbers. Will biological safety cabinets or isolators be exhausted to the outside (they should be)?

  - Storage requirements for supplies and finished preparations.

  - Personnel types and numbers.

  - Materials logistics.

  - Communication systems (e.g., intercom, email, telephones, overhead paging).

  - Services expected from other departments (e.g., IV solution deliveries, housekeeping).

  - Security (e.g., locked doors, access control systems, video cameras).

  - Utilities (e.g., lighting, electrical outlets, plumbing, computer lines, floor drains.)

  - Environmental quality control (i.e., ISO Class 5 or 7 or 8).

  - Housekeeping and cleaning routines.

  - Environmental monitoring routines (e.g., laminar air-flow workbench testing, surface microbial counts, air particulate counts, settle plate colony counts).

Preparing the Request for Information (RFI)

Before you ask a cleanroom vendor to bid on building a cleanroom in your facility, evaluate potential vendors by asking for information about their abilities and resources; solicit financials or Dun and Bradstreet reports and ask for a listing of recently completed projects in facilities like yours. Call for references or visit some of these facilities. Ask the vendor to submit a set of design plans for a similar project and resumes for the proposed project team. Select three to five vendors to whom you will submit a request for proposal.

Handling the Request for Proposal (RFP)

Together, the pharmacist and institutional engineer or architect should prepare the RFP and select the potential vendors most likely to serve the facility's needs. The request for proposal can follow these guidelines[36]:

1. Supply potential vendors with pertinent information to meet the requirements but not so detailed as to stifle their creativity.

2. Provide a general overview of the facility and its requirements, e.g., the type of work to be done, hours of operation.

3. Present the scope of work to be provided by the vendor, i.e., design, construction, electrical, heating, ventilation and air conditioning (HVAC), institutional or vendor-supplied connections for electrical, ventilation, gases, etc.

4. Ask for a proposed project schedule, floor plan, ceiling plan, elevations, equipment location plan, and air balance schematic, as well as details and catalog cuts of preparations and materials used as the basis of the design. Ask for heat load calculations and rough power requirements. Must construction and service personnel be union members? Use all this information to compare proposals and for interviews with potential vendors.

5. Show taxable status of the project so the vendor knows what to include or not include as regards permits, stamps, and fees.

6. Specify whether your cleanroom is to be ISO Class 5 or 7 or 8 for airborne particles, temperature (e.g., 68°F), humidity (e.g., 45% relative humidity), air pressure gradients between the cleanroom and anteroom and the anteroom and surrounding area and air exchanges per hour (e.g., 20 air exchanges per hour in the anteroom).[37] HVAC control is the biggest issue in cleanroom design, because garb, workbenches and refrigerators increase warmth for people in cleanrooms. The number of people in the cleanroom will also add heat and moisture to the environment.

7. Supply a basic floor plan or bubble diagram, equipment list, material pathways, ceiling height (slab to slab), current floor construction, and any seismic or structural issues so the vendor can accurately

assess construction requirements. What cleaning agents will be used on ceilings, walls, and floors in the cleanroom and the anteroom? Are windows or viewing panels required? If so, where should they be in the cleanroom and anteroom? Are pass-through chambers required? If so, where and what size should they be in the cleanroom and anteroom? Where are doors to be located in the cleanroom and anteroom? What type of door (e.g., swing or sliding) should be installed? Do perimeter walls require fire rating? If so, identify rating in hours for the cleanroom and anteroom. Are temperature recording and monitoring required for the cleanroom and anteroom?

8. Present a utility plan. Will additional electrical power be needed? Hospital personnel can usually bring the power source to a single point of connection at a lower cost than having the cleanroom vendor arrange the power source. You may wish to have energy-saving setback controls if the cleanroom is not operating 24 hours per day, 7 days per week. What lighting levels are needed (in footcandles) at 30 inches from the floor in the cleanroom (e.g., 140) and anteroom (e.g., 100)? Requirements for a sprinkler system in the cleanroom are dependent on the occupancy code and use, as well as local building codes. Sprinkler heads should be flush with the ceiling. How far away is the tie-in point for sprinkler water supply? Will the water supply be shut down or will it need to operate during the tie-in process? What are the insurance policy requirements for the sprinkler system? Will smoke or fire alarms be needed in the cleanroom and anteroom? Are hot and cold water available for the anteroom? Can a sink drain be installed without threat to cleanliness? Who will remove waste material? How will hazardous and nonhazardous waste be handled?

9. Require the vendor to do an onsite inspection of your facility before developing a quotation.

10. Ask for the vendor to train your personnel who will use and maintain the cleanroom, e.g., engineers, housekeeping, pharmacy personnel.

11. Ask for a price breakdown, per building trade, allowing you to evaluate where there are differences in proposals. Is payment or performance bonding required?

12. Develop an evaluation matrix to compare proposals. Interview the two or three vendors who look most promising, based on criteria that you have set for your institution. Discuss architecture, mechanical systems, heat load calculations including wall insulation, and electrical and lighting systems.

13. Arrange to have the completed cleanroom evaluated by an independent source based on your RFP performance criteria. Determine who will pay for the final evaluation.

14. Negotiate the schedule that protects both parties from unforeseen delays and costs.

15. Ask what you, as the owner, will have to do to operate the cleanroom after the vendor's work is complete.

16. Finally, have the institution's pharmacist, engineer, administrator and lawyer select the best cleanroom vendor. Lawyers for the vendor and institution will finalize the contract for the administrator's approval.

Building the Cleanroom

Whether planning custom-built or modular, everyone involved in constructing a cleanroom should understand that this is no ordinary building project.[26] The microbial contamination potential of all activities should be reviewed before they are begun. Institutional staff should monitor vendor personnel to ensure that they follow proper techniques so as not to build contamination into the cleanroom or its surroundings. Issues should be resolved with the vendor onsite, not after construction is complete.

Materials for walls, floors, and ceilings should never be stored outdoors. Packaging materials (usually doubled) cannot be torn or removed until the cleanroom vendor is ready for installation. A general wipe down of building materials with clean wipes is recommended both before and after installation.[26] After any cutting or drilling operation, the resealing should be done as soon as possible to prevent oxidation or deep contamination of building materials.

Once the floor is laid, construction workers should wear gowns and shoe covers to reduce contamination and prevent damage to the floor. No eating, smoking, chewing, etc., should be allowed in the area. All spills, filings, etc., should be cleaned up immediately. After walls and ceilings are in place (even before the air supply is turned on), the area should be restricted to authorized personnel. Finally, once the air supply is on, construction workers should be gowned like the operators will be.[26]

Evaluating the Installation

Final steps are inspecting and approving the new facility, installing and evaluating equipment, moving supplies, assessing workflow, and following up on needed changes (which are inevitable). Use of an independent testing agency is recommended to assure unbiased test results

The pharmacist in charge of the project must be sure that air quality (balance and particle levels), surface conditions, environmental requirements (temperature and humidity), and working conditions (e.g., space, sound, and lighting levels) are as specified in the original bidding process.

These requirements must be satisfied before any equipment or supplies are moved into the anteroom or cleanroom. The vendor should supply an operation and maintenance manual that will help identify problems and possible solutions. This manual should also provide scheduling for maintenance and parts replacement.

Furthermore, the institution's facilities management personnel must check that all policies regarding electrical fixtures, heating, ventilation, etc., have been met. An agreement must be reached with the vendor to rectify deficiencies before the contract can be considered satisfied.

Facility Maintenance

Clearly, planning, building, and implementing a cleanroom facility is a detailed process. All that preparation, however, must be preserved with proper maintenance. Preventive maintenance of cleanroom and anteroom prefilters, HEPA filters, and ducts should be arranged with appropriate maintenance personnel or a service vendor. Similarly, lighting should be checked periodically and/or bulbs should be changed.

Cleanroom

Each day, work surfaces near the workbench (e.g., counter tops and carts) should be wiped clean with a freshly prepared mild detergent solution followed by a sanitizing agent approved by the pharmacist in charge. Sufficient time must be allowed for the agent to exert its antimicrobial effect. Furthermore, storage shelving should be emptied of all supplies, cleaned, and sanitized at least weekly. Recleaning should be performed if spillage or other events indicate the need.[2]

When no aseptic operations are in progress, floors should be mopped once daily by trained and supervised custodial personnel. Floors should not be waxed because dried, worn wax adds to airborne particulates.[25] All cleaning and sanitizing agents should be approved, with careful consideration of compatibilities, effectiveness, and inappropriate or toxic residues. In addition, all cleaning tools (e.g., wipers, sponges, and mops) should be nonshedding and used only in the cleanroom (first) and anteroom.

Most wipers should be discarded after one use. If cleaning tools are reused, their cleanliness should be maintained by thorough rinsing and sanitizing and by storage in a clean environment.[2] Ceilings and walls should be cleaned monthly with a mild detergent solution followed by an approved sanitizing agent.

Trash should be collected in suitable plastic bags and removed with minimal agitation. Routine monitoring is used to control the quality of the air and surfaces in the cleanroom (see Chapter 18).

Anteroom

In the anteroom, supplies and equipment removed from shipping cartons should be wiped with a sanitizing agent, such as 70% isopropyl alcohol; this agent should be checked periodically for contamination. (Since 70% isopropyl alcohol may harbor resistant microbial spores, it should be filtered through a 0.2-micron hydrophobic filter before being used in aseptic areas.) Alternatively, if supplies are in sealed pouches (e.g., syringes), the pouches can be removed when the supplies are introduced into the cleanroom, obviating the need to sanitize individual items. No shipping or other cartons should be taken into the cleanroom.[2]

The anteroom should be cleaned and sanitized at least weekly by trained and supervised custodial personnel. However, floors must be cleaned and sanitized daily, always proceeding from the cleanroom to the anteroom. Storage shelving in the anteroom (including refrigerator interior) should be emptied of all supplies, cleaned, and sanitized at planned intervals, preferably monthly.[2] Walls and ceilings should be cleaned and sanitized at least quarterly.

Major Cleanroom Equipment

This section discusses the regulatory standards, justification, purchasing, installation and maintenance of major equipment, like laminar-airflow workbenches, isolators and automated compounding devices. The description and use of this equipment appears in Chapter 3. Environmental monitoring devices such as air particulate counters are covered in Chapter 18. Cleanroom garb is discussed in Chapter 5. Sterilization devices are described in Chapter 13. Cleaning materials such as wipers, detergent and sanitizing solutions, and mops are not covered here because this information is generally available through your institution's purchasing, infection control or housekeeping departments. Equipment such as personal computers, monitors, keyboards and printers should not be placed in cleanrooms because they are too difficult to clean. Printers and paper add too much to air particulate counts.

Purchasing Major Equipment

While workbenches, isolators and compounding devices are major purchases, the purchasing process is not as complicated as that for cleanrooms. The vendor market and their individual pieces of equipment change continually; so it is not practical to list vendors and products here. Nor does this text endorse any specific vendors or products.

To determine what is on the market, go to www.cleanrooms.com or www.a2c2.com and search the buyer's guide. Alternatively, your group purchasing organization may have agreements with a few vendors to help save on capital purchases. Select several vendors and ask your staff or other pharmacists for their experience with these vendors. Contact vendor representatives via vendor websites and ask them for their product that fits your needs. Vendor representatives are trained on product features and can provide specifications, drawings, viable options, and detailed price quotations. Be sure to consider costs for shipping and installation, delivery schedule, and customer support.

Laminar-Airflow Workbenches

These workbenches (or hoods) are not magic boxes. At best, they are designed to maintain the sterility of objects that are already clean and sterile. They do not sanitize or sterilize objects that are introduced into the critical area within them. They should be easy to clean, both inside and outside. User ergonomics should be excellent, e.g., work height and size. Accessories such as hooks and bars should be available in easy-to-reach locations within the critical area.

Horizontal laminar-airflow workbenches

Horizontal laminar-airflow workbenches are suitable for non-hazardous drug compounding such as TPN solutions. ASHP[1] and USP[2] standards require that horizontal laminar-airflow workbenches produce an environment that is ISO Class 5. Horizontal models are available in a variety of widths (2 ft to 8 ft) and with different electrical requirements (120 or 220 volts). Work surfaces are of either high-density laminated composition board or stainless steel. Some models are for use on counter tops, others are stand-alone floor units. Even at the purchasing stage, pharmacists should be familiar with issues related to horizontal workbench certification.[38]

Vertical laminar-airflow workbenches (biological safety cabinets)

Biological safety cabinets (BSCs) can be used for hazardous (e.g., chemotherapy) or non-hazardous sterile drug preparation. BSCs are classified as to their ability to protect personnel from hazardous agents handled inside the BSC, to protect the drug from hazardous (including microbial) particles in the air and/or to protect the environment outside the BSC from hazardous contamination. (Table 17-6.)

ASHP[1] and USP[2] standards require that BSCs produce an internal environment that is ISO Class 5 to maintain proper aseptic technique. The National Institute for Occupational Safety and Health (NIOSH) states,

> When mixing, preparing or otherwise manipulating hazardous drugs, including counting or crushing of tablets, com-

Table 17-6.

Classification of Biological Safety Cabinets

NSF Classification	Biosafety Level	General Description	GeneralApplications *
Class I	Low to moderate risk biological agents	100% room air (dirty) enters cabinet front; exhaust is HEPA filtered to outside or into room	Protects personnel and outside environmental from particles. No product protection from air particles. No personnel protection from volatile toxic chemicals and volatile radionucleotides
Class II, Type A1 (formerly, Type A)	Low to moderate risk biological agents	70% air recirculated inside cabinet; 30% exhausted from a common plenum to the room; exhaust is HEPA filtered to outside or into room	Protects product, personnel and environment from air particles. Exhaust HEPA filtered air is both recirculated into the room and to the outdoors. No protection from volatile toxic chemicals and volatile radionucleotides
Class II, Type A2 (formerly, Type B3)	Low to moderate risk biological agents	70% air recirculated; 30% exhausted from a common plenum through HEPA filter & pulled through dedicated exhaust duct into facility exhaust system to outside or into room	Protects product, personnel and environment from air particles. Better protection from volatile toxic chemicals and volatile radionucleotides
Class II, Type B1	Low to moderate risk biological agents	30% air recirculated inside cabinet; 70% exhausted from cabinet through HEPA filter & pulled through dedicated exhaust duct into facility exhaust system to outside	Protects product, personnel and environment from air particles. Limited protection from volatile toxic chemicals and volatile radionucleotides
Class II, Type B2 (total exhaust)	Low to moderate risk biological agents	0% air recirculated; 100% exhausted from cabinet through HEPA filter & pulled through dedicated exhaust duct into facility exhaust system to outside	Protects product, personnel and environment from air particles. HEPA filtered air is totally exhausted to the outdoors. Best protection from volatile toxic chemicals and volatile radionucleotides.
Class III (total enclosure)	High risk biological agents (Safety Level 4)	Total containment of environment within BSC in which operations are conducted through attached rubber gloves. Exhaust air is treated by double HEPA filtration or single HEPA filtration/ incineration.	Totally protects product, personnel and environment. Used for dangerous microbes, handling carcinogens or equipment generating hazardous vapors or gases.

* NIOSH recommends Class II, Type B2 or Class III BSCs for handling hazardous drugs.

pounding powders, or pouring of liquid drugs, these tasks should be conducted within a ventilated cabinet designed specifically to prevent hazardous drugs from being released into the surrounding environment. NIOSH recognizes that aseptic technique is an important requirement for many applications regarding hazardous drugs in order to protect them from possible contamination . . . When asepsis is required or is the recommended work practice, the use of ventilated cabinets designed for both hazardous drug containment and aseptic processing is recommended . . . When aseptic technique is required, the recommended ventilated cabinets include Class II (Type B2 preferred, Type A2 & B1 allowed under certain conditions) and Class III BSC's as well as isolators intended for asepsis and containment ("Aseptic Containment Isolators"). Each ventilated cabinet should be equipped with a continuous monitoring device to allow confirmation of adequate airflow prior to each use. The exhaust from these controls should be HEPA filtered and preferably exhausted 100% to the outside. The outside exhaust should be installed to avoid re-entrainment by the building envelope or HVAC systems. Fan placement should be downstream of the HEPA filter so that contaminated ducts are maintained under negative pressure. A ventilated cabinet with air recirculation, either within the cabinet or to the room environment, should only be used if the hazardous drug(s) in use will not volatilize during process manipulation or after capture by the HEPA filter . . . Ventilated cabinets require both routine and unscheduled maintenance by building facility personnel or outside contractors. All maintenance activities performed on ventilated cabinets and exhaust systems associated with hazardous drug procedures should be reviewed, in advance, by a health and safety representative familiar with the potential exposures and their associated hazards. A written safety plan should be developed for all routine maintenance activities performed on equipment potentially contaminated with hazardous drugs. Individuals performing the maintenance operations should be familiar with the applicable safety plans, warned of the potential hazards, and trained on the appropriate work techniques and PPE necessary to minimize exposure. . . all hazardous drugs and chemicals should

be removed and the ventilated cabinet decontaminated prior to initiating the maintenance activity.[39]

In addition, biological safety cabinets are standardized by NSF International. The standard includes basic requirements for design, construction, and performance that are intended to provide personnel, product, and environmental protection, reliable operation, durability, cleanability, noise level and illumination control, limitation on temperature rise, vibration control, and electrical leakage and ground circuit resistance and polarity.[40] Any biological safety cabinet purchased should meet the voluntary NSF standards. NSF Standard 49 *Class II (Laminar Flow) Biohazard Cabinetry* applies to Class II biological safety cabinets only, as designed to minimize the hazards inherent in working with agents assigned to biosafety levels 1, 2, or 3. The standard defines the tests that a cabinet must comply with to become NSF Certified.

Isolators

This chapter uses the term "isolator" rather than barrier/isolator because a barrier system is an open system that can exchange contaminants with the surrounding area.[41] Pharmacists are finding that isolators can be used in special situations (e.g., Risk Level 3 compounding, hazardous drug compounding) to upgrade their facility (see Chapter 4 and Figure 17-6). An isolator is no substitute for a cleanroom; the USP states that a well-designed positive pressure isolator supported by adequate procedures for its maintenance, monitoring and control, may offer an acceptable alternative to the use of conventional laminar air-flow workbenches in cleanrooms for aseptic processing.[2] USP further states, "It is preferred, but not necessary, to locate isolators within buffer air quality areas." And the Parenteral Drug Association states,

> There need not be a specific particulate clean air classification requirement for the room surrounding isolators. Regardless of their specific usage, properly designed isolators do not allow the exchange of contaminants with the surrounding environment. Therefore, the quality of the surrounding room is a very minor consideration relative to the quality of the internal environment of the isolator.[4]

Practically speaking it very difficult not to drag microbes from outside an isolation through the transfer port into the critical area of the isolator.[43] So the cleaner the environment outside the isolator, the fewer microbes that will be introduced into the isolator.

Isolator technology was developed to remove people from the environment in which sterile and/or hazardous preparations are compounded. Removing the person from the environment eliminates the primary source of microbial contamination of the drug. Good aseptic technique in the handling of preparations and support materials is still required, with the notable exception of placement restrictions relative to laminar-airflow within the isolator.[44]

Pharmacists should use closed isolators intended for aseptic operations and hazardous drug containment. Such isolators adhere to the following principles[40]:

- They must not exchange air with the surrounding environment except when that air passes through a HEPA filter.

- They must be regularly decontaminated in a reproducible and quantifiable manner.

- All work or handling of materials within the isolator must be accomplished remotely; no human operator can directly reach into the isolator during operation.

- All materials that enter the isolator must be decontaminated or sterilized and must enter either directly through a decontaminating or sterilizing system, or via a rapid transfer port (RTP).

- Isolators are intended to meet ISO Class 5 total particulate levels during operation.

- All materials exiting the isolator must be cleaned or contained in such a way that hazardous materials are not released to the surrounding environment.

- Isolators must be regularly cleaned in a reproducible and quantifiable manner.

Pilong and Moore found that converting from laminar-airflow workbenches to isolators in a pharmacy sterile preparations area allowed the institution to comply with regulatory requirements, meet administrative and cost objectives, and satisfy employee requests for a better working environment.[45] See Tables 17-7 and 17-8. Other advantages of isolators are their usefulness in limited space, the need for fewer HVAC additions, greater flexibility when adding isolators as work increases, and portability when the compounding area must be relocated.

Isolators do have disadvantages as compared to biological safety cabinets. Users require more training; certain operations may be slower (e.g., stat dose preparation); users can not move around as readily (some facilities use two operators, one to supply and re-

Table 17-7.

Comparison of Capital Costs of Sterile Preparations*

Cost Item	Conventional Preparation	Cleanroom	Isolator Workstations
Demolition	$4,000	$7,500	0
New construction	50,000	70,000	$1,000
Equipment	15,000	15,000	75,000**
Temporary facilities	12,000	12,000	0
Total	$81,000	$102,500	$76,000

* Modified from Pilong A and Moore M. Conversion to isolators in a sterile preparation area. *Am J Health-Syst Pharm.* 1999;56:1978–80.

** This includes 3 isolators in 1999 dollars; so isolators can be expected to cost more now.

Table 17-8.

Comparison of Annual Operating Cost of Cleanroom versus Isolators in 1999 Dollars*

Cost Factors	Cleanroom	Isolators (Three)
Energy	$13,400	$525
Disposable items	4,400	2,000
Filter maintenance	2,400	325
Efficiency (lower number represents higher efficiency)	1,800	0
Annual operating costs	$22,000	$2850
Annual savings		$19,150

* Modified from Pilong A and Moore M. Conversion to isolators in a sterile preparation area. *Am J Health-Syst Pharm.* 1999;56:1978–80.

move preparations from transfer ports and the other to do the compounding); isolators require periodic leak testing to assure their containment ability; isolators require a different sequence in cleaning technique.[40] In fact, glove and sleeve leaks are significant in isolator technology.[46]

Automated Compounders

Automated compounding devices can help pharmacists achieve accuracy and efficiency in compounding sterile preparations; however, they have been associated with serious medication errors that have harmed patients. (See Chapter 1.) While cleanrooms, laminar-airflow workbenches, and isolators help maintain aseptic technique, automated compounder use also affects the identity of ingredients, the compatibility of ingredients and the accuracy of ingredient measurement, all of which are riskier processes than maintaining sterility.

Standards for automated compounding devices

ASHP requires that, "Methods should be established for calibrating and verifying the accuracy and sterility of automated compounding methods used in aseptic processing."[1] USP presents a variety of methods to verify the accuracy and precision of automated compounding devices.[2] A.S.P.E.N. has the following practice guideline:

> Manufacturers of automated methods of parenteral nutrition compounding should provide an additive sequence that ensures the safety of the compounding device. This compounding sequence should be reviewed with the manufacturer of the parenteral nutrient products used by institution. As most institutions in the United States are represented by buying groups with many participants, such buying groups should not only ensure the safety and support of the automated compounding device, but should avoid splitting parenteral nutrition contracts (mixing brands of amino acids, dextrose and IFEs) unless such combinations have adequate physiochemical data that ensure the stability, compatibility, and safety of the final formulations commensurate with the data for single-source parenteral nutrition preparations.[47]

Thus, professional standards require that automated compounding devices maintain accuracy of measurement of ingredients, compatibility of ingredients, and sterility of ingredients. These standards apply to parenteral nutrition compounders as well as other compounded sterile preparations such as cardioplegia solutions, dialysis solutions, batch syringe filling and pump reservoir filling.

Justification for automated compounding devices

ASHP lists specific advantages related to cost justification of automated compounding devices[48]:

1. Enhanced efficacy and worker safety during the parenteral nutrition compounding process and patient safety with parenteral use.

2. Reduction in labor associated with manually compounded parenteral nutrition admixtures. Assessment of the overall labor and material costs associated with the current manual compounding methods should include hidden costs such as pharmacists' time to perform calculations, quality assurance checks, and compounder set-up, as well as staff training (initial and ongoing).

3. Reduction in waste through more efficient use of base solutions and additives. Inventory can often be reduced by consolidating source solutions to a few high-concentration, large-volume additives.

Performance requirements

With regard to automated devices for compounding parenteral nutrition admixtures, ASHP says[46]:

> The use of automated devices for compounding parenteral nutrition admixtures should be clearly defined by the health care organization and the manufacturer. This includes the ongoing responsibilities of the pharmacy department and those of the manufacturer during and after implementation of the compounder in the pharmacy practice setting.

Three areas need to be clearly defined before choosing an automated compounding system: (1) the system's performance requirements, (2) the manufacturer's responsibilities, and (3) the pharmacy department's responsibilities. The performance requirements of the automated compounding system should ensure that:

1. The compounder exceeds the level of accuracy achieved with manual compounding. The automated compounding device should be accurate to within 5% of the amount programmed, with verification of the amount pumped versus the programmed amount for each ingredient.

2. The automated compounding device has inherent safeguards, including the ability to detect situations that could result in inaccurate deliveries, such as occluded transfer-set tubing and empty source containers; and the ability to keep incompatible source solutions separate.

3. The automated compounding software alerts the user when formulation issues arise.

4. The automated compounding software meets the standards of the American Society for Parenteral and Enteral Nutrition for parenteral nutrition label formats.[47]

5. The automated compounding software assists the pharmacist in producing physicochemically compatible parenteral nutrition formulations.

6. The automated compounding software provides useful clinical information.

7. The automated compounding software integrates with existing pharmacy programs whenever possible to optimize patient care and avoid therapeutic duplication.

The contractual agreement with the manufacturer should provide continuous support of the compounder and software, including information updates, problem solving, and emergency coverage. FDA considers all automated compounding devices class II devices,[49] and as such they must comply with federal regulations. The manufacturer's responsibilities are as follows:

1. The manufacturer should supply, and the pharmacist should verify, that the device is 510K cleared as evidence of compliance with regulatory requirements; that the device meets the fire and safety standards established by Underwriters Laboratories (i.e., is UL-approved); that the operator's manual and other documentation support recommendations for use; and that

accuracy statements and manufacturer claims are valid.

2. The manufacturer should provide 24-hour support for the compounder and its software throughout the life of the contract.

3. The manufacturer should routinely provide the latest version of the compounder software in a timely manner.

4. The manufacturer should ensure adequate availability of compounding supplies.

5. The manufacturer should provide detailed information and instructions on the appropriate use of the compounder and its software. References should be provided when appropriate.

6. The manufacturer should comply with FDA requirements for reporting adverse events."

Planning for automated compounders

ASHP recommends[47]

Within the pharmacy department, specific policies and procedures should be developed that address responsibilities for compounder operations and maintenance, staff training, and monitoring compounder performance at all times. Before selecting and implementing an automated compounder process, the pharmacy department should

1. Define and agree on automated compounding system needs and performance requirements.

2. Develop an implementation team with a lead person.

3. Develop a set of policies and procedures.

Morris et al. found that 32% of hospital pharmacies already use automatic compounding devices but that only 83% of those pharmacies actually have policies and procedures for the use of their automatic compounders.[10]

Summary

Facilities used for sterile compounding play an integral role in guaranteeing sterility, as does proper aseptic technique. Therefore, pharmacy departments should assess their current facilities and, if needed, upgrade or replace them. Once facilities have been brought up to current standards, a proper maintenance program for both the cleanroom and anteroom must be followed.

Major equipment placed in cleanrooms requires planning to assess needs, determine specifications, assign responsibilities, prepare policies and procedures, train staff, oversee purchasing and installation of equipment and monitor equipment performance according to manufacturer specifications and pharmacy procedures.

References

1. American Society of Health-System Pharmacists. ASHP Guidelines on quality assurance for pharmacy-prepared sterile products. *Am J Health-Syst Pharm.* 2000;57:1150–69.

2. Pharmaceutical compounding—sterile preparations. United States pharmacopeia, 27th ed./national formulary, 22nd rev. (First supplement). Rockville, MD: United States Pharmacopeial Convention. Available at: www.uspnf.com.

3. Federal standard airborne particulate cleanliness classes in cleanrooms and clean zones. Washington, DC: U.S. General Services Administration; 1992 (Sept):1–48.

4. DeSorbo MA. Fed-Std-209 shelved, ISO reigns. *Cleanrooms,* 2002;16:1, 45.

5. International Organization for Standardization Standard 14644-1 *Cleanrooms and associated environments – Part 1: Classification of air cleanliness.* 1st ed. Switzerland, 1999. Available at: www.iso.ch.

6. Federal Food, Drug and Cosmetic Act. Section 501(a)(2)(B) of Act [21 U.S.C. 351(a)(2)(B)]. *Fed Register.* 1978;43:45076–7.

7. Joint Commission on Accreditation of Healthcare Organizations. Standard MM.4.20 and 4.40 under Medication Management. 2004 Automated *Comprehensive Accreditation Manual for Hospital (CAMH).* Available at: www.jcaho.org/. Accessed January 2004.

8. Rich DS. Ask the Joint Commission: Class 100 environment for IV preparation. *Hosp Pharm.* 2001;36:340.

9. Thompson CA. News: USP publishes enforcable chapter on sterile compounding. *Am J Health-Syst Pharm.* 2003;60:1814–7.

10. Morris AM, Schneider PJ, Pederson CA, et al. National survey of quality assurance activities for pharmacy-compounded sterile preparations. *Am J Hosp Pharm.* 2003;60:2567–76.

11. Allen EL, Barker KN, Severson RW, et al. Design and evaluation of a sterile compounding facility. *Am J Health-Syst Pharm.* 1995;52:1421–7.

12. Mangum D, Assistant Director of Pharmacy, and Severson J, Director of Pharmacy, University Hospital, Augusta, GA. September 1994. Personal communications.

13. Barker KN, Allan EL, Lin AC, et al. Facility planning and design. In: Brown TR, ed. *Handbook of Institutional Pharmacy Practice.* 3rd ed. Bethesda, MD: American Society of Hospital Pharmacists; 1992:149–63.

14. Crawford SY, Narducci WA, Augustine SC. National survey of quality assurance activities for pharmacy-prepared sterile products in hospitals. *Am J Hosp Pharm.* 1991;48:2398–413.

15. Griner J. What the HEPA can and cannot do. *Cleanrooms.* 1994;7:29.

16. Miller WA, Smith GL, Latiolais CJ. A comparative evaluation of compounding costs and contamination rates of intravenous admixture systems. *Drug Intell Clin Pharm.* 1971;5:51–60.

17. Poretz DM, Guynn JB Jr, Duma RJ, et al. Microbial contamination of glass bottle (open-vented) and plastic bag (closed-nonvented) intravenous fluid delivery systems. *Am J Hosp Pharm.* 1974;31:726–32.

18. McAllister JC, Buchanan EC, Skolaut MW. A comparison of the safety and efficiency of three intermittent intravenous therapy systems—the mini-bottle, the minibag and the inline burette. *Am J Hosp Pharm.* 1974;31:961–7.

19. Frieben WR. Control of aseptic processing environment. *Am J Hosp Pharm.* 1983;40:1928–35.

20. Ravin R, Bahr J, Luscomb F, et al. Program for bacterial surveillance of intravenous admixtures. *Am J Hosp Pharm.* 1974;31:340–7.

21. Guynn JB Jr, Poretz DM, Duma RJ. Growth of various bacteria in a variety of intravenous fluids. *Am J Hosp Pharm.* 1973;30:321–5.

22. Thur MP, Miller WA, Latiolais CJ. Medication errors in a nurse-controlled parenteral admixture program. *Am J Hosp Pharm.* 1972;29:298–304.

23. Lin AC. *Study of variables affecting floor space requirements for intravenous admixture compounding areas in hospitals: a computer simulation approach* [doctoral dissertation]. Auburn, AL: Auburn University; 1992:281–342, 359–90. Available from University Microfilms, Ann Arbor, MI, Publication DA9237193.

24. Buchanan TL, Barker KN, Gibson JT, et al. Illumination and errors in dispensing. *Am J Hosp Pharm.* 1991;48:2137–45.

25. Kraft R. Cleanroom-construction concerns. *Am J Hosp Pharm.* 1994;51:935. Letter.

26. Kozicki M, Hoenig S, Robinson P. *Cleanrooms Facilities and Practices.* New York, NY: Van Nostrand Reinhold; 1991:49–79.

27. Rose R, Director of Pharmacy, Memorial Hospital, Carthage, IL. Aug 11, 1994. Personal communication.

28. Gingerich K. When is a modular cleanroom right for you? *Cleanrooms.* 2003;17:12, 22.

29. Kuster LM, Snyder GA. The future of hospital-based IV compounding. *Hosp Pharm Times.* 1993;59:38HPT.

30. Samuelson DE, Clark T. Pharmacy preparation meets the contamination control challenge. *Cleanrooms.* 1993;7(8): 126.

31. Clark T, Director of Pharmacy, University of Illinois Hospital, Chicago, IL. Aug 1994. Personal communication.

32. Schumock GT, Kafka PS, Tormo VJ. Design, construction, implementation, and cost of a hospital pharmacy cleanroom. *Am J Health-Syst Pharm.* 1998;55:458–63.

33. Lau D, Shane R, Yen J. Quality assurance for sterile products: simple changes can help. *Am J Hosp Pharm.* 1994; 51:1353. Letter.

34. Chandler SW, Trissel LA, Wamsley LM, et al. Evaluation of air quality in a sterile-drug preparation area with an electronic particle counter. *Am J Hosp Pharm.* 1993;50:2330–4.

35. International Organization for Standardization. International Standard 14644-4 *Cleanrooms and associated controlled environments – Part 4: Design, construction and start-up. 1st ed.* Switzerland, 2001. Available at: www.iso.ch.

36. Loughran T, Burton J. How to write a design/build specification. *Cleanrooms.* 1999;14:19–21.

37. Food and Drug Administration. *Guidance for Industry Sterile drug products produced by aseptic processing¾ Current good manufacturing practice draft.* Food and Drug Administration. August, 2003. Available at: www.fda.gov/cber/gdlns/steraseptic.pdf. Accessed February 2, 2004.

38. Bryan D, Marback R. Laminar-airflow equipment certification: What the pharmacist needs to know. *Am J Hosp Pharm.* 1984;41:1343–9.

39. National Institute for Occupational Safety and Health. Prepublication Copy—Preventing Occupational Exposures to Antineoplastic and Other Hazardous Drugs in Healthcare Settings, June 7, 2004. www.cdc.gov/niosh/docs/2004-HazDrugAlert/pdfs/2004-HazDrugAlert.pdf Accessed July 16, 2004.

40. NSF International. Available at www.nsf.org/standards/. Accessed February 2, 2004.

41. Agalloco J. Barriers, isolators and microbial control. *PDA J Pharm Sci and Technol.* 1999; 53:48–53.

42. Parenteral Drug Association. Design and validation of isolator systems for the manufacturing and testing of health care products: Technical Report No.34. *PDA J Pharm Sci and Technol.* 2001;Sept/Oct:supplement TR34;55.

43. Landry C, Bussieres JF, Lebel P, et al. Factors affecting the sterility of work areas in barrier isolators and a biological safety cabinet. *Am J Health-Syst Pharm.* 2001;58:1009–14.

44. Rahe H. Understanding the critical components of a successful cleanroom and barrier isolator project. *Am J Health-Syst Pharm.* 2000;57:346–50.

45. Pilong A, Moore M. Conversion to isolators in a sterile preparation area. *Am J Health-Syst Pharm.* 1999;56:1978–80.

46. Akers J. Contamination control in isolators. *Advancing Applications in Contamination Control.* 2001;4:19–24.

47. American Society for Parenteral and Enteral Nutrition National Advisory Group on Standards and Practice Guidelines for Parenteral Nutrition. Safe practices for parenteral nutrition formulations. *J*

Parenter Enteral Nutr. 1998;22:49–66.

48. American Society of Health-System Pharmacists. Guidelines on the safe use of automated compounding Devices for the preparation of parenteral nutrition admixtures. *Am J Health-Syst Pharm.*

2000;57:1343–8.

49. Trautmen KA. *The FDA and Worldwide Quality System Requirements Guidebook for Medical Devices.* Milwaukee, WI: ASQ Quality Press; 1997.

18 | Environmental Monitoring

Eric S. Kastango*

*The author acknowledges Philip Schneider, who authored this chapter in the first edition of this text.

Introduction and Requirements

A good quality management program seeks to identify problems before they occur. Although there are several critical elements to consider when working in or managing a sterile compounding operation, environmental monitoring has received minimal consideration in hospital pharmacy practice.[1] In other industries, great attention is placed on the influence and impact that the operating environment has on the quality of the product. It is widely accepted in the pharmaceutical industry that production facility design, environment, and personnel have a direct effect on the sterility of aseptically prepared products. As such, it is essential to ensure that quality be built into sterile products before they are distributed.

Proper sterile compounding requires "A strict design regime, not only on the process area, but on the interactions with surrounding areas and the movement of people, materials and equipment so as not to compromise the aseptic conditions."[2] One of the general principles that is crucial in ensuring that quality is built into compounded sterile preparations is that the environment where sterile preparations are compounded is suitable for its intended purposes.[3] The intended purpose of the compounding environment is to control both human and non-human factors that can affect sterility or stability. There are several interconnected and dynamic variables that form the foundation of a solid environmental monitoring program (Figure 18-1). Failing to understand, maintain, and monitor the compounding environment has resulted in significant patient injury and death.[3-6] Engineering controls (anterooms, cleanrooms, horizontal and vertical airflow work benches, biological safety cabinets and isolators) and the associated controlled environments are utilized to prevent, reduce, and control potential contaminants from being introduced into compounded sterile preparations and to support environmental control programs.

In order to ascertain whether the cleanroom, the processes, and the employees are producing the desired results, data must be routinely and systematically gathered. By integrating monitoring and data collection into compounding processes, "management by facts" can take place versus "management by opinion." Facts are not known until they are identified through the systematic collection of data. From the data, conclusions can be drawn and decisions can be made that are far more likely

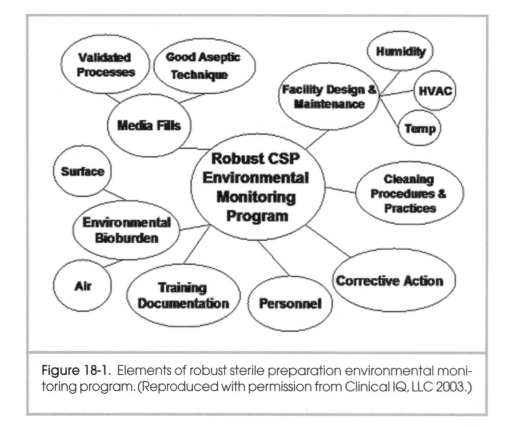

Figure 18-1. Elements of robust sterile preparation environmental monitoring program. (Reproduced with permission from Clinical IQ, LLC 2003.)

to result in desired outcomes. Establishing a comprehensive and robust environmental monitoring (EM) program will provide information on elements of a sterile compounding operation, which can[7]:

- Identify trends and address issues before they become critical. For example, environmental air and surface sampling can identify shifts in microbial bioburden that will stimulate assessment of potential points of failure such as improper employee gowning and gloving, improper cleaning procedures related to changes in maintenance personnel, or problems with HEPA filtration units.

- Facilitate a reflective process whereby an evidence-based assessment of potential points of failure can be identified, processes can be modified, and prevented from recurring.

USP <797> requires each risk level of operation to have a written environmental quality and control plan.[2] One of the most common areas of concern for pharmaceutical and medical device manufacturers that have received FDA warnings for violating good manufacturing practices involves environmental controls and monitoring.[8] Examples of citations are:

1. Facilities are not appropriately designed to minimize microbial contamination

2. Validation of environmental control systems are inadequate

3. Procedures intended to prevent microbial contamination are inadequate

4. Gowning procedures and its training program are not shown to be effective in minimizing microbial contamination of compounded preparations

5. Failure to initiate and achieve corrective action in response to out-of-limits situations secondary to environmental monitoring excursions

Over last several years, almost everyone has been affected by drug shortages and discontinuation of drug products. Many of these shortages and discontinuations have been caused by plant closures resulting from FDA citations involving environmental control and monitoring programs. The FDA takes these matters very seriously and with the passage of USP <797>, the state boards of pharmacy will also be moving to react in kind.

A comprehensive quality management program should include five elements:

1. Personnel controls

2. Environmental requirements and controls

3. Process validation testing (PVT)

4. End product testing

5. Staff education (both initially and on an ongoing basis).

This chapter focuses on environmental requirements and controls to assist in the development and implementation of an environmental monitoring program. It is important to ensure that environmentally controlled work areas operate within exacting specifications and are adequate for the functions being performed in them. These controls should be monitored in the following ways[9]:

- Semi-annual ISO classified work area testing and certification

- Routine environmental airborne particulates and microbiological monitoring

- Routine monitoring of operating temperatures and humidity

- Continuous positive pressure and pressure differentials or gradients between clean areas

- Continuous HEPA filtered air

- Maintaining environmentally zoned areas based on critical activities (i.e., ISO Class 5, 7, or 8)

- Routine cleaning of work areas

- Limiting access to environmentally controlled areas

Physical Plant Definitions

USP <797> requires that the environments where pharmacy activities (warehousing and storage, preparation and staging, and aseptic processing) occur be set up in such a manner as to provide the highest level of cleanliness possible. This is achieved through tiered "zones" of cleanliness, where the closer you are to the critical aseptic processing, the cleaner the environment (air and surfaces). Levels of cleanliness are achieved through various personnel- and engineering-related processes. The personnel-related processes include hand washing, gowning, masking, gloving and process and preparation work flows; the engineering-related processes include HEPA filtered air, laminar-airflow workbenches or isolators, room air exchanges, and positive pressure differentials between the various "zones" of cleanliness. It is important to define the physical plant areas (the "zones" of cleanliness) in the pharmacy that will meet USP <797> standards. They include the following areas:

Anteroom or controlled area

An anteroom or controlled area is any area adjacent to a buffer or a cleanroom where unsterilized products, in-process components, materials, and containers are handled. The supply air may or may not be controlled, but should be constructed and placed relative to the critical aseptic compounding areas so as to minimize personnel traffic and the introduction, generation, and retention of particulates. This area may be a common warehouse or storage/drug room next to the pharmacy compounding area. Temperature and humidity control are necessary. The area must be ISO Class 8 (FS209 Class 100,000) or ISO Class 9 (Class 1,000,000-Fed Std 209E).

Buffer zone or cleanroom

This space is designated for compounding sterile preparations. This room has a controlled number of airborne particles and is constructed and used in such a manner to minimize the introduction, generation and retention of particles inside the room, and to assure other critical operating factors such as temperature, humidity, and air pressure, are controlled as required by the facility design and type of compounding activities being performed (e.g., high-risk level). The laminar-airflow workbench or other engineering controls must be located in the buffer zone or cleanroom as stipulated by USP <797>.[2,10,11] Minimum ISO classification for this type of area as required by USP <797> is ISO Class 8.

Critical area

This area is where sterile products, solutions, preparations, containers or closures are manipulated and exposed to the environment. This environment is typically found within laminar-airflow workbenches or other engineering controls designed specifically to achieve a minimum ISO classification (as required by USP chapter 797) of ISO Class 5 or better.

In addition to the ISO standards, the American Society of Heating, Refrigeration and Air-Conditioning Engineers (AHRAE) has published guidelines that help further define these operating requirements in terms of air exchange rates and airflow velocities.

General Pharmacy Area

Temperature should be controlled in the range between 59° F and 86° F, with a limited number of extreme temperature conditions, especially in the warm months of the year. In order to control mold, mildew, electrostatic charges, the relative humidity (RH) of this area should be in the 30%–60% range (Figure 18-2). This area does not need to be classified with respect to air cleanliness.

Anteroom or Controlled Area

Table 18-1 summarizes the environmental requirements for anterooms. Temperature should be 72° F ± 5° F. In order to control mold, mildew, electrostatic charges, the RH of this area should be in the 30%–60% range. This room is considered clean and supports hand washing, gowning and gloving procedures. This area must have a classification of ISO Class 8 or better.

Buffer zones or cleanrooms

Table 18-2 summarizes the environmental requirements for buffer zones. Temperature should be 72° F ± 5° F, while RH should be in the 30%–60% range. Ideally, the volume of air in a controlled area should be exchanged at least 20 times per hour,[13] with the exception of isolators (see Chapter 4). To avoid particulates and contaminants from entering this area, positive air pressure must be maintained relative to adjacent support areas. The minimum industry standard for buffer zones and cleanrooms is no less than + 0.05 inches of water (WC). (WC is an acronym for inches of water [column] and is the unit of measurement commonly used to measure the difference between high and low pressures in controlled compounding environments). This will prevent "dirtier" air, which has large amounts of particulate matter, from entering cleaner areas (see Figure 18-3).

USP <797> states that buffer zones or cleanroom areas must meet ISO Class 8 (Class 100,000) standards or better. In addition to meeting an air particle standard, classified ar-

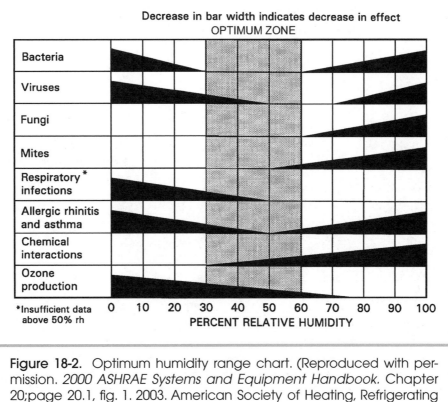

Figure 18-2. Optimum humidity range chart. (Reproduced with permission. *2000 ASHRAE Systems and Equipment Handbook.* Chapter 20;page 20.1, fig. 1. 2003. American Society of Heating, Refrigerating and Air-Conditioning Engineers, Inc.)

Table 18-1.

Environmental Requirements for Anterooms

Parameter	Requirement
Temperature	72° F ± 5° F
Relative humidity	30%–60%
Air exchange	20/hr
Percentage fresh air	5%–20%
Pressure differential	0.01 in of water
Air quality	
● Particulates	100,000 of ≥ 0.5 microns/cu ft
● Environmental bioburden	2.5 CFUs/cu ft

(The following tables are a composite of references from the first edition, ISO 14644-X Cleanroom standards and USP chapter 1206.)

Table 18-2.

Buffer Zone—Cleanrooms (Class ISO 8 (Fed Std 209E Class 100,000)[3]

Parameter	Requirement
Temperature	72° F ± 5° F
Relative humidity	0%–60%
Air exchange	20/hr
Percentage fresh air	5%–20%
Pressure differential	0.05 in of water to adjacent areas
Air quality	
● Particulates	100,000 of ≥ 0.5 microns/cu ft
● Environmental bioburden	2.5 CFU /cu ft

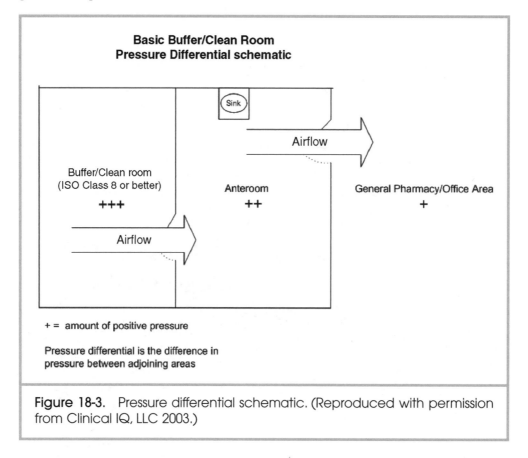

Figure 18-3. Pressure differential schematic. (Reproduced with permission from Clinical IQ, LLC 2003.)

eas within the pharmacy need to be environmentally monitored. The procedures and the methods used to collect air and surface microbial sampling data will be discussed later in the chapter.

Critical area

Table 18-3 summarizes the environmental requirements for critical areas. Because sterile components are manipulated in the critical areas in the process of compounding final sterile preparations, the requirements for the critical areas are more stringent than those for controlled areas. USP <797> requires ISO Class 5 environment or better. Air particle counts for ISO Class 5 conditions call for no more than 100 particles 0.5 µm or larger per cubic foot.

The key operating condition within a laminar-airflow workbench or isolator is HEPA filtered air moving at a velocity sufficient to remove particulate matter that might be introduced by either compounding personnel, components/component containers, or equipment. The recommended airflow velocity across the entire work surface should be maintained at 90 ft/min (±20%) for workbenches,

Table 18-3.

Critical Areas (ISO Class 5 (Fed Std 209E Class 100) Cleanrooms)

Parameter	Requirement
Temperature	N/A for engineered controls (workbenches or isolators)
	72° F ± 5° F
Relative humidity	30%–60%
Air velocity	45–55 fpm (feet per minute)
Air exchanges	450–525 fpm
Percentage fresh air	5%–20%
Pressure differential	0.05 in of water to adjacent areas
Air quality	
• Particulates	100 of ≥ 0.5 microns/cu ft
• Environmental bioburden	0.1 CFU/cu ft

Table 18-4.

Environmental Requirements for Critical Areas (ISO Class 5[Fed Std 209E Class 100] Engineering Controls)

Parameter	Requirement
Temperature	72° F ± 5° F
Relative humidity	30%–60%
Airflow	90 ft/min ± 20%
Air quality	
● Particulates	100 of ≥ 0.5 microns/cu ft
● Environmental bioburden	0.1 CFUs/cu ft

Table 18-5.

Recommended Testing Certification Intervals (ISO 14644-2)

Classification	Maximum Time Interval
Particle concentration limits	
≤ ISO Class 5	6 months
> ISO Class 5	12 months*
Airflow volume or airflow velocity	12 months
Air pressure differential	12 months

*(USP <797> requires max interval of 6 months.)

but may be lower for isolators. This operating condition is pre-engineered into the equipment being used, but needs to be routinely monitored to ensure that airflow velocity is being maintained. It is absolutely critical that any engineering control (workbench or isolator) be turned on and allowed to run for at least 15–30 minutes prior to starting aseptic compounding activities. All work surfaces must be sanitized with 3% hydrogen peroxide or 70% isopropyl alcohol prior to starting aseptic compounding. It is best to leave all engineering controls running continually, so that the critical aseptic compounding environment is maintained and that workbenches positively contribute to the cleanliness of the area and decrease the amount of circulating particulate matter in the air.

Equipment Testing And Certification

In order to verify proper operating condition and equipment functionality, engineering controls need to be tested and certified on a regular basis. There are three different operating phases in which classified areas can be tested and certified. They are[10]:

● As-built: This condition exists when the installation of the cleanroom is complete and the all of the utilities are functional but the room does not have any equipment and supplies present and/or people working.

● At-rest: This condition exists when the installation of the cleanroom or isolator is complete, the room has all supplies and equipment in place and is operational, but there are no people working in it. This is typically the condition that engineering controls and cleanrooms are tested and certified under.

● Operational: This condition exists when the room or isolator is operational and people are present and working.

Each piece of equipment will have specific manufacturer recommendations on testing and maintenance. It is recommended that semi-annual cleanroom or isolator certification include the measurement and documentation of the following[10,14]:

● Airflow volume and velocity (room air exchanges) tests

● Containment leakage test

● Aerosol challenge leakage test (for HEPA filters)

● Particle count

● Room pressurization test

Workbenches can be certified at the same time and the following tests should be performed:

● Aerosol challenge installation leak test

● Containment leakage test

● Particle count

● Velocity profile

● Backstreaming/induction leak test

● HEPA filter pressure drop

USP <797> requires bi-annual (twice a year) certification of the ISO classified rooms and engineering controls. Testing and certification should only be performed by a trained and qualified vendor. Routine particle counts can be done by trained pharmacy personnel as part of an ongoing environmental monitoring program.

Air particulate matter can be measured by two techniques: an electronic particle counter or aerosol challenge test. Particle counters are used to quantify the number of particles in classified but are not acceptable to certify ISO Class 5 environments (e.g., laminar-airflow workbenches or isolators). To classify a room as meeting a specific ISO classification, a number of sampling locations have to be surveyed by the vendor to generate a room classification. The number of sample locations is calculated by the size of room and the height of ceilings against the desired classification. Buffer zones or cleanrooms must be certified no less than every 6 months or whenever room modifications occur.

To verify the operating conditions of the HEPA filter under ISO Class 5 conditions, especially those found in engineering controls, an aerosol challenge test should be employed. This testing procedure involves heating liquid poly alpha olefin (PAO) and generating a polydispersed aerosol with a light scattering mean droplet diameter of 0.3-microns.[13] A known quantity of the PAO aerosol is introduced (pumped into the airflow cabinet) upstream (before) of the high-efficiency particulate air (HEPA) filter. A photometer probe is used to scan the entire filter face in an effort to detect any traces of PAO. A single probe reading equivalent to 0.01% of the upstream challenge indicates a significant leak in the HEPA filter. Depending on the severity of the leakage, HEPA filter holes can be sealed with RTV silicone. It the event the leak can be repaired and filter continues to fail the aerosol challenge, it will not meet ISO Class 5 particulate requirements, is unusable and has to be replaced.

Particle counters, which are available from a number of cleanroom vendors, are best used

Table 18-6.

Environmental Microbial Monitoring Program

Site	Baseline Colony-Forming Units	Low-Risk Action Level	High-Risk Action Level
Settling plates[a]			
A	0	3	2
STA or impaction[b] sampler			
A	0	3	2
Contact plates			
B1	2,3	6	4
C	5	10	7

[a]Based on 3-hr exposure, except 1 hr for A.
[b]Based on 10-cu ft samples.
Sterile drug products for home use. United States pharmacopeia, 24th rev./national formulary, 19th ed. Rockville, MD: United States Pharmacopeial Convention; 2000: 2130–2143.

to verify the number of particles in a room. Pharmacists should have their engineering controls (e.g., laminar-airflow workbenches) tested and certified by a qualified vendor who can perform the aerosol challenge test, along with other tests. ISO Class 5 environments should be certified no less than every 6 months or whenever the piece of equipment is moved.

Airflow velocity and/or volume (cubic feet per minute or CFM) is the speed of air blowing from the face of the HEPA filter and is 6–12 inches from the face of the workbench.[14] The recommended velocity is 90 feet per minute average, with uniformity within ± 20% across the entire work area. This has been interpreted to mean the air velocity averages between 72–108 feet per minute.[9,11,12] As the air travels, its velocity decreases and pockets of turbulence can be generated, potentially causing a backdraft of higher particulate air to enter the critical work areas. This is the reason why it is important to work within 6 inches from the edge of the laminar-airflow workbench. Airflow velocity is measured with an anemometer.

Pressurization is the measurement of air pressures between two adjoining areas where the air pressure in the more stringently classified area is higher than the pressure of the next classified area. Average pressure differentials between two adjoining areas (i.e., ISO 5 area to ISO 7 area) is typically + 0.05 inches WC. Pressure differential is measured with an electronic micromanometer.

Airflow visualization is done via a smoke-stick test to observe airflow patterns over critical work surfaces and to identify areas of air turbulence that could be reservoirs of excessive particles or bioburden. Hand-held small volume smoke generators (e.g., smoke sticks) containing titanium tetrachloride generate dense white smoke that can be used to observe airflow patterns.

Temperature and RH can be measured using inexpensive thermometers and hygrometers, respectively. They are readily available from cleanroom suppliers. More expensive devices offer printing capabilities for documenting environmental requirements.

Table 18-7 summarizes the schedule of test parameters required to be performed and their respective time intervals.

Air and Surface Environmental Testing

It is important to monitor the microbial bioburden of controlled work areas by collecting air and surface samples routinely. The total amount of airborne particles (viable and nonviable) should be determined twice a year during routine workbench and cleanroom certification. This is referred to as a "room particle count." Routine ongoing environmental monitoring involves establishing baseline data for the microbial bioburden of the controlled work areas. Bioburden monitoring provides an inexpensive but effective method of tracking and trending viable contaminants in the controlled pharmacy compounding areas. Bioburden monitoring also provides a good way to monitor the effectiveness of cleaning and sanitizing procedures. Several locations within the airflow workbench, cleanroom and anteroom should be identified as sampling sites. These sampling sites, and their associated frequency of sampling, should reflect an understanding of the relationship of the location to the overall operation being performed (e.g., sterile compounding, gowning and gloving, labeling). Focusing on sample sites that pose the greatest potential hazard of introducing contamination allows for the rapid identification of a potentially significant contamination source. Otherwise, an emerging or existing source of contamination may be missed, or an excessive amount of time may elapse before a serious problem is detected.

Table 18-7.

Recommended Environmental Monitoring Program

Element	Frequency		
	Low-risk	Medium-risk	High-risk
Temperatures	Daily	Daily	Daily
Humidity	Daily	Daily	Daily
Pressure differentials	Daily	Daily	Daily
HEPA filter aerosol challenge leakage test	Semi-annual	Semi-annual	Semi-annual
Room particle certification	Semi-annual	Semi-annual	Semi-annual
Airflow volume and velocity (room air exchanges) tests	Semi-annual	Semi-annual	Semi-annual
Containment leakage test	Annual	Annual	Semi-annual
Room pressurization test	Annual	Annual	Semi-annual
Environmental bioburden monitoring:			
Air	Monthly	Monthly	Weekly
Surface	Monthly	Monthly	Weekly

ISO 14644-2:2000 – "Specification for Testing Cleanrooms and Associated Controlled Environments to Prove Continued Compliance" International Organization for Standardization. 2000.

An effective environmental bioburden testing program required by USP <797> for sterile compounding is based upon the use of various methods for collecting air and surface environmental sample on a nutrient culture medium, incubating at a temperature and for a time period conducive to the growth of discrete colonies of growth. The count, reported as colony forming units (CFUs), is a measurement of microbial contamination of the environment at the time and under the conditions of sampling.[15]

Air and surface sampling involve collecting environmental "snapshots" of microorganisms present at various sample locations in a measured volume of air on tryptic soy broth (TSB)/ agar (TSA) plates that support the growth of many types of microorganisms. Per Figure 18-4, various locations are identified as potential sampling sites. Sampling sites should be chosen by the criticality of compounding that occurs at those locations. All environmental monitoring should occur under dynamic conditions. Dynamic conditions are under normal operating conditions, during regular work activity, and ideally conducted towards the end of the day to monitor "worst case conditions," when the environmental bioburden and particulate matter should be at its highest level. It should be done routinely to generate operating data that can be used to identify shifts in control and trends. A baseline, sample should also occur under at-rest or static conditions. At-rest environmental bioburden monitoring can evaluate the operating status of engineering controls, operating equipment, and the effectiveness of cleaning and sanitizing procedures.

Each location is assigned three values: baseline (ideal), alert, and action limit (Table 18-1). Before the baseline is determined, the controlled area should be thoroughly cleaned with a disinfecting detergent. After the cleaned areas are dry, locations from which samples are obtained should be tested. In ISO 5 environments (workbenches or isolators), the ideal CFU baseline should be zero. The integrity of ISO 5 environments is closely correlated with the sterility of compounded sterile preparations.

Air sampling

Environmental air microbial bioburden can be measured by either passive or active air sampling. Both of these approaches have a role in monitoring the sterile compounding environment.

For passive air sampling, TSA settling plates are used that are 100 mm in diameter. They should be exposed to room air for a period of from 1 hour to 3 hours. Exposure of longer than 3 hours causes the agar to dry out. Air sampling is a cost-effective way of obtaining quantitative data relative to the viable microbial particles expected to settle from the air at each sampling site. CFUs isolated on TSA plates should be sent for microbiological identification of the microbial flora.

For active air sampling, a large volume of air is drawn over the growth medium. Three different devices can be used.

Monitoring devices

Reuter centrifugal sampler—This device draws up to 40 L/min of air through rotary blades, forcing particles against a nutrient agar strip by centrifugal force. It is the most convenient and least expensive of the three devices and is readily available.

Slit-to-agar impaction sampler—This device employs a revolving plate containing the growth medium under a fixed-slot orifice. Air is drawn through the slot over the medium by vacuum. With this device, a concentration-time relationship can be established.

Liquid impingement—With this device, air is drawn into the unit by vacuum. The volume of air is determined by the orifice size. Particles and microorganisms are "impinged" onto the liquid, which is then filtered. The filters are placed on nutrient media and monitored for microbial growth.

Surface sampling

Environmental surface microbial bioburden can be measured by three techniques, which include Rodac contact plates, swabs and paddles.

Rodac Contact Plates: Surface sampling can be performed with raised TSA plates that are 60 mm in diameter (Rodac plates). The TSA in Rodac plates is mixed with polysorbate 80 and lecithin, which inactivates many residual disinfectants.[16] Polysorbate 80 neutralizes phenols, hexachlorophene, and formalin, and lecithin inactivates quaternary ammonium compounds. During sampling, a Rodac plate is pressed onto the area to be tested. Any microorganisms on the surface of the area tested

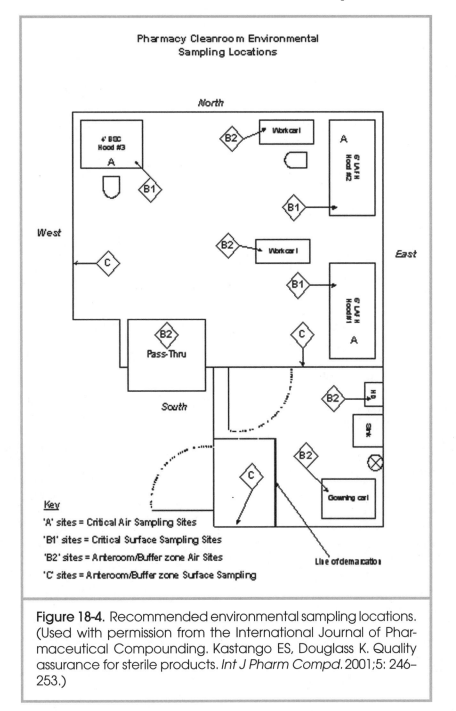

Figure 18-4. Recommended environmental sampling locations. (Used with permission from the International Journal of Pharmaceutical Compounding. Kastango ES, Douglass K. Quality assurance for sterile products. *Int J Pharm Compd.* 2001;5: 246–253.)

(which should ideally be flat) are transferred onto the Rodac plate. After the sample has been obtained, the area tested should be wiped down with isopropyl alcohol to remove any residue left by the Rodac plate. These plates are prepared with an appropriate TSA whose surface is higher than the sides of the plate. Then the plate is incubated. This device is suitable for monitoring flat surfaces such as laminar-airflow workbenches, floors, and walls. Contact plates can be employed to establish and monitor the efficacy of disinfec-

tants and/or cleaning techniques.

Swabs: By aseptic technique, swabs are rubbed over a test surface and immersed in a liquid medium. If the surface is contaminated, there will be growth in the medium. Swabs are suited to irregular surfaces, and results are more qualitative than with contact plates.

Agar paddles: Like Rodac contact plates, plastic paddles are layered with TSA and used to sample various surface and are ideal for surfaces that are not flat.

Surface testing materials may be obtained from the microbiology laboratory or infection surveillance department of most hospitals. Alternatively, these supplies are available from a number of vendors.

Buffer zones have the recommended number of viable microorganisms, per cubic foot (or cubic meter) of air. In an ISO Class 7 (FS 209 Class 10,000) environment, the requirement is no more than 0.5 CFU per cu ft of air.[17]

The number of viable microorganism as measured by either air or surface sampling should be no more than 0.1 CFU per cubic feet of air. Ideally, the count should be zero since sterile fluid pathways (vials, needles, open ampules, etc.) are exposed to the air in the area.

In addition to air quality, recommended standards have been established for surface cleanliness and the maximum number of CFU per sampled area. In an ISO Class 5 environment, the number is 3 CFU per contact plate (24-30 cm^2). The sample site is either critical work surfaces within airflow workbench or the floor. In an ISO Class 7 environment, the number is 5 CFU per Rodac plate (24-30 cm^2) for all surfaces except the floor. The maximum number for the floor is 10 CFU.

It is critical to understand that the environmental bioburden testing, especially of those critical areas like the ISO Class 5 workbench surfaces should not be considered as a surrogate sterility test (i.e., a positive test on a critical surface test does not mean that the compounded preparation is sterile.[18]

Recommended Environmental Monitoring Program

Like the FDA cGMPs, USP <797> is ambiguous in the exact details of how to implement the requirements. Pharmacists must be able demonstrate that their sterile preparation compounding program is "under control." With some planning and constant vigilance in ensuring that the critical elements of a robust environmental monitoring program are performed and documented regularly, environmental control can be easily demonstrated and monitored. Sources of environmental monitoring equipment include www.cleanrooms.com, www.a2cs.com. Search the buyer's guide on either website.

Summary

Current standards of practice warrant a comprehensive environmental monitoring program that will exceed the historical annual workbench certification. By routinely monitoring the critical operating parameters of aseptic compounding environment, a robust program can be created with some investment that can demonstrate the environment is functioning properly and being maintained.

References

1. International Society of Professional Engineers. *ISPE Sterile Manufacturing Facilities Guide*. Volume 3. ISPE Publications. January 1999.
2. Pharmaceutical Compounding—Sterile Preparations. In: United States pharmacopeia, rev./national formulary, Rockville, MD: United States Pharmacopeial Convention; in press.
3. Hallissy E, Russell S. Who's mixing your drugs? Bad medicine: Pharmacy mix-ups a recipe for misery; some drugstores operate with very little oversight. *San Francisco Chronicle*. June 23, 2002.
4. Officials to Shut Pharmacy [transcript]. KTVU news. July 6, 2001. Available at: http://www.bayinsider.com/partners/ktvu/news/2001/07/06/meningitis.html. Accessed July 6, 2002.
5. North Carolina Department of Health and Human Services. Painkiller suspected in fourth N.C. meningitis case. Available at: www.dhhs.state.nc.us/ pressrel/10-18-02.htm. Accessed September 14, 2003.
6. Centers for Disease Control and Prevention. *Exophiala* infection from contaminated injectable steroids prepared by a compounding pharmacy—United States, July–November 2002. Available at: http://www.cdc.gov/mmwr/preview/mmwrhtml/mm5149a1.htm. Accessed October 5, 2003.
7. Kastango ES, Douglass, K. *Good Compounding Practices, ICALM™ Training Series* (multimedia CD-ROM). Denver, CO: Coram Healthcare; 1999.
8. FDA/PDA meeting. "An industry perspective on environmental monitoring presentation." September 2002. Available at: http://www.pda-it.org/legnani.pdf.

Accessed September 3, 2003

9. Kastango ES, DeMarco S. Pharmacy cleanroom project management considerations: an experience-based perspective. *Int J Pharm Compd.* 2001;5:221–5

10. International Organization for Standardization Standard 14644-1 *Cleanrooms and associated environments—Part 1: Classification of air cleanliness.* 1st ed. Switzerland, 1999. Available at: www.iso.ch.

11. American Society of Health-System Pharmacists. ASHP Guidelines on quality assurance for pharmacy-prepared sterile products. *Am J Health-Syst Pharm.* 2000; 57:1150–69.

12. International Organization for Standardization Standard 14644-2 *Cleanrooms and associated environments—Part 2: Specifications for testing and monitoring to prove continued compliance with ISO-14644-1.* 1st ed. Switzerland, 2000. Available at: www.iso.ch.

13. International Organization for Standardization Draft Standard 14644-3 *Cleanrooms and associated environments – Part 3:Metrology and test methods.* 1st

ed. Switzerland, 2002. Available at: www.iso.ch.

14. Institute of Environmental Sciences and Technology. *IEST-RP-CC006.2:Testing Cleanrooms.* Mount Prospect, Ill: IEST; 2000.

15. Sterile drug products for home use. United States pharmacopeia, 24th rev./ national formulary, 19th ed. Rockville, MD: United States Pharmacopeial Convention; 2000: 2130–2143

16. Brummer, B. Influence of possible disinfectant transfer on s*taphylococcus aureus* plate counts after agar contact sampling. *Appl. Environ. Microbiol.* 1976;32:80–4.

17. Block SS. AAMI steam sterilization and sterility assurance in health care facilities. In: Block SS, ed. *Disinfection, Sterilization, and Preservation.* 5th ed. Philadelphia, PA: Lippincott Williams & Wilkins; 2000:22.

18. Food and Drug Administration. *FDA's concept paper on sterile drug products.* Bethesda, MD: PDA letter (January 2003); volume 39, number 1:page 7.

19 | Dealing with Latex Allergies

*Stephen K. Hetey**

*The author acknowledges Philip Schneider, who authored this chapter in the first edition of this text.

Background

Documentation of natural rubber latex (NRL) allergy among healthcare workers was first noted in 1984.[1] Although earlier reports do exist, this was the first to document anaphylactic reactions among healthcare workers to surgical gloves. Latex allergy has, therefore, been coined as a "new disease." The prevalence of this allergy has reached "epidemic" proportions in highly exposed populations since 1983. Estimates of the incidence of latex allergy throughout the general population range from 1%–6%,[2] while certain pediatric populations range from 18%–73%.[3,4] Among healthcare workers, the projected incidence of NRL allergy is between 8% and 17%.[5-7] Additionally, there has been a corresponding increase in public awareness of latex allergy. The incidence data on latex allergy vary according to skin test methods used, small sample populations, and the use of selected populations.[7]

History

Latex Origins and Uses

The oldest rubber artifacts have been found in Veracruz, Mexico, and were carbon dated back to 1600 B.C.[8] These early Mesoamerican artifacts were made from a latex derived from the *Castilla elastica* tree. This *Castilla* latex was too brittle to retain its shape and had to be processed with juice from a morning glory vine to create a more malleable and elastic product.[8]

Today, nearly all commercial latex is a natural product derived from the latex sap of *Hevea brasiliensis* tree. The latex derived from this tree contains rubber particles referred to as natural rubber latex (NRL) which is widely used in the manufacturing of medical devices as well as everyday articles. When processed, this NRL has the highly desirable properties with which we are all familiar.[1]

Source of Latex Allergens

The two basic manufacturing types of NRL products are molded and dipped. Molded rubber products are comprised of dried rubber and coagulated latex. These products are made rigid through compression. Items falling into this category include drug vial stoppers, syringe plungers and intravascular injection ports used in virtually all healthcare settings.

Dipped rubber products are, as the name implies, manufactured through a process of dipping a mold into NRL. Examples of these types of products include surgical gloves, coatings for tool handles, and condoms.

The distinction between these two types of manufacturing processes is critical to antigenicity. Molded rubber products do not leach antigens to any appreciable extent, whereas dipped rubber products leach antigens in abundance.[9,10] Additionally, dipped rubber products, e.g., surgical gloves, are often manufactured with a dry lubricant such as corn starch which serves as a potent vehicle for the aerosolization of NRL antigens. NRL antigens are ubiquitous in nature and can be detected in NRL products, foods, spices, pollen and plants. This ubiquity raises the possibility that sensitization can occur from multiple sources and may be difficult to determine in individual patients. Certain fruits such as bananas, chestnuts, kiwi, avocado, and tomato show cross-reactivity, presumably due to resemblance to a latex protein component.[9] Hence, the term *latex-fruit syndrome*.[11] Sensitization may, therefore, actually occur from nonrubber products.

Allergic Reactions

People with allergies experience hypersensitive immune system responses to substances called allergens. Common allergens include dust, pollen and pet dander. Allergens are a type of antigen, which is any foreign substance that triggers an immune response. These allergens include substances that are innocuous to non-allergic subjects as well as generally harmful such as viruses and bacteria. Allergic reactions have been classified as Types I, II, III or IV. Each type has unique characteristics and time of onset. Allergic reactions can involve most of the components of the immune system including cellular, immunoglobulins, complement and cytokines.

Type I reactions (IgE mediated) are also referred to as immediate and anaphylactic reactions. These generally occur within 30 minutes of exposure to the antigen (e.g., protein in NRL) and are the most severe reaction. On initial exposure, allergen from NRL binds to immuno-

Table 19-1.

Type I Reactions to Latex

Cardiovascular	Hypotension, sinus tachycardia, arrhythmias, cardiac arrest
Gastrointestinal	Nausea, vomiting, diarrhea, abdominal cramping
Respiratory	Shortness of breath, wheezing, bronchospasm, cyanosis, laryngeal edema, respiratory arrest
Skin	Flushing, urticaria, pruritis, rash
Systemic	Faintness, general edema, feeling of "impending doom"

Reprinted with permission from *J Intrave Nurs* 1999;22:281-291. Lippincott Williams & Wilkins, Baltimore.

globulin E on the basophils or mast cells. During this initial exposure to the NRL antigen, predisposed individuals produce IgE specific for this antigen. On subsequent exposure to the antigen, an IgE-antigen complex is formed and binds to the basophil or mast cell. This binding results in the release of inflammatory mediators such as histamine, serotonin, chemotactic factors, bradykinin, etc. Systemic and anaphylactic reactions to NRL are mediated through Type I allergic reactions.

Type II or cytotoxic reactions are characterized by cell destruction (usually blood elements) secondary to cell-associated antigen initiated cytolysis and usually occurs within 5–12 hours. Type II allergic reactions are mediated by IgG or IgM.

Type III or immune complex reactions are caused by antigen-antibody complexes that deposit on blood vessel walls and activate complement resulting in local or disseminated inflammatory reactions. Type III allergic reactions typically manifest in 3–8 hours.

Type IV or cell mediated or delayed hypersensitivity reactions occur within 24–48 hours and are caused by antigen activation of lymphocytes (T cells) which in turn release inflammatory mediators. Clinical hallmarks include erythema, scaling and vesiculation.[12] This is generally an allergic contact dermatitis and is much more common among latex sensitive individuals than Type I reactions and is not life threatening (see Table 19-1).[13]

Identification of NRL Allergens

NRL contains more than 200 different proteins.[14] Ten of these proteins bind IgE of individuals who are allergic to latex and have been recognized by the International Union of Immunological Societies as being relevant to latex allergy. These are labeled *Hevea brasiliensis* latex protein allergens (HEV b 1 through 10).[14] Studies that detected the presence of IgE antibody to the HEV b allergens among various groups of latex sensitive individuals have identified different sensitizing antigens for each group (see Table 19-2).[14] The relevance of these data suggest different mechanisms of acquired sensitivity to NRL. For example, health care workers are exposed to airborne NRL allergens or contact with latex gloves. The antigens to which this group is sensitive are water soluble, whereas children with spina bifida recognize hydrophobic proteins that are tightly bound to other particles. Exposure to hydrophobic proteins probably occurs during the multiple surgical procedures encountered by children with spina bifida.[14]

Diagnosis of Latex Allergy

The diagnosis of latex allergy is based on a focused medical history and physical examination along with positive *in vitro* testing.[2,15,16] Risk factors for latex allergy (Table 19-3)[14] must be considered in the diagnosis.

Serological testing involves the quantitative measurement of serum-specific IgE antibodies to latex using a radioallergosorbent test (RAST). Currently, there are no commercially available latex extract skin testing reagents in the United States.[17] However, various scientific studies[2,11,18] have demonstrated the sensitivity, specificity and safety of a skin-prick test using ammoniated latex, nonammoniated

Table 19-2.

Sensitizing Antigens in NRL (HEVb 1-7)

- Spina bifida (1, 2, 3)
- Health workers (1, 5, 6)
- Children (6)
- Kiwi (5)
- Potato/tomato (7)
- Avocado, chestnut, banana (6)

HEVb, *Hevea brasiliensis* latex protein allergen. Ten NRL proteins bind IgE of latex allergic individuals have been recognized by the International Union of Immunological Societies; these are labeled *Hevea brasiliensis* latex protein allergens (HEV b 1 through 10).

Adapted with permission from Table 1 and Table IV, *Journal of Allergy and Clinical Immunology;*110:S107-S110. John J Condemi, ©2002 American Academy of Allergy, Asthma and Immunology.

latex and extracts from latex gloves. Hamilton and Adkinson,[15] in a skin-prick study of 358 adults, found that none of the subjects with a history of latex allergy developed an episode of systemic anaphylaxis. Some subjects did develop signs of mild systemic reactions such as pruritis, rash, rhinitis, ocular itch or urticaria after skin testing.

Data

There is some controversy around the best practice for latex avoidance in the preparation of sterile products. Manufacturers of parenteral products continue to minimize or eliminate latex from components of their drug containers. The only definitive way to ascertain the latex content of parenteral products is through communication with individual manufacturers. Inquiries should specifically identify products by lot number. Additionally, data regarding latex content may change as manufacturers change.

Yunginger et al.[10] developed an inhibition immunoassay using latex-specific human IgE. The limit of latex protein detection of the immunoassay is 250 ng/mL. Thomsen and Burke,[19] using this inhibition immunoassay technique, performed a quantitative analysis of latex allergen contamination of solutions

Table 19-3.

Risk Factors for the Development of NRL Sensitivity

- Health care worker
- Rubber industry worker who manufactures latex products
- Spinal cord abnormalities
- Multiple surgical procedures
- Multiple catheterizations
- Atopy
- Food allergy

Adapted with permission from Table 1 and Table IV, *Journal of Allergy and Clinical Immunology;*110:S107-S110. John J. Condemi, ©2002 American Academy of Allergy, Asthma and Immunology.

from vials with NRL stoppers. Their data indicate no detectable difference in latex allergen concentrations between standard and latex allergy precaution preparation methods. Therefore, manipulation of the vial to remove vial stoppers had no detectable effect on the amount of latex allergen in the medication. Manipulation did, however, result in 1 of 20 vials supporting bacterial growth. These findings were further corroborated by my personal communication with Dr. John Yunginger (Allergic Diseases Research Laboratory, Mayo Clinic, 2000 September 18) whose laboratory has performed extensive basic science and clinical research in the area of latex allergy. His data support the Thomsen study.

Another study by Primeau et al.[18] performed *in vivo* and *in vitro* analyses on a series of standard solutions in pharmaceutical-grade vials capped with either NRL (2 types) or a synthetic (3 types), nonrubber closure. All vials were stored inverted at room temperature until their use within a 9-month period. Vial closures were subjected to either no punctures (0P) or 40 punctures (40P) using a 21-gauge needle. A total of 23 subjects (12 latex allergic and 11 without latex allergy) were challenged in a double-blind fashion with puncture (prick) skin tests and intradermal skin tests. All subjects were negative to the puncture skin test. Results of the intradermal skin test reactions with 0P and 40P solutions were all negative in the 11 subjects without latex allergy. In the latex allergic group, 2 subjects had positive reactions to solutions from 0P natural rubber closure containing vials. In the latex allergic group, 5 subjects experienced a positive reaction to the 40P solutions containing a natural rubber closure. Additionally, 2 subjects from the latex allergic group exhibited positive intradermal skin test reaction to 0P and 40P solutions from vials with a synthetic closure. Upon rechallenge both subjects had negative results. The blind was broken to perform *in vitro* analyses. Inhibition analysis results of the 2 natural rubber closures (95.3% and 66% natural rubber) detected 6 and 7 Allergen Units (AU) of latex allergen per gram. No allergen (<0.5AU/g) was detected in extracts from synthetic closures or any of the solutions stored in 0P or 40P vials. These data are concordant with the results of the Thomsen and Burke[19] study in which only extracted closures and not solutions stored in vials with punctured closures contained detectable latex allergen.

Significance of the Data

Data from the Primeau[18] study support the fact that latex allergen can be released into pharmaceutical solutions through direct contact during manufacture and storage in vials with NRL closures. Since there is no known method by which these allergenic proteins can be removed from these solutions, there is no rationale for removing the closure prior to withdrawal of the pharmaceutical. Multiple needle penetrations of NRL vial closures seem to increase the chance of a positive intradermal response from latex allergic patients; allergen units per ml of solution in all vials was below the *in vitro* test threshold (<0.5 AU/ml). Another confounding factor was the fact that solution from one of the synthetic (bromobutyl rubber) closure vials resulted in a positive intradermal skin test in 2 different subjects, one after the no puncture method and the other after the 40 puncture method. One hypothesis for this "idiosyncratic" reaction is that accelerator chemicals or other ingredients in bromobutyl rubber may induce immediate-type hypersensitivity reactions in the skin. This hypothesis is not supported by data in the literature and requires further clinical study. Therefore, using a "one-stick" rule for vial closures does not provide adequate protection against intradermal response in patients who are latex allergic and supports the

need for pharmaceutical manufacturers to provide latex-free packaging, including closures. Additionally, pharmaceutical manufacturers should provide full disclosure of latex content on all labeling. The data also validate the fact that there is no correlation between latex-specific IgE titer and intradermal response. One of the 12 latex allergic subjects with the highest latex-specific IgE titer was negative in all tests. Although these data provide valuable information for latex allergy management, additional studies are required to address some of the apparent inconsistencies.

Best Practices and Guidelines

Sensitization to latex allergens is an on-going concern for all segments of the population, especially among healthcare workers and children with spina bifida and those who have had multiple surgeries early in life. Current management of latex allergy or sensitivity involves avoidance and reduction of cumulative exposure. Health systems should create an environment that is as free of NRL as possible. Even though more and more pharmaceutical manufacturers are eliminating NRL from their products, practitioners often have no easy method for determining which contain NRL. Frequently, pharmaceutical manufacturers do not have this information.

Since leaching of latex allergens from closures containing NRL has been demonstrated, the allergen source should be removed from pharmaceutical products at the point of manufacture because suitable latex-free substitutes are readily available.[5,15,18]

The single greatest threat to latex-allergic patients and healthcare givers in the healthcare environment is the use of powdered latex gloves.[17] With the availability of various synthetic copolymer and nitrile compounds used in the manufacture of latex-free, powder-free, sterile surgical and exam gloves, there is no reason for the continued use of latex.[15]

Management

Guidelines for the management of latex allergy should include:

- Asking all patients and employees about latex sensitivity; using a screening questionnaire if relevant.

- Including latex allergy information on patients' charts and identification bracelets.

- Identifying patient room as "latex precaution" and entering in all relevant areas of signage, notes and databases.

- Distributing latex allergy protocol and lists of latex-free substitutes for latex-containing materials that may contact patients or employees.

- Eliminating all latex products from the environment.

- Using intravenous tubing made of polyvinyl chloride (PVC).

- Checking adhesives and tapes, including electrocardiography electrodes and dressing supplies for latex content, where available.

- Stocking all crash carts with latex-free supplies.

- Notifying dietary staff of relevant food allergies and latex cross-allergenic fruits such as bananas, chestnuts, kiwi, avocado, tomato, etc.; also, eliminating the use of powdered, latex gloves in food handling.

- Advising pharmacy staff to use standard aseptic technique in the preparation of parenteral products without removing vial closures.

- As an extra precaution for the highly sensitive individual, recommending that ampules of drug be used whenever possible in the preparation of parenteral products.

Areas for Future Developments and Therapies

Currently, the diagnosis of latex allergy is problematic since no FDA-licensed skin test reagent is available.[9,15,17] *In vitro* tests for latex IgE show relatively low sensitivity and inconsistent results. The development of standardized or recombinant latex allergen test reagents may increase testing accuracy.[17]

Clinical trials of specific immunotherapy using a standardized latex extract are very limited at this time. Preliminary studies showed promising results in healthcare workers with occupational exposure. A study by Leynadier et al.[20] was the first multi-center, randomized, double-blind, placebo-controlled trial on this subject. The clinical benefits observed during this study included a significant improvement of rhinitis, conjunctivitis and cutaneous symptoms. Immunotherapy also decreased allergen-specific conjunctival reactivity. Results appear promising, but will require further trials on a larger number of patients.

Genomics is an additional area for future research that may identify therapies that can effectively block the IgE-mediated Type I anaphylactoid reactions. Variants in many different genes form the basis for the genetic contribution to disease across the spectrum.[21]

Summary

The predisposing and causative factors for latex sensitivity and allergy are very complex. The relatively "recent" awareness of this allergy has been attributed, at least in part, to the 1987 publication of the Centers for Disease Control guidelines for universal precautions in the spread of HIV and Hepatitis B.[1,15] These guidelines precipitated a significant increase in the use of protective gloves, all of which were latex at that time. Consequently, predisposed healthcare workers and patients became sensitized and, in some cases, developed a bona fide allergy. As demonstrated by the studies presented in this chapter, pharmacy personnel may actually do more harm than good by removing vial closures through the risk of bacterial contamination. Health-system pharmacies that use latex-free syringes, tubing and devices for parenteral compounding are practicing latex avoidance for all patients. Manufacturers can and should remove all latex from drug packaging and label accordingly. As of September 30, 1998, all medical devices or medical device packaging containing natural rubber latex have been required to be labeled accordingly by the FDA.[22] The ultimate barometer of latex or any other allergy is the human body. Patients or employees who are exquisitely sensitive to latex may require additional precautions (e.g., using ampules of drug whenever possible) to insure their safety.

References

1. Ownby DR. A history of latex allergy. *J Allergy Clin Immunol.* 2002;110:S27–S31.
2. Poley GE, Slater JE. Latex allergy. *J Al-*

lergy Clin Immunol. 2000;105:1054–62.

3. Anonymous. Latex allergy fact sheet for patients with spina bifida and those who undergo multiple invasive procedures [press release]. *Am Assoc Nurse Anesth.* April 11, 2002.

4. Slater JE, Mostello LA, Shaer C. Rubber-specific IgE in children with spina bifida. *J Urol.* 1991;146:578–9.

5. American Society of Health-System Pharmacists. ASHP latex allergy resource center. Available at: www.ashp.org. Accessed February 11, 2003.

6. Liss GM, Sussman GL, Deal K, et al. Latex allergy: epidemiological study of 1351 hospital workers. *Occup Environ Med.* 1997;54:335–42.

7. Yunginger JW. Latex allergy in the workplace: an overview of where we are. *Ann Allergy Asthma Immunol.* 1999;83:630–33.

8. Hosler D, Burkett SL, Tarkanian MJ. Prehistoric polymers: rubber processing in ancient Mesoamerica. *Science.* 1999;284:1988–91.

9. Sumana R. Latex allergy. *Am Family Physician.* 1998;57:93–100.

10. Yunginger JW, Jones RT, Fransway AF, et al. Extractable latex allergens and proteins in disposable medical gloves and other rubber products. *J Allergy Clin Immunol.* 1994;93:836–42.

11. Niggemann B, Breiteneder H. Latex allergy in children. *Int Arch Allergy Immunol.* 2000;121:98–107.

12. American Academy of Dermatology. Position paper on latex allergy. *J Am Acad Dermatol.* 1998:39:98–106.

13. Gritter M. Latex allergy: Prevention is the key. *J Intraven Nurs.* 1999;22:281–91.

14. Condemi JJ. Allergic reactions to natural rubber latex at home, to rubber products, and to cross-reacting foods. *J Allergy Clin Immunol.* 2002;110:S107–S110.

15. Hepner DL, Castells MC. Latex allergy: an update. *Anesth Analg.* 2003;96:1219–29.

16. Hunt LW, Kelkar P, Reed CE, et al. Management of occupational allergy to natural rubber latex in a medical center: The importance of quantitative latex allergen measurement and objective follow-up. *J Allergy Clin Immunol.* 2002; 110:S96–S106.

17. Charous BL, Blanco C, Tarlo S, et al. Natural rubber latex allergy after 12 years: Recommendations and perspectives. *J Allergy Clin Immunol.* 2002; 109:31–4.

18. Primeau MN, Adkinson NF, Hamilton RG. Natural rubber pharmaceutical vial closures release latex allergens that produce skin reactions. *J Allergy Clin_Immunol.* 2001;107:958–62.

19. Thomsen DJ, Burke TG. Lack of latex allergen contamination of solutions withdrawn from vials with natural rubber stoppers. *Am J Health-Syst Pharm.* 2000;57:44–7.

20. Leynadier F, Herman D, Vervloet D, et al. Specific immunotherapy with a standardized latex extract versus placebo in allergic healthcare workers. *J Allergy_Clin Immunol.* 2000;106:585–90.

21. Burke W. Genomics as a probe for disease biology. *N Engl J Med.* 2003; 349:969–74.

22. Anonymous. Natural rubber-containing medical devices: user labeling. Food and Drug Administration. *Federal Register.* 1997; 62:51021–31.

20 | Process Validation

*Eric S. Kastango**

*The author acknowledges Philip Schneider, who authored this chapter in the first edition.

This chapter is based on requirements detailed in USP <797>, which is more extensive than the ASHP Guidelines on Quality Assurance for Pharmacy-Prepared Sterile Products. Process validation is evidence-based science that is used extensively in other industries like pharmaceutical manufacturers, semiconductors and aerospace to ensure quality.

Principles of Process Validation

The sterility and quality of compounded sterile preparations is dependent on a number of factors, including the types of components (sterile vs. nonsterile), the methods of compounding (open vs. closed systems), compounding environment, the controls during compounding, and final preparation testing. Due to the complexity of compounded sterile preparations, routine final preparation testing alone often is not sufficient to assure sterility and quality, for several reasons.[1] These include:

- Insufficient sensitivity to verify sterility and quality of the compounded preparation (e.g., antibiotics or cytotoxic agents)

- Destructive testing would be required to show that compounding produced a sterile and correct preparation. Absolute sterility cannot be practically demonstrated without testing every unit within a batch.[2]

- Poor compounding technique or error can yield false-positive results rather than detect a nonsterile preparation.

- Routine final preparation tests do not reveal all variations in quality and sterility (e.g., visually inspecting TPN or other compounded preparations).

Process validation involves establishing documented evidence that a specific compounding procedure will consistently result in a final compounded preparation that meets its pre-determined specifications of sterility with a high degree of confidence.[3] It is critical to understand the principles of sterility by understanding the difference between sterility assurance levels (SAL) and rates of contamination.[4] The definition of sterility is the absence of all viable microorganisms. Rates of contamination involve the number of compounded preparations that are nonsterile within a batch after preparation. SAL is defined as the probability of an item being nonsterile after it has been exposed to a validated sterilization process (steam, ionizing radiation, or ethylene oxide). Terminally sterilized preparations typically have a SAL of 10^{-6} (the probability of one in a million items being nonsterile). Preparations compounded via aseptic procedure (no final filtration) can claim a SAL of no more than 10^{-3} (the probability of one in a thousand items being nonsterile), assuming that a robust process validation procedure had been conducted. This is why it is important to have processes that have been validated through media fills. SAL is product-related and contamination rates are process-related.[4]

An effective method of performing a process validation is through process simulation testing (media fill). A media fill mimics an actual and entire compounding procedure using a suitable growth medium such as tryptic soy broth (TSB) instead of using ingredients to prepare a finished compounded preparation. Media fills can be used to evaluate the capabilities of aseptic compounding procedures and can be used to identify any weaknesses in the procedures that could contribute to the inaccuracy and/or contamination of the compounded sterile preparation.[4] Using the PDA Technical Report No. 22 as a basis, a properly designed media fill will be able to[5]:

- Demonstrate the capability of the aseptic procedures to result in a sterile preparations.

- Qualify, certify, and validate the aseptic technique of all pharmacy compounding personnel (anyone who prepares compounded sterile preparations must be validated).

- Meet the validation and sterility testing requirements for compounded sterile preparations as detailed in USP <797>.

USP <797> states that all aseptic processing operations and configurations be adequately established by media-fill validation.[6] Microbial contamination of sterile preparations compounded aseptically (without further sterilization such as filtration) is mainly caused by human factors.[7] In fact, from 1980 to 2000, most of FDA regulated products recalled for nonsterility or lack of sterility assurance were prepared by aseptic processing.[8] Through careful process validation design and validation of both the compounding procedure and the compounding checks and controls, quality (accuracy and sterility) can be significantly improved. This assumes that all compounding personnel utilize and adhere to the same compounding procedures, checks, and controls that were validated in the media fill procedure. Professional distinction between compounders (e.g., assuming that everyone has their own way of compounding sterile preparations) is not acceptable. When different procedures are followed by different people, compounding consistency cannot be realized. It is only out of consistency that quality can be assured.[5]

One tool that is particularly useful in organizing the overall validation effort is a Hazard Analysis, Critical Control Points (HACCP). A HACCP plan involves analyzing the compounding process and flow charting it to ensure that it reflects the actual procedure that is performed. Once the procedure has been clearly identified, the hazards within the procedures are identified. They can be one of three different types of hazards: chemical, biological, or physical. Out of the hazards, critical control points (CCP) can be identified. A CCP can be a practice, procedure, process, or location at or by which preventive or control measures can be exercised that will eliminate, prevent, or minimize the identified hazards. An example of a chemical hazard during the compounding of parenteral nutrition solutions (TPN) is incorrect source containers (amino acids, dextrose, or water) being spiked on the wrong compounding device solution lead. The CCP for this hazard would be to double-check and document the initial compounding device setup and subsequent source container changes during the day. As each CCP is addressed, the controls are documented. The end result is a control plan and procedure. By knowing where failures can occur in a process and by controlling and monitoring those critical control points of failure, the likelihood of compounding a quality preparation consistently is better than all other methods. Quality cannot be inspected into final preparation; quality must be built in.[9] This is the level of detail that can assure that compounded sterile preparations are accurate and sterile.

A successfully validated process can reduce the dependence upon final testing for some types of compounded sterile preparations (low- and medium-risk preparations). Final preparation testing must play a major role in assuring that quality for high-risk compounded sterile preparations. Note that media fills and end-product testing are not mutually exclusive activities.

To properly conduct a media fill, a written protocol must be prepared which specifies the procedures to be followed and the data to be collected.[5] The data generated from the media fill procedure must reflect the actual procedure methods and activities that occurred during the validation procedure. This would include activity during the incubation period (e.g., daily room or incubator temperatures, the signature of person inspecting the media fill units [MFUs]).

The process simulation test should also specify a sufficient number of media fills repeated over several days in order to demonstrate reproducibility and provide an accurate measure of variability among repeated media fills. The duration (number of days) and the number of media fills required to meet USP <797> media fill requirements is not clearly defined. Generally, in the medical device and pharmaceutical manufacturing industry, media fills are conducted for three consecutive runs (days) in order to be successfully validate a process. Again, validation is conducted to demonstrate process consistency. The principle behind conducting three consecutive runs is to ensure repeatability and eliminate any possible Hawthorne Effect[10] (the stimulation to output or accomplishment that results from the mere fact of being under observation).

Another critical principle that must be considered during process validation is the concept of "worst case." "Worst case" scenarios occur when compounding operations are at their greatest risk of introducing contamination into sterile preparations. These conditions typically occur at the end of compounding days, during high-volume periods and inherently when using suitable growth media versus typical ingredients. Media fills should not be performed during normal compounding activities in order to prevent possible cross-contamination and/or dispensing errors.

Analysis of the data collected from monitoring and inspecting the media fills will establish the variability of compounding parameters for individual media fill runs and will establish whether or not the equipment, personnel training, physical plant, and process controls are adequate to maintain control that contributes to the assurance that the sterility of sterile product preparations can be met.

Sampling Techniques

Process validation of aseptic technique and aseptic procedures is based on the concept that, when contaminated, a growth medium will support the organisms introduced by the operator. Therefore, a suitable growth medium used (e.g., soybean casein digest media or TSB) must support the types of microbes typically found in operator-contaminated sterile preparations. TSB is a good "all-purpose" medium that will support the growth of pathogenic organisms. Any purchased TSB should have with it a certificate of analysis (COA) and a growth promotion certificate. A certificate of analysis certifies the contents of the solution and the growth promotion certificate certifies that the medium will able to support the growth microorganisms such as staph, E. coli and others. All TSB must be handled to mimic the range of activities performed during the compounding of sterile preparations. Depending on the type of compounding activities performed at the pharmacy (low-risk, medium-risk, or high-risk), TSB is available in a variety of different formulations (ready-to-use, sterile solution, or non-sterile powder). The completed media fill units have to be properly incubated according to USP guidelines to insure proper detect of microbial contamination. A number of commercially available kits are available that can be used to validate personnel and procedures.

Commercial Kits

Several aseptic technique validation kits are currently available. Some are limited to the use of only ampules, vials, and syringes. Although those kits produce a valid representation of aseptic technique for ampule and vial transfer activities, many do not include aseptic manipulations performed in most pharmacy operations. Other methods may be required to mimic the range of activities performed in pharmacies that compound sterile preparations. This would include the use and sterilization of nonsterile tryptic soy powder to mimic the compounding of a sterile preparation from powder (narcotics and/or anesthesia formulations such as morphine, baclofen, buvipicaine, fentanyl, and any combination). Ideally, a media-fill procedure should incorporate multiple manipulations with syringes, ampules, vials, media-fill bags, transfer tubing, and empty bags for the administration of intravenous medication.

Validation of compounding equipment

Manufacturers validate the volumetric and/or gravimetric delivery capability of their equipment to accurately measure components from source containers but not the aseptic capability to produce a sterile preparation. Rates of contamination are procedure related and how and where automated compounding equipment is used can have a direct impact of the sterility of the preparation. Validating the ability of each type of equipment used to compound sterile preparations according to written policy is required by USP. Changes in the environmental factors in which equipment for sterile compounding is used requires revalidation.[11] If for example, a syringe-filler or automated TPN compounder is relocated to a different type or size of hood (e.g., from a horizontal laminar-airflow hood to a vertical laminar-airflow hood), revalidation is required. Environmental factors (e.g., type of laminar-airflow workbench or isolator) can adversely affect the aseptic operation of compounding equipment.

The initial validation procedure for all pieces of equipment should be consistent. TSB should be used as the source solution during equipment validation, during which the entire compounding process must be mimicked. Ten MFUs should be prepared and incubated for 7 days at room temperature followed by 7 days in the incubator (the minimum incubation period is at least 14 days and temperatures can be anywhere between 20° C to 35° C[5]). Evidence of no growth is usually sufficient to validate equipment. After successful validation, an automated device can be used to compound sterile preparations. This process validates only the capability of the automated compounder to produce sterile products and does not replace the need for its daily calibration, which is necessary to ensure the delivery accuracy of the preparations compounded.

Although a specific number of validation tests cannot be recommended for a sterile preparations program, a facility should be evaluated when it first opens and be revalidated at least twice a year. Validation is necessary not only for the personnel compounding sterile preparations but also for the processes, procedures, and facility.[11] Any media fill produced as part of an individual qualification test can be also counted towards a facility validation procedure.

When the process validation method is selected, the number of aseptic manipulations required for the test must be considered. In no case should this number be less than the number required to prepare the most complex product being produced. Typical antibiotic preparations involve 10–20 aseptic manipulations and parenteral nutrition preparations may involve as many as 100 aseptic manipulations. Pharmacists need to use good professional judgment when selecting the validation procedure, the number of procedures per time interval, and the frequency of testing.

Sampling Plan and Size

Initially, process validation was developed for the manufacture of large quantities of products. Therefore, sample size recommendations used by industry that are based on statistical sampling plans are not statistically significant for compounding most sterile preparations. The number of different procedures involved and the relatively small number of admixtures prepared per batch renders statistical sampling inappropriate. The minimum number of media fill units required to demonstrate a contamination rate of no more than 0.1% (SAL 10^{-3}: 1 nonsterile preparation per 1000 units compounded) with a 95% confidence interval is 3000.[2,5] This statistic uses the principle of Poisson distribution. The Poisson distribution is a discrete distribution which takes on the values X = 0, 1, 2, 3 and is often used as a model for the number of events, such as the number of positive media fills during a process validation in a specific time period.

One appropriate method has been described for determining the number of test samples needed to monitor the sterility of compounded sterile preparations.[12] It uses cumulative sum control charts to determine sample size given acceptable and rejectable quality levels. Thus, with a maximum acceptable contamination rate of 3% and a rejectable quality level of 12%, a sampling of 5% of output is recommended to monitor the aseptic technique of a person compounding sterile preparations.[13] For example, if a technician compounds 800 admixtures per month, 40 validation samples need to be tested. Previous reports suggested that 40 tests are statistically appropriate for initial validation, based on the anticipated potential for contaminating an IV admixture drug preparation.[13,14] Furthermore, 10 samples per

month per technician were recommended to detect a shift from the acceptable to the rejectable level of quality.[13]

Other recommendations indicate that sample size should be based on[1,5]:

- The number of preparations normally compounded during a given fill period or maximum batch size compounded.
- The number of preparations per unit of time based on compounding speed. (Sample size could be based on the number of IV admixtures compounded in 30 min, for example.)

Frequency of Process Validation

In USP <797>, there are recommendations on how often personnel should perform media fills.[6] These recommendations are based on the complexity of the products. Table 20-1 details a sample validation plan. Follow-up monitoring of staff technique should take place quarterly thereafter unless a media fill is contaminated during quarterly validation, the procedures change significantly, or there is evidence that a person has contaminated a preparation. In this case, the person should be retrained and retested.

Psychomotor Skill Assessment and Competency

In addition to using process simulation procedures to validate aseptic processes and compounder technique, visual observation of actual aseptic technique (psychomotor skills) should occur every 6 months. Psychomotor skills are coordinated muscular movements that are typified by smoothness and precise timing. Psychomotor abilities are very important because they work hand in hand with cognitive thinking. The skills it requires are physical in nature and each individual must think about what he/she is doing. Proper aseptic technique requires the compounder to be aware of where their hands are at all times. Figure 20-1 details a sample psychomotor skill assessment and competency checklist.

Low-Risk Compounded Sterile Preparations

Manipulations that are limited to aseptically opening ampules, penetrating sterile stoppers

Table 20-1.

Sample Validation Plan

Program Validation	Minimum Validation Requirements	
Validation Purpose	Low-and Medium-Risk Preparations	High-Risk Preparations
Initial aseptic validation	*Personnel validation*	*Process validation*
● Must be successfully completed before compounding is permitted	3 consecutive daily media-fill runs*	3 consecutive daily media-fill runs
Revalidation after a positive media fill		
● Must be completed if one media-positive bag occurs during the initial validation or two media-positive bags during ongoing revalidation	3 consecutive daily media-fill runs	3 consecutive daily media-fill runs
Ongoing revalidation		
● Must be successfully completed quarterly	1 media-fill run	Annual media fill run

*A media-fill run is defined as 10 MFUs per day.

on vials with sterile needles and syringes, and transferring sterile liquids in sterile syringes to sterile administration devices and packages of other sterile products, are considered low-risk compounding activities.

Example of a media-fill test procedure for low-risk preparations

This or an equivalent test is performed at least annually by each person authorized to compound low-risk level preparations under conditions that closely simulate the most challenging or stressful conditions encountered during compounding of low-risk level compounded sterile preparations. Once begun, this test is completed without interruption. Within an ISO Class 5 (Class 100) air quality environment, three sets of four 5-mL aliquots of sterile Soybean-Casein Digest Medium are transferred with the same sterile 10-mL syringe and vented needle combination into separate sealed empty sterile 30-mL clear vials, i.e., four 5-mL aliquots into each of three 30-mL vials. Sterile adhesive seals are aseptically affixed to the rubber closures on the three filled vials, and then the vials are incubated for 14 days at 25°–35°.

Medium-Risk Compounded Sterile Preparations

Manipulations that involve multiple individual or small doses of sterile products that are combined or pooled to compound the compounded sterile preparation that will be administered to either multiple patients or to one patient on multiple occasions, and compounding procedures that include complex aseptic manipulations other than the single-volume transfers are considered medium-risk compounding activities.

Example of a media-fill test procedure for medium-risk preparations

This or an equivalent test is performed under conditions that closely simulate the most challenging or stressful conditions encountered during compounding, but does not include compounding performed on automated compounding devices (ACDs). This test must be completed without interruption within an ISO Class 5 air quality environment. Six 100-mL aliquots of sterile Soybean-Casein Digest Medium are aseptically transferred by gravity through separate tubing sets into separate

Employee Name: _____   Job: _____

Date of Evaluation: _____   Name of Evaluator: _____   Title: _____

Type of Evaluation: _____ Initial Assessment

_____ Quarterly Re-certification

_____ Other (specify): _____

Observations must be made by qualified pharmacy staff. Please indicate performance in the appropriate box. Any skill marked "unmet" requires instruction and practice until standard is met. Document remedial activities in Comments section. Key: M = met; U = unmet.

SKILL	M	U	COMMENTS
Proper gowning procedure			
Remove jewelry from hands and wrists.			
Donned proper garments (booties, headcover, gown, mask, gloves).			
Scrubbed nails, hands and arms to midforearm with disinfecting agent for at least 30 seconds.			
Protected outer surfaces of garment items.			
Donned special chemoprotective gown and gloves as appropriate.			
Entry into cleanroom performed with minimal contamination of hands and uniform.			
Preparation of aseptic work area.			
Remove any supply items not needed from hood. No extraneous articles (pens, labels, scissors) are placed in hood.			
Clean all hood work surfaces and bar at the start of each workday. Side to side, back to front motion, with Kim Wipe and IPA. Record hood cleaning.			
Collected and introduced supply items into aseptic work area in proper manner.			
Collected from cart all supply items needed for order(s). Items are inspected for expiration date and defects.			
Wiped with IPA all items introduced intact into hood which are stored in raw cardboard.			
Removed outer wrap, where appropriate, at edge of aseptic work area and placed them in hood.			
Arranged items more than 6 inches within aseptic work area and 3 inches from each side, in a manner not to disrupt clean air flow.			
Arranged items for efficient operation.			

Figure 20-1. Personnel Assessment for Good Aseptic Practices (GAP).

(Continued next page)

evacuated sterile containers. The six containers are then arranged as three pairs, and a sterile 10-mL syringe and 18-gauge needle combination is used to exchange two 5-mL aliquots of medium from one container to the other container in the pair. For example, after a 5-mL aliquot from the first container is added to the second container in the pair, the second container is agitated for 10 seconds, then a 5-mL aliquot is removed and returned to the first container in the pair. The first container is then agitated for 10 seconds, and the next 5-mL aliquot is transferred from it back to the second container in the pair. Following the two 5-mL aliquot exchanges in each pair of containers, a 5-mL aliquot of medium from each container is aseptically injected into a sealed empty sterile 10-mL clear vial using a sterile 10-mL syringe and vented needle. Sterile adhesive seals are aseptically affixed to the

(Continued)

SKILL	M	U	COMMENTS
Aseptic Operations			
Meticulously conducted aseptic operations so that exposed critical sites were always directed into the HEPA filtered air stream.			
Manipulated syringes so as to not touch the tip or plunger.			
Swabbed all rubber stoppers and ampule necks with IPA before puncturing or breaking open.			
Injected proper amount of air into vials before withdrawing solution (when appropriate)			
Checked graduations on syringes, bags, and bottles carefully; relative to amount of drug ordered.			
Opened ampules with a firm snapping motion and pointed towards the side of the hood.			
Filtered solutions taken from ampules and any other solutions with visible particles.			
Made all syringe and tubing connections aseptically, expertly, and securely.			
Performed all aseptic manipulations in a manner showing obvious effort to prevent touch contamination.			
If contamination was suspected from the procedure or otherwise, the product was discarded.			
Inspected product for visible particulate matter, evidence of incompatibility or other defects.			
Removed waste or unused supplies with minimal in-and-out motion. Partially used multidose vials are dated and initialed.			
Cleaned and sanitized aseptic work area between each batch.			
All technician work is checked by a pharmacist.			
Additional procedures are used with antineoplastic drug compounding.			
A plastic backed absorbent drape is placed on the work surface during all preparation procedures.			
No venting or splashing of drug occurs through use of special needles or guards.			
All disposable items used during drug preparation except needles are disposed of in chemo waste.			
Chemo gown donned prior to compounding.			
Chemo gloves or double latex gloves donned prior to compounding.			
Process Simulation Testing			
All compounded products are sterile.			

Figure 20-1. Personnel Assessment for Good Aseptic Practices (GAP).

rubber closures on the three filled vials, and then the vials are incubated for 14 days at 25°–35°. Media fill procedure for ACDs should be mimic how parenteral nutrition solutions are prepared. LVP bags of Soybean-Casein Digest Medium must hang on the ACD like amino acids, dextrose, sterile water, and lipid typically would be. Manually program a volume of 100 mL for each station, with each solution have a specific gravity of 1.00. The micro-additive (e.g., electrolytes, vitamins, trace elements) will be substituted with vials of TSB and either injected as individual components in the pumped bag of broth or pooled into an evacuated bottle and transferred by means of a repeater pump or some other type of mechanical pump.

High-Risk Compounded Sterile Preparations

Manipulations that involve the handling of nonsterile ingredients, including manufactured products, for routes of administration that include baths and soaks for live organs and tissues, implants, inhalations, injections, powders for injections, irrigations, metered sprays and ophthalmic and otic preparations are considered high-risk compounding activities. Also included are sterile ingredients, components, devices, and mixtures that are exposed to air quality inferior to ISO Class 5.

Example of a media-fill test procedure for high-risk sterile preparations

This or an equivalent test is performed under conditions that closely simulate the most challenging or stressful conditions encountered when compounding high-risk level compounded sterile preparations. This test is completed without interruption in the following sequence:

1. Dissolve 3 g of nonsterile commercially available Soybean-Casein Digest Medium in 100-mL of non-bacteriostatic water to make a 3% solution.

2. Draw 25 mL of the medium into each of three 30-mL sterile syringes. Transfer 5 mL from each syringe into separate sterile 10-mL vials. These vials are the controls and they generate exponential microbial growth, indicated by visible turbidity upon incubation.

3. Under aseptic conditions, using aseptic technique, affix a sterile 0.2-micron porosity filter unit and a 20-gauge needle to each syringe. Inject the next 10 mL from each syringe into three separate 10-mL sterile vials. Repeat the process into three more vials. Label all vials and affix sterile adhesive seals to the closure of the nine vials and incubate for 14 days at 25°–35°.

Acceptance Criteria

Ideally, MFUs should be read daily, but must be read on days 7 (the last day of room temperature incubation) and 14 (the last day of incubator incubation), if two separate incubation temperatures are employed. Personnel should successfully pass an initial aseptic process simulation test (three media fill runs) before compounding. Compounded sterile preparations. Passing is considered having zero growth in any of the MFUs demonstrating that no contamination occurs in three consecutive media fills. Cloudiness or turbidity in any MFU is indicative of a media-positive or contaminated bag. Policies on the type and frequency of aseptic technique validation is required for compounding staff must also be in place.[6]

Summary

In some situations, when final preparation sterility testing is not feasible, a properly designed and executed process validation could meet the sterility release check requirements of USP <797> as a quality-control measure for sterile preparation compounding programs. Process validation or process simulation tests using media fills are internationally recognized by various compendia such as the United States Pharmacoepeia, European Union Good Manufacturing Practices, Japanese Pharmacoepeia, and ISO-13408-1. In addition to media fills, visual observation, and the use of psychomotor skills, checklists are considered the best methods for evaluating aseptic compounding operations.[8] A number of commercially available media-fill containers and kits are on the market that can facilitate the process validation requirements detailed in USP <797>. Unfortunately, available scientific methods are not practical for selecting a sample size or determining the frequency of testing. Pharmacists need to review the various published recommendations to determine a robust and defendable sample size and frequency that demonstrate quality control. Process validation must become an important part of every sterile preparation compounding program.

References

1. Food and Drug Administration. *Guidelines on General Principle for Process Validation.* Rockville, MD: FDA; 1987.

2. Microbiological evaluation of clean rooms and other controlled environments. United States pharmacopeia, 27th rev./ national formulary 22nd ed. Rockville, MD: United States Pharmacopeial Convention. Available at: www.uspnf.com. Accessed January 19, 2004.

3. Medical Devices; Current Good Manufacturing Practice (CGMP) Final Rule; Quality System Regulation. 21C.F.R Parts 808, 812, and 820. 1996.

4. Halls NA. Practicalities of setting acceptance criteria for media fill trials. *PDA J Pharm Sci Technol.* 2000;54:247–52.

5. *Process Simulation Testing for Aseptically Filled Products. Technical Report No. 22.* Philadelphia, PA: Parenteral Drug Association; 1996 supplement; vol 50: number S1.

6. Pharmaceutical compounding—sterile preparations. United States pharmacopeia, 27th rev./ national formulary, 22nd, ed (first supplement). Rockville, MD: United States Pharmacopeial Convention; 2004.

7. Kastango ES, Douglass K. Improving the management, operations and cost effectiveness of sterile-product compounding—improve the ability to predict employee efficiency, cost of service and product wastage while simultaneously improving quality. *Int J Pharm Compound.* 1999; 3:253–8.

8. Kawamura K, Abe H. Consideration of media fill tests for evaluation and control of aseptic processes: a statistical approach to quality criteria. *PDA J Pharm Sci Technol.* 2002;56:235–41.

9. Kastango, ES, Trissel, LA, Bradshaw, B. An ounce of prevention: controlling hazards in extemporaneous compounding practices. *Int J Pharm Compound.* 2003; 5:401–16.

10. Merriam-Webster website. Available at: www.m-w.com. Accessed October 21, 2003.

11. Kastango, ES, Douglass, K. Quality assurance for sterile products. *Int J Pharm Compound.* 2001;5: 246–53.

12. Sanford RL. Cumulative sum control charts for admixture quality control. *Am J Hosp Pharm.* 1980;37:655–9.

13. Brier KL. Evaluating aseptic technique of pharmacy personnel. *Am J Hosp Pharm.* 1983;40:400–3.

14. Morris BG, Avis KE, Bowles GC. Quality control plan for intravenous admixture programs. II: Validation of operator technique. *Am J Hosp Pharm.* 1980;37:668–72.

21 | End-Preparation Evaluation

*Eric S. Kastango**

*The author acknowledges Philip Schneider, who authored this chapter in the first edition of this text.

Introduction

Since 1990, the Food and Drug Administration (FDA) has become aware of more than 55 quality problems associated with compounded preparations, many of which resulted in recalls, patient injury and deaths.[1-12] In 2001, FDA's Division of Prescription Drug Compliance and Surveillance conducted a limited survey of preparations compounded by a group of community pharmacies located throughout the United States. The goal of the survey was to gather information on the quality, purity, and potency of compounded drug preparations in the marketplace. The compounded preparations included in the survey were selected from a cross-section of commonly compounded dosage forms based on FDA's assessment of the potential health risks resulting from improper compounding. The analytical testing failure rate for these sampled compounded preparations was thirty-four percent (34%), which is higher than the analytical failure rate (2%) of drug products from commercial FDA-registered manufacturers.[1]

Regulatory and public concern about the quality of pharmacist-compounded sterile preparations has prompted quasi-governmental organizations like the United States Pharmacopeial Convention, Inc. (USP) to take action in order to ensure that pharmacy-compounded sterile preparations meet a pre-defined set of qualifications.

The USP <797>, Pharmaceutical Compounding—Sterile Preparations, now requires some form of final preparation testing before release of pharmacy-compounded sterile preparations. The analytical portion of any release testing procedure demonstrates that the sample was representative of the compounded lot. A statistically appropriate sampling plan should assure that a valid analytical portion is evaluated. The following example provides an illustration of the sampling problem. The FDA regulations for raw peanut lots specify a 25 parts per billion (ppb) aflatoxin action level. If a 20-ton lot of peanuts were evaluated, the limit would be exceeded if four peanut-equivalents of the approximately 700,000,000 peanuts in the lot were present as aflatoxin. How does one obtain a representative analytical portion to determine if a box car full of peanuts will meet the limit or "how do you find a needle in a haystack?"[13]

Sterility and final preparation testing has scientific and practical limitations which are well known. Some of these are[14]:

1. The statistical limitations of the sample size used for testing in any testing program also applies to sterility testing.

2. Final preparation testing may not been a definitive and useful method of assuring quality.

3. Sterility tests will only detect viable microorganisms present at the time of the test.

4. Viable organisms present at the time of the test can only be detected if they are capable of growth in the specified culture media.

5. Sterility and pyrogen tests may be subject to potential interference from drug concentrations.

6. Adventitious microbial contamination introduced at the time of testing, may result in false positive readings.

7. Sterility tests are always destructive of the samples tested and do not offer the opportunity to reexamine the same samples in the event of either positive or negative findings.

The USP Sterility Test is limited in its ability to detect whether a batch contains contaminated units, with a threshold sensitivity of fifteen percent (15%). To detect contaminated units in a batch, 15% of batch would have to be contaminated and 30% of the batch have to be tested for the sample size.[13,15,16] The drug product lot from an FDA-registered manufacturer would fail the USP test requirement if any microbial growth is found and the test is not invalidated. The USP states that a manufacturer should not perform a sterility retest without evidence that a positive sterility test can be attributed to contamination introduced by the laboratory operator technique.[15]

With these limitations and challenges, how does one meet the requirements set forth in USP <797> or in state board pharmacy practice acts?

This chapter will review critical points of evaluation that compounders can use for sterile preparations. In addition to microbial and pyrogen testing, final preparation evaluation should include physical and analytical testing. Techniques now being used include weight, refractometry, pH, and laboratory analyses.

Component Standards

If the compounding process is analyzed for critical control points (CCPs) that can influence the quality (sterility, purity, strength, and identity) of the compounded sterile preparation, the type of component must be considered. Ideally, pharmacists, should use components prepared by FDA-registered firms that have done all of the necessary release testing to ensure the integrity of their components. Often pharmacists are required to seek other sources of components that are not finished sterile final products in order to meet a sterile preparation need of the patient. Raw components (e.g., nonsterile powders) are supplied in many levels of purity. Table 21-1 summarizes purity classifications applied to chemicals.[17] The USP <797> requires that USP or NF grade be lowest grade of purity used in compounding. If that grade is not available, then higher grades of purity can be used if deemed acceptable by the pharmacist.

Two very important ways to assure the quality of raw components is to purchase them only from FDA-registered manufacturers or repackagers and only accept the raw components if manufacturers provide with a Certificate of Analysis (COA). A COA provides the truest measure of component purity and provides information about "how clean" the component really is. It is a document, often required by an importer or governmental authorities like USP, attesting to the quality or purity of component.

Physical Inspection (Organoleptic Method)

Physical inspection provides some very basic information about the compounded sterile preparation. The primary concern is that the actual preparation contains the ingredients specified in the original prescription. If the clinical and therapeutic appropriateness of drug, dose, and formulation have been evaluated for the patient, the final preparation still should be evaluated for:

- Container leaks and integrity: physical examination of the final prepared container visually inspected for leaks, holes or other container-closure breaches.

- Particulates in solution: physical examination of the solution for the presence of mobile, randomly sourced, extraneous substances other than gas bubbles.[18] The use of Light/Dark Background Observation Device is an effective tool for performing a thorough visual inspection for particulates.[19]

Table 21-1.

Summary of Purity Classifications Applied to Chemicals

Grade of Chemical	Description
Technical (commercial)	Commercial or industrial quality, generally of indeterminate quality
CP (chemically pure)	More refined than technical grade, but still of unknown quality; only partial analytical information available
USP/NF	Meets standards set by the USP/NF
FCC	Meets specifications of Food Chemical Codex
ACS reagent	High purity; meets specifications of the Reagent Chemicals Committee of the American Chemical Society
AR (analytical reagent)	Very high purity
HPLC	Very high purity; used in high pressure liquid chromatography
Spectroscopic grade	Very high purity
Primary standard	Highest purity; used in standard solutions for analytical purposes

Used with permission. Allen, LV, Jr. General guidelines for the use of chemicals for prescription compounding. *International Journal of Pharmaceutical Compounding.* 1997;1:46.

- Solution color, volume, and odor (if possible).

- Phase separation (oiling, creaming, or cracking).

- Clear, legible, and correct labeling, including proper ancillary or auxiliary labeling.

Good Documentation Practices

Good documentation ensures that all procedures and actions performed before, during and after compounding actually occurred. It is the only proof that written policies and procedures were followed. Good documentation is another component of final preparation evaluation. It provides a means of tracing or recreating a set of events that can be investigated and acted upon. Good documentation is critical to ensure the quality of a preparation. It will:

- Provide enough of the right information to "stand on its own" without the person documenting being present to justify or explain the entries. It will note:

  - Who performed the task

  - When the task was performed

  - How the task was performed

- Serve as a control for quality and final preparation evaluation. It allows others to verify and validate recorded actions that occurred during compounding.

- Be correct, accurate, legible, exact, and free of unnecessary information.

- Capture the original observations that are critical to preparation integrity.

- Exhibit the following characteristics:

Preparation traceability: Preparation traceability is an essential element of any sterile preparation compounding program. Proper documentation follows the final preparation back to source providing the necessary assurance as to the configuration, characteristics and integrity of the preparation.

Preparation recallability: preparation traceability forward through distribution channels is essential element for an effective and targeted preparation withdrawal and/or recall, if and when necessary.

Use as a risk management tool: The expression: "If it isn't documented, it didn't happen" is an expression that is routinely used to stress the importance of proper documentation practices. Documentation becomes evidence and can be used to prove that the final preparation was prepared properly.

Use as a quality assurance tool: Good documentation serves as a product acceptability measure. It allows compounded sterile preparations to be released for patient use because it met all of the requirements for acceptability and fitness for use.

Proper documentation practices: Proper documentation practices are only fostered by active participation and review from management. People generally respect what others inspect. If documentation activities are just exercises with no value in monitoring and improving the procedures, it should not be done. Besides direct observation, a quality system that is in control can only be supported by the degree of documentation that occurs from compounding activities. Documentation in and of itself is not good if it is not used to ensure quality, but more importantly that it is used proactively to identify problems and allow for correction. Documentation of past events does not prevent future errors. Documentation serves as a means of detecting and correcting of conditions or situations that affect quality.

There are a few cardinal rules for proper documentation: They are:

1. Observations are considered original data and as such should be immediately documented (e.g., temperature or pressure reading). If you didn't observe the data, you shouldn't document it.

2. All documentation should be performed in such manner as to allow it to be read in days, months, or years to come and still to be understood.

A pharmacist should verify that the final preparation was compounded accurately according to the compounding batch record or worksheet with respect to:

1. Proper components were checked prior to compounding and used (vials, ampuls, and final solution container).

2. Proper compounding methods (reconstitution, solution transfer quantities) were

used. In some instances, the use of the "syringe plunger pull-back method" is acceptable.[20]

3. Proper quantities of components were used when compared to desired batch yields versus actual batch yields (10-1 gram antibiotic syringes were expected and 10 syringes were prepared using 1-10 gram source vial of antibiotic with no residual solution in the source container).

4. Correct and proper number of labels (The right label for the right compounded sterile preparation for the correct patient), labeled in a manner to allow for unencumbered administration (obstructed volume graduation of syringes, etc.).

Weight Verification

Weight verification can be an effective final preparation evaluation test when using sterile, final released components from FDA registered firms. It is a method that is often used to evaluate preparations compounded from ingredients with different specific gravities such as total parenteral nutrition (TPN) and cardioplegia solutions. Per the ASHP Guidelines on the Safe Use of Automated Compounding Devices for the Preparation of Parenteral Nutrition Admixtures, the use of gravimetric measurement allows the operator the ability to evaluate the accuracy of the automated compounding device.[21] Using the gravimetric method, measurement of fluid volume delivered from the source container to the final container is determined by weighing the fluid transferred and dividing the weight by the solution's known specific gravity, thereby converting weight to volume.[21] Knowing the specific gravity of each solution and the desired volume, the final bag weight of the compounded sterile preparation can be calculated and used as a method of ensuring that the final preparation was compounded correctly. It is critical that the automated compounding device be properly calibrated daily or per the manufacturers recommendations to ensure proper operating conditions. Also, hanging the proper source container on the assigned pumping channel or solution lead is crucial, since hanging the wrong solution on the wrong pumping channel or lead can yield devastating results. This can be best controlled through double-checking the initial automated compounding device setup and anytime the source container is changed. With most automated compounding devices, the final solu-

tion can be weighed on the load cell or some other type of electronic scale connected to the device. Sensitive electronic balances also can be used to compare actual to calculated weights.

Refractometry Verification (Refractive Index)

Refractometry is another method that can be used to qualitatively evaluate compounded sterile preparations quickly but not with a lot of specificity. It is not a quantitative test of a solution's actual concentration of components. The unit of measure for refractometry verification is Brix units. The Brix scale describes percentage concentration of soluble solids in a water solution. The soluble solid content is the total of all the solids dissolved in the water, beginning with sugar, protein, acids, etc. The Brix reading is the value of the sum total of those solutes in solvent. It directly correlates to the refractive index (nD) scale and is calibrated to the number of grams of cane sugar (sucrose) contained in 100 ml of water.[22]

25 Brix = 25 g solids/100 g of solution

The refractive index differs for various solutions. Lactated Ringers has a refractive index of 1 Brix unit but dextrose 5% water and Lactated Ringers has a refractive index of 5.5 Brix units.[23] The difference is reflected by the presence of dextrose plus electrolytes.

In the 1980s and early 1990s, this technique was applied to the analysis of controlled substances, particularly to monitor for diversion,[24-27,29] and parenteral nutrition solutions.[28] Refractometry verification can only be used for solutions containing an organic compound (e.g., a drug or dextrose). It cannot be used for opaque products (e.g., total nutrient admixtures containing fat emulsion) or solutions of inorganic compounds (e.g., electrolytes).[22]

pH Testing

The pH of the final solution can be measured using an electronic pH device or even simple pH paper. Then the measured pH can be compared to published values[23] as one indicator of proper product preparation and its intended physical and biological state. Depending on the placement or use of the compounded sterile preparation (vascular vs. ophthalmic use), the final pH can have a significant impact on patient morbidity and mortality.

Laboratory Analysis (Purity, Potency, and Strength)

To evaluate the contents of a compounded sterile preparation, analytical techniques also may be needed. This type of testing can provide both quantitative and qualitative analysis of the final preparation. This method is recommended for any preparation that falls into the high-risk category and when nonsterile bulk components are used. Analytical testing will provide information necessary to validate that the compounding procedures, formulation and the operator are capable of creating the preparation meeting the desired concentration and sterility. Laboratory analysis is also required to establish appropriate beyond-use dating for compounded preparations using nonsterile bulk components. This type of testing should only be performed by qualified personnel using instrumentation designed and validated to determine the concentration of the various components in the compounded sterile preparation. For example, traditional physical inspection techniques may not be reliable for preparations compounded using automated compounding devices.

Microbial Testing

As noted earlier in this chapter, final preparation sterility testing (microbial testing) as a quality release standard has many limitations. Notwithstanding these limitations, USP standards and state board of pharmacy regulations require some form of sterility (microbial) testing.

Despite the limitations, microbial testing has two roles in a sterile preparation compounding program:

- Testing of preparations suspected of contamination.
- Testing of batch-compounded preparations that are quarantined before use.

There are two official methods of microbial testing: (1) direct transfer of a sample to sterile culture media, and (2) membrane filtration.

These methods are described in the *United States Pharmacopeia/National Formulary (USP/NF)*.[30,31] All testing for microbial contamination must occur in ISO Class 5 (FS209e Class 100) environments using aseptic technique to prevent unintended environmental and operator contamination.

Sterile Culture Media

Microbial growth in incubated testing media indicates that the parenteral preparation is contaminated. Identification of the contaminant often can indicate its source. The most common method for sterile growth media testing is direct transfer. A sample aliquot of a compounded parenteral preparation is aseptically transferred into two sterile culture media. One medium, Fluid Thioglycollate, is incubated at 32° C for 14 days. The other medium, soybean casein digest, is incubated at 22° C for 14 days. Positive (intentionally contaminated samples with known organisms) and negative (no contamination) controls are incubated with the test samples. Any sample that becomes turbid during the incubation period is a positive test.

This technique can detect only *grossly* contaminated preparations. It might be used to test a quarantined batch compounded significantly in advance of use or a suspected preparation several days after compounding. Sterile culture media testing is of limited use for evaluating individual IV admixtures within a few hours of compounding.

Membrane Filtration

Parenteral preparations also can be tested using membrane filters. This technique is recommended if the preparation contains preservatives or is a compound with intrinsic bacteriostatic activity (e.g., an antibiotic). It also is useful if preparation testing is needed within hours of compounding.

For this method, the entire preparation is filtered through a sterile, 0.45-micron filter. Then the membrane is washed with a sterile fluid to remove compounds having a bacteriostatic effect. The membrane is aseptically divided and placed into thioglycollate medium and soybean casein digest and incubated at 32° and 22°C, respectively. Both positive and negative controls are used. Turbidity during a 7-day incubation is a positive test.[32]

Commercial kits are available to assist pharmacists in using the membrane filter technique for final preparation sterility testing.

Total Nutrient Admixture Testing

Total nutrient admixture preparations pose a new challenge for sterility testing. Since they are not aqueous solutions, turbidity cannot be used as an endpoint for a positive test. However, a technique used for culturing blood has been applied; the system uses a culture bottle containing 70 ml of trypticase soy broth (TSB) and a plastic cylinder with an agar-coated slide unit. The total nutrient admixture sample is first cultured in TSB and then subcultured in the TSB after the broth is washed over the agar surface. Growth on the agar surface reflects a positive test.[33]

Pyrogen and Bacterial Endotoxin Testing

Pyrogens and bacterial endotoxins are metabolic products of living microorganisms or the dead microorganisms themselves. When present in parenterals administered to patients, they can cause fever and chills. Contaminated preparations for intrathecal use have the capacity to cause both septic and aseptic meningitis and aseptic shock.[34-38] For the same reasons as microbial testing, both pyrogen and endotoxin testing have limited applicability for sterile preparation compounding programs. Compounded sterile preparations compounded from nonsterile bulk components are required to be tested for pyrogens/endotoxins. Most preparations injected into vascular or central nervous systems that exceeded storage conditions published in USP <797> must be tested to ensure that they do not contain excessive bacterial endotoxins. The maximum allowable amount of endotoxin units (EU) per hour per kilogram of body weight for most compounded sterile preparations is 0.25–0.5 EU, depending on the USP monograph. It is recommend that USP <85>, Bacterial Endotoxin Tests, be reviewed for more information regarding this requirement. Using glassware or other compounding equipment that comes into direct contact with the compounded sterile preparations should also be devoid of pyrogens. A preparation can be sterile but still be pyrogenic. Sterility and pyrogenicity are two distinct and exclusive concepts. It is recommended to use a positive-charged endotoxin retaining 0.22-micron or better filter when compounding preparations using nonsterile bulk components to ensure that pyrogens have been removed. It is important that any filter used to terminally sterilize compounded preparations be certified by the manufacturer to retain at least 10^7 microorganisms of a strain *Brevundimonas diminuta* and be approved for human-use applications in sterilizing pharmaceutical fluids. Not all 0.2-micron filters meet this requirement.

Two tests are used for pyrogens and bacterial endotoxins in parenteral preparations: the rabbit test and the limulus amebocyte lysate test. Detailed descriptions of these methods appear in the USP/NF.[28,36]

Rabbit Test

Since the rabbit is very sensitive to pyrogens, it is used in the official test for them. Samples of a parenteral product are injected into the ear veins of three rabbits, and their body temperatures are monitored. An increase indicates the presence of pyrogens. In pharmacy practice, other more sensitivity and acceptable methods should be used other than the rabbit test.

Limulus Amebocyte Lysate Test

The limulus amebocyte lysate (LAL) test was recognized recently by the USP as a test for bacterial endotoxins. Because it is less expensive and faster than the rabbit test, it has more applicability to pharmacy practice settings. Amebocyte lysate is a lyophilized powder derived from red blood cells of horseshoe crabs. These cells contain a protein that clots in the presence of certain quantities of bacterial endotoxins. When a solution with bacterial endotoxins is added to the LAL reagent solution, the lysate causes the solution to gel within 1 hr. This method is considered the most accurate and sensitive procedure for testing and least expensive method of testing the finished compounded sterile preparation for pyrogens or the compounding systems used.[39] It is important to understand the LAL reagent can be inactivated or inhibited by concentrated drug products and may produce a false-negative test result. As such, it is important that a validated method for testing medication for pyrogens be established.[40] More sensitive pyrogen testing methods using turbidimetric, colorimetric, and chromogenic assays are available but are more expensive, are quicker but may be more prone to laboratory, operator or other errors. They also require proper training and initial and ongoing validation. Unless volume testing is required, these methods are not the most desirable methods for testing for endotoxins.

Summary

Final preparation evaluation in pharmacy practice often requires a quick physical check so that a dose is available for a patient when needed. When compounded sterile preparations that fall in the medium-risk level category, such as complex procedures associated with compounding parenteral nutrition formulations, additional analytical testing (such as refractometry, or bag weight verification) should be employed. For high-risk level compounded sterile preparations, especially those prepared using bulk, nonsterile components, more sophisticated evaluation procedures, (such as microbial, pyrogen, and potency testing) should be used. Final preparation evaluation should complement the quality control systems that focus on identifying and preventing errors before they occur.

References

1. U.S. Food and Drug Administration. *Report: Limited FDA Survey of Compounded Drugs.* Available at: http://www.fda.gov/cder/pharmcomp/survey.htm. Accessed on January 3, 2004.
2. Hallissy E, Russell S. Who's mixing your drugs? Bad medicine: pharmacy mix-ups a recipe for misery; some drugstores operate with very little oversight. *San Francisco Chronicle.* June 23, 2002.
3. United States Department of Justice, Federal Bureau of Investigation. Available at: http://kansascity.fbi.gov/kcmostate042202.htm. Accessed on July 6, 2002.
4. Officials to shut pharmacy, July 6, 2001. KTVU News website. Available at: http://www.bayinsider.com/partners/ktvu/news/2001/07/06/meningitis.html. Accessed July 6, 2002.
5. Solomon SL, Khabbaz RF, Parker RH, et al. An outbreak of *Candida parapsilosis* bloodstream infections in patients receiving parenteral nutrition. *J Infect Dis.* 1984;49:98–102.
6. Hughes CF, Grant AF, Leckie BD, et al. Cardioplegia solution: a contamination crisis. *J Thorac Cardiovasc Surg.* 1986;91:296–302.
7. Associated Press. Pittsburgh woman loses eye to tainted drug; 12 hurt. *Baltimore Sun.* November 9, 1990:3A.
8. Dugleaux G, Coutour XL, Hecquard C, et al. Septicemia caused by contaminated parenteral nutrition pouches: the refrigerator as an unusual cause. *J Parenter Enteral Nutr.* 1991;15:474–475.
9. Perrin J. Unsafe activities of compounding pharmacists. *Am J Health Syst Pharm.* 1995;52:2827–8.
10. Pierce LR, Gaines A, Varricchio R, et al. Hemolysis and renal failure associated with use of sterile water for injection to dilute 25% human albumin solution. *Am J Health Syst Pharm.* 1998;55:1057–70.
11. Food and Drug Administration. Hazards of precipitation with parenteral nutrition. *Am J Health Syst Pharm.* 1994; 51:427–8.
12. Myers CE. Needed: Serious attention to sterile products. *Am J Health Syst Pharm.* 1996;53:2582.
13. Layoff TP. Parametric release in lieu of drug end-product testing: can we get there from here? *American Genomic/Proteomic Technology,* 2002 (May/June);2, #3:14–17.
14. 21 C.F.R. part 820: Quality System Regulation. Government Printing Office. Bethesda, MD: 1 April 2003.
15. Food and Drug Administration. *Human Drug cGMP Notes.* Vol. 7;2:June 1999.
16. In a conversation between Harold Blackwood, FDA Inspector, Columbia, SC, and Ray Burns, Pharmacist, Columbia, SC. November, 2002.
17. Allen, LV, Jr. General guidelines for the use of chemicals for prescription compounding. *Int J of Pharm Comp.* 1997; 1:46.
18. Particulate matter in injections. United States pharmacopeia, 27th rev/national formulary, 22nd ed. Rockville, MD: United States Pharmacopeial Convention; 2004: In press.
19. Standard operating procedure for particulate testing for sterile products. *Int J Pharm Comp.* 1998;2:78.

20. Pharmaceutical considerations-sterile drugs. United States pharmacopeia, 27th rev/national formulary, 22nd ed. Rockville, MD: United States Pharmacopeial Convention; 2004: In press.

21. ASHP guidelines on the safe use of automated compounding devices for the preparation of parenteral nutrition admixtures. *Am J Health-Syst Pharm.* 2000;57:1343–8.

22. Purdue University, Agricultural and Engineering. Available at: http://pasture.ecn.purdue.edu/~mmorgan/Refractometry2_18_02.ppt. Accessed November 5, 2003.

23. Trissel LA. *Handbook on Injectable Drugs*, 12th ed. Bethesda, MD: American Society of Hospital Pharmacists; 2002.

24. Gill DL Jr, Goodwin SR, Knudsen AK, et al. Refractometer screening of controlled substances in an operating room satellite pharmacy. *Am J Hosp Pharm.* 1990; 47:817–8.

25. Cheung JF, Chong S, Kitrenos JG, et al. Use of refractometers to detect controlled substance tampering. *Am J Hosp Pharm.* 1991;48:1488–92.

26. Frankenfield DL, Johnson RE. Refractometry of controlled substances. *Am J Hosp Pharm.* 1991;48:2120–30.

27. Donnelly AJ, Petryna HM, Newman LM, et al. A simple, reliable, inexpensive method to aid in the detection of diversion of controlled substances by operating room personnel. *Anesthesiology.* 1990;73:A1053. Abstract.

28. Meyer GE, Novelli KA, Smith JE. Use of refractive index measurement for quality assurance of pediatric parenteral nutrient solutions. *Am J Hosp Pharm.* 1987; 44:1617–20.

29. Donnelly AJ, Newman LM, Petryna HM, et al. Refractometric testing of alfentanil hydrochloride, fentanyl citrate, sufentanil citrate and midazolam hydrochloride. *Am J Hosp Pharm.* 1993;50:298–300.

30. Sterility test. United States pharmacopeia, 27th rev/national formulary, 22nd ed. Rockville, MD: United States Pharmacopeial Convention; 2004: In press.

31. Sterilization and sterility assurance of compendial articles. United States pharmacopeia, 27th rev/national formulary, 22nd. Rockville, MD: United States Pharmacopeial Convention; 2004:In press.

32. Akers MJ, Wright GE, Carlson KA. Sterility testing of antimicrobial-containing injectable solutions prepared in the pharmacy. *Am J Hosp Pharm.* 1991;48:241–8.

33. Murray PR, Sandrock MJ. Sterility testing of a total nutrient admixture with a biphasic blood culture system. *Am J Hosp Pharm.* 1991;48:2419–21.

34. Cooper JF, Harbert JC. Endotoxin as a cause of aseptic meningitis after radionuclide cisternography. *J Nucl Med.* 1975;16:809–13.

35. Alderson PO, Siegel BA. Adverse reactions following In-DTPA cisternography. *J. Nucl Med.* 1973;14:609–11.

36. Food and Drug Administration. *Inspection Technical Guides.* Bacterial endotoxins/pyrogens. Rockville, MD: Office of Regulatory Affairs; March 20, 1985. ITG No. 40.

37. Jones TD, Feler CA, Simmons BP, et al. Neurological complications including paralysis after a medication error involving implanted intrathecal catheters. *Am J Med.* 2002; 112:31–6.

38. Pyrogen test. United States pharmacopeia, 27th rev/national formulary, 22nd ed. Rockville, MD: United States Pharmacopeial Convention; 2004:In press.

39. Joiner TJ, Kraus PF, Kupiec TC. Comparison of endotoxin testing methods for pharmaceutical products. *Int J Pharm Comp.* 2002;6:408–9.

40. Cooper JF, Thoma LA. Screening extemporaneously compounded intraspinal injections with the bacterial endotoxins test. *Am J Health-Sys Pharm.* 2002;59: 2426-33.

22 | Policies and Procedures for Compounding Sterile Preparations

E. Clyde Buchanan

A good policy and procedure manual can promote the safe, efficient, and uniform performance of all departmental functions.[1] Each department involved in compounding sterile preparations should have its own policies and procedures based on specific circumstances.[2] Procedures should be organized (e.g., numbered under headings) so that they are easy for a new employee to find. Compounding procedures can be available either in written form or electronically stored with printable documentation. The USP stipulates what makes for good compounding practices whether for sterile or non-sterile preparations.[3] Policies and procedures specific to compounding sterile preparations are available commercially.[4,5]

A policy—the general statement—provides a basis for decision-making. It addresses what must be done and, sometimes, why and when. A procedure—the "how to" document—provides methods for carrying out a policy. Procedures outline the complete cycle of a task, step by step, and assign responsibility to specific personnel.

Written policies and procedures can lead to numerous benefits[1]:

- Establishment of practice standards for both administrative and professional activities, in compliance with regulatory accrediting and certifying bodies.

- Coordination of resources (personnel, supplies, and equipment) for delivery of efficient and economic services.

- Reduction in waste (time and materials) resulting from errors, inexperience, and lack of supervision.

- Improvement in intradepartmental communications.

- Reduction in errors associated with oral transmission of information.

- Improvement in employees' security, job satisfaction, and productivity.

- Rapid detection of inefficient or inferior personnel performance.

- Establishment of means to evaluate the quality of services.

- Consistency in orienting and training new personnel.

The ASHP Guidelines[6] state that policies and procedures should be available to all involved personnel (see Appendix A). These policies and procedures should be updated at least annually, by the designated pharmacist and department head, to reflect current standards. Revisions then should be communicated to affected personnel. Before compounding sterile preparations, personnel should read the policies and procedures and verify (by signature) having done so.

This chapter notes the topics pertinent to compounding sterile preparations that should be covered in a pharmacy's policy and procedure manual. These same topics are presented in detail throughout this book and the appendices.

Personnel Training and Evaluation and Training

Job Description

Complete job descriptions for personnel compounding sterile preparations are essential to the hiring and orientation process. Job descriptions should include

- Basic qualifications (e.g., education level, certification, registration, and length and type of experience).

- Physical requirements (e.g., ability to lift moderately heavy weights, push carts, and perform rapid, repetitive, and accurate manipulations).

- Working conditions (e.g., shifts, environment, and garb).

- Responsibilities and competencies (e.g., ability to compound a pharmaceutical preparation that is free of errors of content and free of microbial, particulate, and pyrogenic contaminants).

Job Orientation

Policies and procedures on orientating new employees to sterile compounding should include their roles and those of coworkers, garb, facilities, equipment, area-specific techniques, and reference books (see Chapters 15 and 16).

Training and Education

Personnel training and continuing education procedures should specify frequency, methods, requirements, and documentation. Educational topics should include (1) aseptic technique and quality control; (2) chemical, pharmaceutical, and clinical properties of drugs; (3) good compounding practices; (4) equipment operation; and (5) preparation handling (see Chapters 15 and 16).

Competency Evaluation

Policies and procedures for competency evaluation should specify the methods of observation and/or testing and the intervals between these evaluations. For example, personnel could be observed continually for aseptic technique, could demonstrate how to use new equipment, or could have periodic written tests of math skills. Perhaps the most important means of demonstrating continued competence is media-fill validation of aseptic technique[7] (see Chapter 20).

Acquisition, Storage, and Handling of Products and Supplies

Acquisition

Policies and procedures for acquisition of sterile and non-sterile ingredients should include (see Chapter 2)

- Ingredient selection by *United States Pharmacopeia/National Formulary (USP/NF)* standards.
- Bulk drug substance dating procedures.
- Repackaging guidelines.
- Identification of ingredients by testing.
- System for purchase of equipment, containers, and closures.

Storage

Policies and procedures concerning storage should be based on USP or manufacturer-specified conditions. Written procedures are needed for temperature monitoring of refrigerators and freezers; light, ventilation, and humidity standards; stock rotation and inspection; and locations of quarantined preparations (both ingredients and end preparations) (see Chapters 2, 11, and 21).

Handling

These policies and procedures should include the removal of outer packaging in the anteroom, handling of pouched supplies (e.g., syringes), decontamination of ampuls and vials, and disposal of used items, hazardous waste, and sharps. Inspection of sterile ingredients and containers just prior to compounding is part of aseptic technique.

Handling policies and procedures for expired drugs and supplies should encompass their removal and quarantine as well as their return or disposal. Preparation recall procedures should detail notification of recalls, removal from stock and nursing areas, and retrieval from patients (see Chapters 11 and 12).

Facilities

Policies and procedures should contain clear rules for cleanliness of work areas, including time periods between cleaning, selection of disinfectants, and cleaning methods. The traffic control policy for work areas should identify authorized personnel and equipment and supply access to the anteroom and cleanroom. If a sterile compounding area is less clean than ISO Class 7 (Class 10,000) for ASHP[6] or ISO Class 8 (Class 100,000) for USP,[7] the preparations that can be compounded there must be specified. Safety features, such as emergency showers and eyewashes, also should be covered (see Chapter 17).

Equipment

These policies and procedures should encompass:

- Location of equipment and supplies in relation to work areas (e.g., prohibition of particle-producing items, such as pencils and paper towels, in the cleanroom).
- Use and cleaning of fixtures and equipment (e.g., sinks, lockers, and carts).
- Cart use on either side of demarcation line in the anteroom.
- Methods for using all laminar-airflow workbenches.
- Traffic near a laminar-airflow workbench.
- Starting, cleaning, stopping, and moving laminar-airflow workbenches.

Clear procedures are especially important for the use of automatic compounders and pumps since they have been implicated in serious errors. Such equipment must be calibrated for accuracy, monitored continually, and recertified periodically (see Chapter 3). Finally, sterilization methods for nonsterile equipment and vessels must be clearly written (see Chapter 13).

Personnel Behavior and Garb

Policies should prohibit staff from eating, drinking, smoking, and wearing makeup and jewelry in the cleanroom and under the hood. Hand-washing and drying rules should be spelled out, as well as regulations dealing with infectious conditions such as skin rashes, sunburn, and coughs. Policies also should prevent pregnant women from exposure to teratogenic preparations.[8]

Garb policies and procedures should describe how to (1) remove outer garments; (2) don coats or gowns; (3) reuse coats and gowns on reentry to the cleanroom; (4) use masks, hair covers, and shoe covers; (5) use gloves for both hazardous and nonhazardous drugs; (6) rinse gloves between operations; and (7) use sticky mats to clean shoes[7] (see Chapters 5 and 7).

Preparation

Written policies and procedures should ensure stability, compatibility, purity, and physiologic norms for all preparations based on pharmaceutical standards and references. Procedures also should cover inspection of ingredients and containers for expiration dates and defects prior to compounding (see Chapter 2).

Aseptic Technique

These policies and procedures should outline the cleaning of containers prior to their introduction into the hood, touch avoidance of critical container areas, use of needles and syringes, manipulations relative to laminar airflow in a hood, and organization of work in the laminar-airflow hood. Furthermore, requirements concerning the identification of cytotoxic and hazardous drugs and equipment and protective garb must be clearly stated. Particulate filtration methods also should be outlined (see Chapters 6 and 13).

Master Work Sheets

Policies and procedures should specify pharmacist verification of ingredients and their amounts, the order of compounding additives and the compounding process, for both manual and automated additives (see Chapter 13). For each preparation, a master work sheet should delineate[3]:

- Ingredients and their quantities.
- Equipment and supplies to assemble prior to preparation.
- Compounding directions.
- Sterilization method.
- Sample label.
- Evaluation and testing requirements.
- Quarantine methods.
- Storage conditions.
- Beyond-use date and time.

Batch Compounding Records

For each batch, these records document the procedures, materials, and personnel involved. A batch compounding record identifies all solutions and ingredients with their corresponding amounts, concentrations, or volumes; manufacturer and lot numbers for each component; and signatures or initials of individuals measuring ingredients.

A unique lot or control number, an expiration date, and the preparation date are assigned to each batch. Personnel who compound or approve the batch are indicated, as are the specific equipment used, end-preparation evaluation and testing specifications, storage requirements, and the actual yield compared to the anticipated yield (see Chapter 14).

Sterilization Methods

Selection

Policies and procedures should state the sterilization method for each type of preparation.[7] Although micropore filtration is used for heat-labile preparations, it cannot assure a pyrogen-free preparation. Autoclaving is preferred for batches of heat-stable preparations; if done properly, all units should be sterile and pyrogen free. Dry heat sterilization is usually reserved for highly heat-stable preparations that must remain in powder form (see Chapter 13).

Specific Requirements

Sterile filtration procedures should indicate both the filter material (e.g., hydrophilic or lipophilic) for different preparation types and methods for ensuring filter integrity. For autoclaving, the arrangement of units, the validation of cycles, and the maintenance of equipment must be described. For dry heat sterilization, procedures must clearly state how the oven heating process is validated and monitored, how the preparation is arranged in the oven, and how the oven is maintained.

Terminally sterilized preparations require quarantine and release procedures (e.g., duration, location, and documentation) (see Chapter 13).

Environmental Monitoring

The designated pharmacist, along with infection control and microbiology personnel, should develop an environmental monitoring plan for cleanroom air, work surfaces, walls, floors, and ceilings.[7] Monitoring devices should be specified. A method for periodic monitoring of particulate matter in the air is mandatory to document cleanroom conditions.

Microbial sampling of the air and surfaces, done by growing viable colony-forming units of bacteria from samples, should be included. Procedures should specify upper limits of microbial counts, required actions when limits are exceeded, and restarting of compounding after an environment has failed (see Chapter 18).

Process Validation

These policies and procedures must specify when and how an operator's ability to compound sterile preparations is to be validated. New staff members must initially establish competence for each preparation type they are to handle (e.g., syringes, TPNs, and batch-reconstituted antibiotics) by use of media fills. Then staff members must be revalidated periodically (e.g., quarterly or annually) and whenever they learn to prepare a different preparation.[7] (See Chapter 20.)

Beyond-Use Dating

Beyond-use dating policies and procedures should cite the methods followed for setting beyond-use dates and the references used for determining preparation stability times, especially when strengths or storage times differ from manufacturer labeling.[7] Expiration times include specific storage temperatures (e.g., 24 hr at room temperature and/or 7 days under refrigeration). The department should have a policy for handling preparations removed from and returned to refrigeration.

To determine an expiration date for preparations not covered by manufacturers' labeling or reliable literature, experimental stability testing is required. Sometimes the institution's laboratory personnel can help pharmacists test a preparation's shelf life (see Chapter 8).

Labeling

Policies and procedures for labeling should outline the required information for:

- Preparations compounded in batches in anticipation of routine orders.
- Preparations dispensed for administration within the institution.
- Patient-use preparations.

Procedures should indicate where labels are obtained and stored in the pharmacy. They should also require sequestration of batch labels with their preparation batch (see Chapter 9).

End-Preparation Evaluation

For all sterile preparations, policies and procedures for evaluating the final preparation should include pharmacist inspection for leaks, container integrity, cloudiness, particulates, color, and volume.[7] Also to be covered is pharmacist verification of ingredients, quantities, containers, reservoirs, and labels versus the drug order or prescription. Furthermore, a policy may specify that certain preparations require doublechecks (e.g., pediatric TPNs). Verification of automatic compounder settings also is extremely important, as is the disposal of defective preparations.[7]

For ASHP[6] Risk Level 3 preparations (USP[7] High Risk), methods for testing and documenting the sterility, nonpyrogenicity, and ingredient concentration (i.e., potency) should be described.

A quality-control program also must be explained, including the separation of responsibility for compounding and quality control; a sampling plan; methods of sterility, pyrogen, and ingredient potency testing; and in-use preparation sterility testing for suspected contamination (see Chapter 21).

Maintaining Quality of Compounded Preparations

Inside the Institution

Policies and procedures should document storage methods that ensure preparation identity, strength, and quality during transport and storage for both unrefrigerated and refrigerated preparations. These policies will differ from those developed for noncompounded preparations.

Special transport procedures for different preparation types also must be outlined. Furthermore, the selection of manual or automated delivery systems should be discussed (see Chapter 11).

Outside the Institution

These policies and procedures should cover packing for transport, in-transit temperatures, precautions for toxic preparation transport[8], commercial carrier expectations, evaluation of shipper performance, and in-home conditions. For the home, procedures should include (1) assurance of proper storage capability; (2) written instructions for storage, use (e.g., hand washing, aseptic technique, site care, etc.), and unsuitability for use; and (3) home visitation and inspection.

Patient and Caregiver Training

Policies and procedures for patient or caregiver training must be formalized (see Chapter 12) and include:

- Understanding of the therapy provided.
- Handling and storage of the sterile preparation.
- Appropriate administration techniques.
- Use and maintenance of any infusion device used.
- Use of printed material.

- Appropriate post-training verbal counselling.[7]

Patient Monitoring and Complaint System

For outcome monitoring, policies and procedures should encompass reporting and handling of patient problems and trending of patient problems regarding sterile preparations.[7]

Housekeeping Procedures

These policies and procedures should cover cleaning and disinfecting of floors, work surfaces, and walls. Intervals between each type of cleaning should be specified, cleaning equipment and supplies should be listed, and the reuse of cleaning supplies should be outlined. When these procedures are developed, the institution's housekeeping department should be consulted.

Brands of disinfectants and changing intervals also should be specified. Infection control personnel can help to develop these policies.

Quality-Assurance Program

The pharmacy should have written policies and procedures for monitoring, evaluating, correcting, and improving sterile preparation activities and processes. These policies and procedures should refer to those on training and education, competency evaluation, preparation compounding, sterilization methods, process validation, and end-preparation evaluation. The program must delineate individual responsibilities for each aspect of the program.

Documentation Records

Policies and procedures concerning documentation records should specify the location of stored records and the required storage time. The following records should be kept, but storage periods will vary according to laws, regulations, and professional standards (see Chapter 10):

- Training records and competence tests scores for each employee (e.g., aseptic technique observation and media fills).

- Refrigerator and freezer temperature logs or charts.

- Certification of laminar-airflow workbenches and scales.

- Batch compounding records.

- Master work sheets.

- Environmental monitoring tests.

- Process validations.

- Drug recalls.

- Product problem reports to manufacturers and USP.

- Adverse drug reaction reports to manufacturers and the Food and Drug Administration.

- Patient complaints and problem handling and outcome.

Summary

The establishment of policies and procedures is a critical step in any sterile preparation program. A thorough policy and procedure manual must be available to all involved personnel. These employees also must show an understanding of each policy and procedure before being allowed to compound sterile preparations. Moreover, their competency in performing these procedures and interpreting each policy should be assessed periodically.

References

1. Hethcox JM. The policy and procedure manual. In: Brown TR, ed. *Handbook of institutional pharmacy practice.* 3rd ed. Bethesda, MD: American Society of Hospital Pharmacists; 1992:53–62.

2. Ginnow WK, King CM Jr. Revision and reorganization of a hospital pharmacy policies and procedures manual. *Am J Hosp Pharm.* 1978;35:698–704.

3. Good compounding practices. United States pharmacopoeia, 27th rev./national formulary, 22nd ed. Rockville, MD: United States Pharmacopeial Convention; 2004. Available at: www.uspnf.com. Accessed January 19, 2004.

4. Lima SND, ed. *Hospital Pharmacy Management Forms, Checklists & Guidelines.* Gaithersburg, MD: Aspen Publishers, Inc. 1997.

5. International Journal of Pharmaceutical Compounding. Available at: www.IJPC.com. Accessed November 24, 2003.

6. American Society of Health-System Pharmacists. ASHP guidelines on quality assurance for pharmacy-prepared sterile preparations. *Am J Health-Syst Pharm.* 2000;57:1150–69.

7. Pharmaceutical compounding—sterile preparations. United States Pharmacopoeia 27th rev./National Formulary 22nd ed (first supplement). Rockville, MD: United States Pharmacopeial Convention; 2004. Available at: www.uspnf.com. Accessed April 1, 2004.

8. American Society of Hospital Pharmacists. ASHP technical assistance bulletin on handling cytotoxic and hazardous drugs. *Am J Hosp Pharm.* 1990;47:1033–49.

23 | Outsourcing the Compounding of Sterile Preparations

E. Clyde Buchanan

In a recent survey, Morris et al. found that 14% of hospitals outsource some of their sterile preparation compounding.[1] Why would so many hospitals choose an outside pharmacy to provide pharmaceutical services to their patients? The reasons are many but include shortages of pharmacist and pharmacy technician staff, costs of space and equipment and lack of expertise within the pharmacy to safely compound the more complex sterile preparations.

National Trends

In the past few years, many sterile pharmaceuticals have become unavailable, e.g., urokinase, methylprednisolone, sincalide, hyaluronidase.[2] Patients and physicians still need the products and require that pharmacists make or buy them.[3] Moreover, patients or physicians may ask pharmacists to make drugs that are available in other countries but not the U.S. Most pharmacists do not have the facilities or expertise to safely compound such products.[1] Even finding USP pharmaceutical grade raw materials to compound these drugs can be difficult or impossible.[2]

Pharmacists and technicians are in short supply as well.[4] Even when available, pharmacists and technicians are poorly trained to compound sterile preparations (see Chapters 15 and 16). Pharmacists are faced with new technologies such as indwelling infusion pumps and continuous renal replacement therapy (CRRT).[5] Future technologies, such as genetically engineered pharmaceuticals and individualized dosing based on pharmacogenomics, look even more imposing to the compounding pharmacist.

New laws, regulations, and professional guidelines make compounding sterile preparations more complex as well (see Chapter 1). In particular, USP <797> will force pharmacies to upgrade garb, procedures, personnel training, equipment and facilities.[6] Otherwise pharmacies will face citations from licensing and accrediting bodies. Future Occupational Safety and Health Administration regulations look daunting as regards the preparation of hazardous drugs, i.e., pharmacies will be required to upgrade personal protective equipment and environmental controls to protect the employees and environment from contamination with hazardous drugs (see Chapter 7).

Faced with these difficulties, pharmacists must consider outsourcing sterile compounding to pharmacies that purport to have the trained staff, facilities, and supply of ingredients to make the pharmaceuticals demanded by patients and physicians (Table 23-1). There are at least two national companies, CAPS[7] and COMPASS,[8] that are eager to provide sterile compounding services. In addition, increasingly more local "compounding pharmacies" claim to be competent to prepare sterile pharmaceuticals.[9]

What responsibilities does a pharmacy director have to assure the quality of sterile preparations compounded in contract pharmacies?

Laws, Regulations, and Standards

An organization's licensed pharmacy director or pharmacist-in-charge must take complete responsibility for patient outcomes from all medication-related activities performed at or for the organization's work sites, whether they are carried out by the organization's or contractor's onsite staff or by the contractor off site.[10] For the purposes of this discussion, the pharmacy to which an organization

Table 23-1.

Outsourcing of Sterile Drug Preparation (Sample n = 513)*

Sterile Preparation Outsourced	Number of Pharmacies	Percentage of Total Pharmacies
Total parenteral nutrition solutions	62	12.1%
Patient-controlled analgesia and epidural analgesia preparations	24	4.7%
I.V. admixtures and small-volume i.v. solutions	23	4.5%
Flushes	17	3.3%

*Modified from Table 19 in Pedersen CA, Schneider PJ, Scheckelhoff DJ. ASHP national survey of pharmacy practice in hospital settings: Dispensing and administration—2002. *Am J Health-Syst Pharm.* 2003;60:52–68.

outsources sterile preparation is referred to as the "contract pharmacy."

Joint Commission on Accreditation of Healthcare Organizations (JCAHO®)

The JCAHO has several standards that apply to compounded sterile pharmaceuticals obtained from contract pharmacies. The contract staff must meet all the competency measures of the staff of the pharmacy that purchases the compounding services.[11] The goal of the human resources function is to ensure that the hospital determines the qualifications and competencies for all staff including contractors or contract employees who provide services in the organization. The new medication management chapter states, "When pharmacy services are provided through a contract, the contract should address responsibility for these standards (Medication Management) and performance expectations. A hospital receiving pharmacy services should monitor the performance of contracted services."[12] A 1999 survey showed that almost 11% of hospitals outsource the preparation of total parenteral nutrition solutions but that only two thirds of those report monitoring quality assurance of the contract pharmacy.[13] Finally, according to JCAHO the contract pharmacy must meet the requirements of USP <797>.[6]

Health Insurance Portability and Accountability Act (HIPAA)

A contract pharmacy is a business associate to the organization in terms of the HIPAA law.[14] This means that the organization pharmacy will be disclosing protected health care information (PHI) to the contract pharmacy (e.g., patient names, identifying numbers, medical information). In order to make such disclosures, the contract pharmacy must sign a business associate agreement that gives the contract pharmacy legal access to the information needed to prepare and label a sterile prescription and requires the contract pharmacy to follow rules to protect patients' PHI. No more medical information can be sent to the contract pharmacy than they need to perform the compounding service. Second, patients must sign a general consent upon hos-

pital admission that their PHI may be used by a third party to provide treatments. Data transmitted in either direction between the organizational pharmacy and the contract pharmacy must be secured by authentication, encryption, alarms, etc.

Food and Drug Administration (FDA)

With respect to 21 U.S. Code 360 (g) (1), the FDA exempts retail pharmacies from registering as pharmaceutical manufacturers.[15] This exemption applies to pharmacies that operate in accord with state laws and dispense drugs upon prescriptions of practitioners licensed to administer such drugs to patients under their care in the course of their professional practice, and which do not manufacture, prepare, propagate, compound, or process drugs or devices at retail.

United State Pharmacopoeia (USP)

The FDA has the authority to require pharmacies to adhere to the national standards published in the current edition of the United State Pharmacopoeia/National Formulary (see Chapter 1). Such standards include:

- Chapter 1075 Good Compounding Practices[16]
- Chapter <797> Pharmaceutical Compounding – Sterile Preparations (Appendix F)
- Chapter 1191 Stability Considerations in Dispensing Practice[17]

Drug Enforcement Administration (DEA)

The DEA requires the use of DEA Form 222 for the transfer of Schedule II controlled drugs between pharmacies. This has implications for compounding narcotics for patient controlled analgesia and epidural analgesia; a recent survey showed that almost 5% of hospitals outsource the preparation of these preparations.[18] The DEA requires record-keeping and security for all schedules of controlled drugs that are purchased by one pharmacy from another pharmacy. Records of purchases, storage, distribution and administration or destruction are required for any controlled drug.[19] In addition, DEA security measures dictate that any transporter of controlled drugs be licensed and bonded. In other words, taxi cabs and most common carriers could not be used to transport controlled drugs.

Antitrust Laws

The Robinson-Patman Act requires that a hospital that purchases drugs at preferential prices (e.g., through an acute care hospital group purchasing organization contract) limit the use of those drugs to their "own use."[20] Contract pharmacies are usually in a different class of trade from hospital pharmacies, for example they may be classed as retail pharmacies as opposed to acute care hospital pharmacies. This difference in class means that the contract pharmacy may not be able to purchase drugs as cheaply. This becomes significant for sterile preparations such as total parenteral nutrition and CRRT. The upshot is that organization pharmacies must find ways to have the contract pharmacy use the institution's pharmaceutical ingredients in compounding. This may require the contract pharmacy to have the organization pharmacy purchase the pharmaceutical ingredients for delivery to the contract pharmacy, which in turn must maintain a separate inventory for each organization that it serves. This practice often increases the inventory cost for the organization pharmacy which must have two inventories of compounding ingredients, one for stat orders within the organization and one in the contract pharmacy for routing compounding. This is not to say that the organization pharmacy and the contract pharmacy accountants and lawyers cannot find other creative ways to purchase and account for "own use" pharmaceutical ingredients.

State Boards of Pharmacy

To compound and dispense medications, the contract pharmacy must be a pharmacy licensed by a state board of pharmacy, usually the state board in the same state in which the patient is receiving such medications. Many states have regulations covering good compounding practices in general and at least five states have regulations pertaining to the compounding of sterile preparations. State Boards regulate compounding, which by definition requires a specific drug order or prescription by a licensed prescriber for each sterile preparation from the contract pharmacy. Therefore, it is difficult for contract pharmacies to prepare batches ahead of a prescription for sterile preparations such as sterile talc injection, cardioplegia solutions, ophthalmics, and inhalations. It is incumbent on the organization's pharmacy director to determine the state board's stance on the legality of the particular sterile preparations to be purchased from a contract pharmacy.

American Society of Health-System Pharmacists (ASHP)

Almost 1100 pharmacy residency programs are accredited by ASHP.[21] To maintain their accreditation, pharmacies with residency programs must meet all ASHP guidelines and, by extension, any contract pharmacy should meet ASHP guidelines. Those ASHP guidelines that pertain to sterile preparation include:

- ASHP Guidelines on Outsourcing Pharmaceutical Services[10]
- ASHP Guidelines on Pharmacy-Prepared Sterile Products (Appendix A)
- ASHP Technical Assistance Bulletin on Pharmacy-Prepared Ophthalmic Products (Appendix B)
- ASHP Guidelines on the Safe Use of Automated Compounding Devices for the Preparation of Parenteral Nutrition Admixtures (Appendix C)
- ASHP Technical Assistance Bulletin on Handling Cytotoxic and Hazardous Drugs (Appendix D)

Organizational Pharmacy Responsibilities in Outsourcing

The pharmacy director is responsible for the legality and quality of pharmaceuticals obtained from contract pharmacies but in addition they have other fiduciary responsibilities to their organization.

Administration

All organizations have cultures. Some favor outsourcing; others do not. One of the first things the pharmacy director should do is to assess the willingness of the chief executive officer to enter into an outsourcing contract. Outsourcing has implications for the organization's patient satisfaction, nursing and medical staff relations and reputation within the community. Sometimes the decision to outsource can be reversed only with great difficulty. Lastly, the administrator may not wish to lose control over decisions about pharmaceutical services.

Fiscal Responsibilities

The pharmacy director must make sure that the organization makes the best decisions to protect the organization's margin. A full cost analysis, pro-forma or business plan is needed before any outsourcing pharmacy contracts are consummated. All direct and indirect costs must be considered, including technical support for information services, computer hardware and connections (e.g., internet service provider and modem lines), and interfaces; legal services and liability insurance; accounting and tax services; medical staff support (e.g., medical director salary); transportation charges, including licensing and bonding; pharmaceutical ingredient inventory at the contract pharmacy and, of course, all product and support fees for the contract pharmacy. All these costs must be compared to performing the same sterile compounding services within the organization. Some organizations have saved money by outsourcing.[22]

Information System Responsibilities

Transmission of prescription orders between pharmacies must be accommodated. The pharmacy director must involve the information services (IS) department early on to ascertain whether IS has the time and resources to support information transfer.

Materials Responsibilities

The pharmacy director must arrange for receiving compounded pharmaceuticals from the contract pharmacy. Do arrangements jibe with the receiving department for hours of service, space, refrigeration, and security for deliveries?

Risk Management

Most organizations have risk management departments. The pharmacy director must get support from the risk manager to use compounded pharmaceuticals from a contract pharmacy. The pharmacy director may have to explain all the liabilities for clarity in the decision-making process.

Contracting for Outsourced Sterile Compounding

Legal contracts are mandatory for a continuing relationship between an organization and a contract pharmacy. Where there is more than one option for the contract pharmacy, the pharmacy director should consider obtaining proposals from different contract pharmacies; i.e., a request-for-proposal (RFP) process.[10] Once a contract pharmacy is chosen, the contract should include at least the following provisions:

- Term of service—how long the contract will last; how it will be renewed and the reasons for which either party can exit the contract before the end of term. Such reasons might include "cause" such as bankruptcy or change of ownership of the contract pharmacy, breech of obligations, market changes, technology changes etc.

- Extent of service—what preparations are to be provided, e.g., total parenteral nutrition, cardioplegia solutions, CRRT, prefilled syringes, etc.

- Level of service—how many deliveries per day, the deadline for deliveries, after-hour services, etc.

- Quality of service—agreement that the contract pharmacy agrees to comply with federal and state laws and regulations and with JCAHO standards; specific compliance with USP <797>.

- Terms of payment—fees for preparations and support services, late payment fees, resolution method for disputed services, special fees for extra deliveries or after-hour deliveries, credit for returns, etc.

- Information transfer—confidentiality of PHI, of proprietary business information,

247

i.e., the business associate agreement; order transmission method along with ownership and maintenance of related hardware and software; drug use evaluation and legal record-keeping and documentation.

- Indemnification—the relationship as to how either party will hold the other harmless in case of lawsuits against a party in the agreement.

- Insurance—how much liability insurance must be carried by either party for single or multiple incidents.

- Force majeure—clause to cover acts of God (e.g., storm damage to either party that interrupts service); labor disputes; legal interruptions of service etc.

- Access to books, documents, and records of subcontractors clause[23]

- Amendments—how to amend the agreement

- Severability of portions of the agreement —how the parties might delete selected portions of the agreement or may not sever any portion.

- Entire agreement—clause stating that there are no other parts to the agreement other than what is stated in the agreement.

- Independent contractor—statement to the effect that the contract party is independent of the organization as to ownership and any obligations outside of the agreement; this clause prevents one party from "steering" business to the other party, an issue in Medicare fraud.

- Dispute resolution—clause stating manner by with disputes are to be resolved by the parties, e.g., independent arbitration, legal channels, etc.

Compounding Pharmacy Relationship

Occasionally pharmacy directors are faced with having a hospital patient use sterile preparations compounded by a retail, home care, or compounding pharmacy. Patients may be admitted while a sterile preparation made elsewhere (e.g., TPN or peritoneal dialysis solution compounded by a home care pharmacy) is being administered. Physicians might bring in sterile preparations that they have obtained from a compounding pharmacy[3] or even from

a foreign country—sterile products that are not FDA-approved. The hospital pharmacy itself might want to obtain a specific product from a compounding pharmacy to deal with a market shortage. Before a sterile preparation is obtained from an outside pharmacy, the pharmacy director should consider the following questions[24]:

1. What are the regulations for using compounded preparations in the state where the purchasing organization is located?

2. Does the organization get informed consent from patients before using a compounded preparation from an outside source?[25] A medical staff committee (e.g., Pharmacy and Therapeutics) should participate in this decision. Some state medical practice acts prohibit physicians from prescribing drugs that have not been approved by the U.S. FDA.

3. Does the organization inform health care professionals (e.g., prescribers, nurses) that a compounded preparation from an outside source will be used, including the possible risks associated with its use?[25] A medical staff committee (e.g., Pharmacy and Therapeutics) should participate in this decision.

4. Does the compounding pharmacy use USP-grade raw materials?

5. What is the source of the raw material (if animal, domestic or imported)? The reason that hyaluronidase was withdrawn from the market was that there was no way to assure the beef origin was free from mad cow disease.

6. Is every batch of raw material, if from an animal source, screened for viral contamination?

7. Is every batch of the compounded preparation tested for purity, potency, sterility and pyrogenicity, and compliance with standards published in the USP?

8. What sterilization process is used for the packaging and the final preparation?

9. Is every batch quarantined for more than 10 days?

10. Is every batch of preparation tested for sterility on days 2 and 10?

11. Is every batch of preparation tested for pyrogens on day 10?

12. Has the compounding pharmacy performed extended stability tests?

13. For each batch of preparation made, does the compounding pharmacy provide a "beyond-use" date after which it should not be used?

Summary

Organizational pharmacies must consider outsourcing sterile preparation compounding to contract pharmacies due to shortages of pharmacist and pharmacy technician staff, of space and equipment and of expertise within the pharmacy to safely compound more complex sterile preparations. However, many obstacles stand in the way of outsourcing, such as the organization's responsibility to assure the same or better quality of compounding as the organization is expected to provide; the many legalities and liabilities of outsourcing compounding services and the finances and logistics of outsourcing.

References

1. Morris AM, Schneider PJ, Pederson CA et al. National survey of quality assurance activities for pharmacy-compounded sterile preparations. *Am J Health-Syst Pharm.* 2003;60:2567–76.
2. Young D. Taking full responsibility. *Am J Health-Syst Pharm.* 2003;60:1209.
3. Young D. Outsourced compounding can be problematic. *Am J Health-Syst Pharm.* 2002:59:2261, 2262, 2264.
4. Gouveia WA. Solutions to pharmacy's staffing crisis. *Am J Health-Syst Pharm.* 2001; 58:807–8.
5. Forni LG, Hilton PJ. Continuous hemofiltration in the treatment of acute renal failure. *New Eng J Med.* 1997;336(18): 1303–9.
6. Thompson CA. USP publishes enforceable chapter on sterile compounding. *Am J Health-Syst Pharm.* 2003;60:1814–7.
7. Central Admixture Pharmacy Service. Available at: http://www.bbraunoem-industrial.com/capabilities/caps.cfm. Accessed March 2, 2004.
8. COMPASS. Available at: www.pharmedium.com. Accessed August 13, 2004.
9. Spencer J, Mathews AW. As druggists mix customized brews, FDA raises alarms. *Wall Street Journal.* February 27, 2004.
10. Council on Administrative Affairs. ASHP Guidelines on outsourcing pharmaceutical services. *Am J Health-Syst Pharm.* 1998;55:1611–7.
11. Joint Commission on Accreditation of Healthcare Organizations. Management of human resources. In: *2004 Comprehensive Accreditation Manual for Hospitals: The Official Handbook (CAMH).* Chicago, IL: Joint Commission on Accreditation of Healthcare Organizations. Available at: www.jcaho.org. Accessed March 3, 2004.
12. Joint Commission on Accreditation of Healthcare Organizations. Hospitals medication management overview. In: *2004 Comprehensive Accreditation Manual for Hospitals: The Official Handbook (CAMH).* Chicago, IL: Joint Commission on Accreditation of Healthcare Organizations. Available at: www.jcaho.org. Accessed March 3, 2004.
13. Ringold DJ, Santell JP, Schneider PJ. ASHP national survey of pharmacy practice in acute care settings: Dispensing and administration—1999. *Am J Health-Syst Pharm.* 2000; 57:1759–75.
14. Tribble DA. The Health Insurance Portability and Accountability Act: Security and privacy requirements. *Am J Health-Syst Pharm.* 2001;58:763–70.
15. Food and Drug Administration. Compliance policy guidance for FDA staff and industry (chapter 4, subchapter 460; section 460.200). Available at: www.fda.gov/ora/compliance_ref/cpg/cpgdrg/cpg460-200.html. Accessed March 3, 2004.
16. Good compounding practices. United States pharmacopeia, 27th rev/national formulary 22nd ed. Rockville, MD: United States Pharmacopeial Convention. Available at: www.uspnf.com. Accessed March 3, 2004.
17. Stability considerations in dispensing practice. United States pharmacopeia, 27th rev/national formulary, 22nd ed. Rockville, MD: United States Pharmacopeial Convention. Available at: www.uspnf.com. Accessed March 3, 2004.
18. Pedersen CA, Schneider PJ, Scheckelhoff DJ. ASHP national survey of pharmacy practice in hospital settings: dispensing and administration—2002. *Am J Health-Syst Pharm.* 2003; 60:52–68.
19. Drug Enforcement Administration. Controlled Substances Act. Available at: http://www.usdoj.gov/dea/pubs/csa.html. Accessed March 3, 2004.

20. Welch CA. Robinson-Patman Act and the own-use exemption in health systems. *Am J Health-Syst Pharm.* 1999;56:990–4.

21. American Society of Health-System Pharmacists (ASHP) website. Available at: http://www.ashp.org/rtp/Seeking/index.cfm?cfid=453742&CFToken=71981316. Accessed March 3, 2004.

22. Gates DM, Smolarek RT, Stevenson JG. Outsourcing the preparation of parenteral nutrient solutions. *Am J Health-Syst Pharm.* 1996;53:2176-8.

23. Medicare program: Access to books, documents, and records of subcontractors. Final rule. *Federal Register.* 47;251: 58260–70, 1982.

24. American Society of Health-System Pharmacists. Tips for working with a compounding pharmacy. *Action Line.* March 2004.

25. Young D. Compounding sterile preparations raises informed-consent issues. *Am J Health-Syst Pharm.* 2003;60:1209–10.

APPENDIXES

Appendix A | ASHP Guidelines on Quality Assurance for Pharmacy-Prepared Sterile Products

Patient morbidity and mortality have resulted from incorrectly prepared or contaminated pharmacy-prepared products.[1-7] Pharmacists seldom know that inaccurate or contaminated products are dispensed when pharmacy quality monitors are inadequate.[8-10] In contemporary health care organizations, more patients are receiving compounded sterile products that are stored for extended periods before use (allowing the growth of a pathological bioload of microorganisms[11]), more patients are seriously ill, and more patients are immunocompromised than ever before.

These ASHP guidelines are intended to help pharmacists and pharmacy technicians prepare sterile products of high quality.[a] The pharmacist is responsible for compounding and dispensing sterile products of correct ingredient identity, purity (freedom from physical contaminants, such as precipitates,[12] and chemical contaminants), strength (including stability[13] and compatibility), and sterility and for dispensing them in appropriate containers, labeled accurately and appropriately for the end user.

Other professional organizations have published useful guidelines on compounding and dispensing sterile products. The United States Pharmacopeia (USP) publishes the official compendium *The United States Pharmacopeia and The National Formulary* (*USP*) and its supplements, all of which may have legal implications for pharmacists.[14,15] The reader would especially benefit from studying the *USP* general information chapter on sterile drug products for home use,[13] which is referred to often in this ASHP guideline. The National Association of Boards of Pharmacy (NABP) has published less detailed model regulations for use by state boards of pharmacy.[16,17] The American Society for Parenteral and Enteral Nutrition (A.S.P.E.N.) recently published a special report on safe practices for parenteral nutrition formulations.[18]

Other governmental and accreditation sources are more general. The Joint Commission on Accreditation of Healthcare Organizations (JCAHO) publishes at least four sets of standards that mention pharmacy compounding. The hospital accreditation standards simply state that the organization adheres to laws, professional licensure, and practice standards governing the safe operation of pharmaceutical services.[19] The JCAHO home care standards require that medications be safely prepared, including "using appropriate techniques for preparing sterile and nonsterile medications and products." For example, the home care standards state that "appropriate quality-control techniques are used to check for preparation accuracy and absence of microbial contamination. Techniques for preparing sterile products follow guidelines established by the American Society of Health-System Pharmacists."[20] The JCAHO standards for long-term-care pharmacies list important conditions for product preparation, such as separate areas for sterile product preparation, use of a laminar-airflow workbench or class 100 cleanroom, and quality control systems to ensure the accuracy and sterility of final products.[21] The JCAHO standard for ambulatory care infusion centers states, among other things, several facility-related standards, for example the use of biological safety cabinets to protect personnel preparing cytotoxic or hazardous medications; work surfaces free of equipment, supplies, records, and labels unrelated to the medication being prepared; and a separate area for preparing sterile products that is constructed to minimize opportunities for particulate and microbial contamination.[22]

The Food and Drug Administration (FDA) publishes regulations on current good manufacturing practices that apply to sterile products made by pharmaceutical manufacturers for shipment in interstate commerce. Pursuant to the FDA Modernization Act of 1997 (FDAMA), Section 503A of the Food, Drug, and Cosmetic Act states that pharmacy compounding must comply with an applicable *USP* monograph, if one exists, and the *USP* chapter on pharmacy compounding[14] or be a component of an FDA-approved drug product; or, if neither of these apply to the ingredient being compounded, the substance must appear on a list of bulk drug substances developed by FDA and must be accompanied by a valid certificate of analysis and be manufactured in an FDA-registered establishment.[23] Inactive ingredients compounded by licensed pharmacies must comply with applicable *USP* monographs, if they exist, and the *USP* chapter on pharmacy compounding.[14] FDAMA prohibits pharmacists from compounding drug products that appear on a list of products that have been withdrawn or removed from the market because they have been found unsafe or ineffective. FDAMA also says that pharmacists may not compound, regularly or in inordinate amounts, drug products that are essentially copies of commercially available drug products; nor may they compound drug products identified by regulation as presenting demonstrable difficulties for compounding that reasonably demonstrate an adverse effect on safety or effectiveness.

The Centers for Disease Control and Prevention (CDC) has published guidelines for hand washing, prevention of intravascular infections, and hospital environmental control.[24,25]

The ASHP Guidelines on Quality Assurance for Pharmacy-Prepared Sterile Products are applicable to pharmaceutical services in various practice settings, including, but not limited to, hospitals, community pharmacies, nursing homes, ambulatory care infusion centers, and home care organizations. ASHP has also published practice standards on handling cytotoxic and hazardous drugs[26] and on pharmacy-prepared ophthalmic products.[27] These ASHP guidelines *do not* apply to the *manufacture* of sterile pharmaceuticals as defined in state and federal laws and regulations, *nor* do they apply to the preparation of medications by pharmacists, nurses, or physicians in emergency situations for *immediate* administration to patients (e.g., cardiopulmonary resuscitation). All guidelines may not be applicable to the preparation of radiopharmaceuticals.

These guidelines are referenced with supporting scientific data when such data exist. In the absence of published supporting data, guidelines are based on expert opinion or generally accepted pharmacy procedures. Pharmacists are urged to use professional judgment in interpreting these guidelines and applying them in practice. It is recognized that, in certain emergency situations, a pharmacist may be requested to compound products under conditions that do not meet these guidelines. In such situations, it is incumbent upon the pharmacist to employ professional judgment in weighing the potential patient risks and benefits associated with the compounding procedure in question.

Objectives

The objectives of these guidelines are to provide

1. Information on quality assurance and quality control activities that should be applied to the preparation of sterile products in pharmacies and

2. A method to match quality assurance and quality control activities with the potential risks to patients posed by various types of products.

Multidisciplinary Input

Pharmacists are urged to participate in the quality or performance improvement, risk management, and infection control programs of their health care organizations, including developing optimal sterile product procedures.

Definitions

Definitions of selected terms, as used in this document, are provided in Appendix A. For brevity in this document, the term *quality assurance* will be used to refer to both quality assurance and quality control (as defined in Appendix A), as befits the circumstances.

Risk-Level Classification

In this document, sterile products are grouped into three levels of risk to the patient, increasing from least (level 1) to greatest (level 3) potential risk based on the danger of exposing multiple patients to inaccurate ingredients or pathogens and based on microbial growth factors influenced by product storage time, temperature and product ability to support microbial growth, surface and time exposure of critical sites, and microbial bioload in the environment. When circumstances make risk-level assignment unclear, guidelines for the higher risk level should prevail. Consideration should be given to factors that increase potential risk to the patient such as high-risk administration sites and immunocompromised status of the patient. A comparison of risk-level attributes appears in Appendix B.

Risk Level 1

Risk level 1 applies to compounded sterile products that exhibit characteristics 1, 2, *and* 3, stated below. All risk level 1 products should be prepared with sterile equipment (e.g., syringes and vials), sterile ingredients and solutions, and sterile contact surfaces for the final product. Risk level 1 includes the following:

1. Products

   a. Stored at room temperature (see Appendix A for temperature definitions) and completely administered within 28 hours after preparation or

b. Stored under refrigeration for 7 days or less before complete administration to a patient over a period not to exceed 24 hours (Table 1) or

c. Frozen for 30 days or less before complete administration to a patient over a period not to exceed 24 hours.

2. Unpreserved sterile products prepared for administration to one patient or batch-prepared products containing suitable preservatives prepared for administration to more than one patient.

3. Products prepared by closed-system aseptic transfer of sterile, nonpyrogenic, finished pharmaceuticals (e.g., from vials or ampuls)[b] obtained from licensed manufacturers into sterile final containers (e.g., syringes, minibags, elastomeric containers, portable infusion-device cassettes) obtained from licensed manufacturers.

Examples of risk level 1 processes include transferring a sterile drug product from a vial into a commercially produced i.v. bag; compounding total parenteral nutrient (TPN) solutions by combining dextrose injection and amino acids injection via gravity transfer into a sterile empty container, with or without the subsequent addition of sterile drug products to the final container with a sterile needle and syringe; and transferring a sterile, preserved drug product into sterile syringes with the aid of a mechanical pump and appropriate sterile transfer tubing device.

Risk Level 2

Risk level 2 sterile products exhibit characteristic 1, 2, *or* 3, stated below. All risk level 2 products should be prepared with sterile equipment, sterile ingredients and solutions, and sterile contact surfaces for the final product and with closed-system transfer methods. Risk level 2 includes the following:

1. Products stored beyond 7 days under refrigeration, stored beyond 30 days frozen, or administered beyond 28 hours after preparation and storage at room temperature (Table 1).

2. Batch-prepared products *without preservatives* (e.g., epidural products) that are intended for use by more than one patient. (Note: Batch-prepared products without preservatives that will be administered to multiple patients carry a greater risk to the patients than products prepared for a single patient because of the potential effect of inaccurate ingredients or product contamination on the health and well-being of a larger patient group.)

3. Products compounded by complex or numerous manipulations of sterile ingredients obtained from licensed manufacturers in a sterile container or reservoir obtained from a licensed manufacturer by using closed-system aseptic transfer; for example, TPN solutions prepared with an automated compounder. (Note: So many risks have been associated with automated compounding of TPN solutions that its complexity requires risk level 2 procedures.[18])

Examples of risk level 2 processes include preparing portable-pump reservoirs for multi-day (i.e., ambient temperature) administration; subdividing the contents of a bulk, sterile injectable (without preservatives) into single-dose syringes; and compounding TPN solutions with an automated compounding device involving repeated attachment of fluid

Table 1.

Assignment of Products to Risk Level 1 or 2 according to Time and Temperature before Completion of Administration

Risk Level	Room Temperature (15–30°C)	No. Days Storage	
		Refrigerator (2–8°C)	Freezer (−20 to −10°C)
1	Completely administered within 28 hr	≤7	≤30
2	Storage and administration exceed 28 hr	>7	>30

containers to proximal openings of the compounder tubing set and of empty final containers to the distal opening, the process concluding with the transfer of additives into the filled final container from individual drug product containers or from a pooled additive solution.

Risk Level 3

Risk level 3 products exhibit either characteristic 1 *or* 2:

1. Products compounded from nonsterile ingredients or compounded with nonsterile components, containers, or equipment before terminal sterilization.

2. Products prepared by combining multiple ingredients—sterile or nonsterile—by using an open-system transfer or open reservoir before terminal sterilization.

Examples of risk level 3 products are calcium levulinate injection, estradiol in oil injection, and morphine sulfate 50-mg/mL injection.[32]

Quality Assurance for Risk Level 1

RL 1.1: Policies and Procedures[33]

Up-to-date policies and procedures for compounding sterile products should be written and available to all personnel involved in these activities. When policies and procedures are changed they should be updated, as necessary, to reflect current standards of practice and quality. Additions, revisions, and deletions should be communicated to all personnel involved in sterile compounding and related activities. These policies and procedures should address personnel education and training requirements, competency evaluation, product acquisition, storage and handling of products and supplies, storage and delivery of final products, use and maintenance of facilities and equipment,[34] appropriate garb and conduct for personnel working in the controlled area, process validation, preparation technique,[35] labeling, documentation, and quality control.[36] Further, written policies and procedures should address personnel access and movement of materials into and near the controlled area. Policies and procedures for monitoring environmental conditions in the con-

trolled area should take into consideration the amount of exposure of the product to the environment during compounding and the environmental control devices used to create the critical area. Sources of information include vendor-supplied inservice programs and multimedia training programs, such as videotapes and Internet-site information. Before compounding sterile products, all personnel involved should read the policies and procedures. Written policies and procedures are required for all environmental control devices used to create the critical area for manipulation of sterile products. Examples of such devices are laminar-airflow workstations, biological safety cabinets, class 100 cleanrooms, and barrier isolator workstations (see Appendix A).[c]

RL 1.2: Personnel Education, Training, and Evaluation

Training is the most important factor in ensuring the quality of sterile products. Pharmacy personnel preparing or dispensing sterile products must receive suitable didactic and experiential training and competency evaluation through demonstration, testing (written or practical), or both. Some aspects that should be included in training programs include aseptic technique; critical-area contamination factors; environmental monitoring; facilities, equipment, and supplies; sterile product calculations and terminology; sterile product compounding documentation; quality assurance procedures; aseptic preparation procedures; proper gowning and gloving technique; and general conduct in the controlled area. In addition to knowledge of chemical, pharmaceutical, and clinical properties of drugs, pharmacists should be knowledgeable about the principles of pharmacy compounding.[14] Videotapes[37,38] and additional information on the essential components of a training, orientation, and evaluation program are described elsewhere.[39,40] All pharmacy and non-pharmacy personnel (e.g., environmental services staff) who work in the controlled area should receive documented train-ing on cleaning, sanitizing, and maintaining equipment used in the controlled area. Training should be specific to the environmental control device and equipment present in the controlled area and should be based on current procedures.

The aseptic technique of each person preparing sterile products should be observed and evaluated as satisfactory during orientation and training and at least annually thereafter.[41] In addition to observation, methods of evaluating the knowledge of personnel include written or practical tests and process validation.[42,43]

RL 1.3: Storage and Handling within the Pharmacy[44]

Solutions, drugs, supplies, and equipment used to prepare or administer sterile products should be stored in accordance with manufacturer or *USP* requirements. Temperatures in refrigerators and freezers used to store ingredients and finished sterile preparations should be monitored and documented daily to ensure that compendial storage requirements are met. Warehouse and other pharmacy storage areas where ingredients are stored should be monitored to ensure that temperature, light, moisture, and ventilation remain within manufacturer and compendial requirements. To permit adequate floor cleaning, drugs, supplies, and compounding equipment should be stored on shelving, cabinets, and carts above the floor. Products that have exceeded their expiration dates should be removed from active storage areas. Before use, each drug, ingredient, and container should be visually inspected for damage, defects, and expiration date.[45]

Unnecessary personnel traffic in the controlled area should be minimized. Particle-generating activities, such as removal of intravenous solutions, drugs, and supplies from cardboard boxes, should not be performed in the controlled area. Products and supplies used in preparing sterile products should be removed from shipping containers outside the controlled area before aseptic processing is begun. Packaging materials and items generating unacceptable amounts of particles (e.g., cardboard boxes, paper towels [unless lint-free], reference books) should not be permitted in the controlled area or critical area. The removal of immediate packaging designed to retain the sterility or stability of a product (e.g., syringe packaging, light-resistant pouches) is an exception; obviously, this type of packaging should not be removed outside the controlled area. Disposal of packaging materials, used syringes, containers, and needles should be performed at least daily, and more often if needed, to enhance sanitation and avoid accumulation in the controlled area.

Trash cans should be below the level of the laminar-airflow workbench and should be removed from the controlled area before being emptied. Sharps containers should be safely placed into the waste stream, according to policies developed by the institution to comply with regulations of the Occupational Safety and Health Administration (OSHA).

In the event of a product recall, there should be a mechanism for tracking and retrieving affected products from specific patients to whom the products were dispensed.

RL 1.4: Facilities[46] and Equipment[47]

The controlled area should be a limited-access area sufficiently separated from other pharmacy operations to minimize the potential for contamination that could result from the unnecessary flow of materials and personnel into and out of the area. The controlled area is a buffer from outside air that is needed because strong air currents from briefly opened doors, personnel walking past the laminar-airflow workbench, or the air stream from the heating, ventilating, and air conditioning system can easily exceed the velocity of air from the laminar-airflow workbench. Also, operators introducing supplies into the laminar-airflow workbench or reaching in with their arms can drag contaminants from the environment surrounding the workbench.[15] Cleanliness of the controlled area can be enhanced by (1) limiting access to those personnel assigned to work in the controlled area, (2) having those personnel wear the appropriate garb, (3) donning and removing garb outside the controlled area, (4) keeping doors to the controlled area closed, (5) limiting storage in the controlled area to items in constant use, (6) using low-particulate shelving, counters, and carts (e.g., stainless steel) in the controlled area, (7) not allowing cardboard and other particle-generating materials in the controlled area, (8) controlling the temperature and humidity inside the room, and (9) implementing a regular cleaning (e.g., nightly floor disinfection) and maintenance schedule.[48]

Barrier isolator workstations are closed systems and are not as sensitive to their external environment as laminar-airflow equipment. It is good practice to (1) place barrier isolator workstations in limited-access areas, (2) control the temperature and humidity of the surrounding area, and (3) clean and sanitize the surrounding area on a routine basis.[49]

Special precautions should be taken to clean equipment and compounding areas meticulously after preparing products that contain allergenic ingredients (e.g., sulfonamides and penicillins). Equipment should be of appropriate design and size for compounding and suitable for the intended uses. Equipment and accessories used in compounding should be inspected, maintained, and cleaned at appropriate intervals to ensure the accuracy and reliability of their performance.[14]

Computer entry, order processing, label generation, and record keeping should be performed outside the critical area. The controlled area should be well organized[50] and lighted[51] and of sufficient size to support sterile compounding activities. For hand washing, a sink with hot and cold running water should be in close proximity to but outside the controlled area. Refrigeration, freezing, ventilation, and room temperature control capabilities appropriate for storage of ingredients, supplies, and pharmacy-prepared sterile products in accordance with manufacturer, USP, and state or federal requirements should exist. The controlled area should be cleaned and disinfected at regular intervals with appropriate agents, according to written policies and procedures.[52] Disinfectants should be alternated periodically to prevent development of resistant microorganisms.[d] The floors of the controlled area should be nonporous and washable to enable regular disinfection. Active work surfaces in the controlled area (e.g., carts, compounding devices, counter surfaces) should be disinfected, in accordance with written procedures. Refrigerators, freezers, shelves, and other areas where pharmacy-prepared sterile products are stored should be kept clean.

Sterile products must be prepared in a class 100 environment (i.e., the critical area).[29] Such an environment exists inside a certified horizontal- or vertical-laminar-airflow workbench, a class 100 cleanroom, or a barrier isolator.[53] Cytotoxic and other hazardous products should be prepared in a vented class II biological safety cabinet or a barrier isolator of appropriate design to meet the personnel exposure limits described in product material safety data sheets (MSDS).[54] Barrier isolators are gaining favor as clean environments, especially for cytotoxic drug compounding.[55-57] Properly maintained barrier isolators provide suitable environments for the preparation of risk level 1, 2, and 3 sterile products.[58]

Laminar-airflow workbenches are designed to be operated continuously. If a laminar-airflow workbench is turned off between aseptic processes, it should be operated long enough to allow complete purging of room air from the critical area (e.g., at least 30 minutes), then disinfected before use. Barrier isolators, because of their closed nature, require less start-up time. If the barrier isolator has been turned off for less than 24 hours, a two-minute start-up time is sufficient. For periods greater than 24 hours, the chamber should be sanitized and the isolator should not be used for a minimum of 10 minutes after application of the sanitizing agent. The critical-area work surface and all accessible interior surfaces of the workbench should be disinfected with an appropriate agent before work begins and periodically thereafter, in accordance with written policies and procedures.[52] The exterior surfaces of the laminar-airflow workbench should be cleaned periodically with a mild detergent or suitable disinfectant; 70% isopropyl alcohol may damage the workbench's clear plastic surfaces. The laminar-airflow workbench should be certified by a qualified contractor[59] every six months[53] or when it is relocated to ensure operational efficiency and integrity. Prefilters in the laminar-airflow workbench should be changed (or cleaned, if they are washable) periodically (e.g., monthly), in accordance with written policies and procedures.

A method should be established for calibrating and verifying the accuracy of automated compounding devices used in aseptic processing (e.g., routine reconstitution of bulk or individual vials, transferring of doses from a bulk container to a minibag, syringe, or other single-dose container).

RL 1.5: Garb[60]

Procedures should require that personnel wear clean gowns or coveralls that generate few particles in the controlled area.[53] Scrub attire by itself is not acceptable (but can, like street clothes, be covered by a gown or coverall). Hand, finger, and wrist jewelry should be minimized or eliminated. Fingernails should be kept clean and trimmed. Head and facial hair should be covered. Masks are recommended because most personnel talk[61] or may cough or sneeze. Gloves are recommended. Personnel who have demonstrated sensitivity to latex should use either powder-free, low-latex protein gloves or, in the case of severe allergy, latex-free (synthetic) gloves.[62,63]

RL 1.6: Aseptic Technique[64,65] and Product Preparation[66]

Sterile products must be prepared with aseptic technique in a class 100 environment. Personnel should scrub their hands and forearms for an appropriate length of time with a suitable antimicrobial skin cleanser at the beginning of each aseptic compounding process and when reentering the controlled area, in accordance with written procedures. Personnel should wear appropriate attire (see RL 1.5: Garb). Eating, drinking, and smoking are prohibited in the controlled area. Talking should be minimized in the critical area during aseptic preparation (even when masks are worn).

Ingredients used to compound sterile products should be determined to be stable, compatible, and appropriate for the product to be prepared, according to manufacturer or USP guidelines or appropriate scientific references. The ingredients of the preparation should be predetermined to result in a final product that meets physiological norms for solution osmolality and pH, as appropriate for the intended route of administration. Each ingredient and container should be inspected for defects, expiration date, and product integrity before use. Expired, inappropriately stored, or defective products must not be used in preparing sterile products. Defective products should be promptly reported to the FDA MedWatch Program.[67]

Only materials essential for preparing the sterile product should be placed in the laminar-airflow workbench or barrier isolator. The surfaces of ampuls, vials, and container closures (e.g., vial stoppers) should be disinfected by swabbing or spraying with an appropriate disinfectant solution (e.g., 70% isopropyl alcohol or 70% ethanol) before placement in the workbench. Materials used in aseptic preparation should be arranged in the critical area (within the laminar-airflow workbench or barrier isolator) in a manner that prevents interruption of the unidirectional airflow between the high-efficiency particulate air (HEPA) filter and critical sites of needles, vials, ampuls, containers, and transfer sets. All aseptic procedures should be performed at least 6 inches inside the front edge of the laminar-airflow workbench, in a clear path of unidirectional airflow between the HEPA filter and work

materials (e.g., needles, closures). The number of personnel preparing sterile products in the workbench at one time should be minimized. Overcrowding of the critical work area may interfere with unidirectional airflow and increase the potential for compounding errors. Likewise, the number of units being prepared in the workbench at one time should allow unobstructed airflow over critical areas. Automated compounding devices and other equipment placed in or adjacent to the critical area should be cleaned, disinfected, and placed to avoid contamination or disruption of the unidirectional airflow between the HEPA filter and sterile surfaces. Closed systems like barrier isolators require less stringent placement of sterile units and equipment because the critical area encompasses the entire work surface. Hand and arm movements are not critical because the walls of the barrier isolator provide protection from the outside environment.[50]

Aseptic technique should be used to avoid touch contamination of sterile needles, syringe parts (e.g., plunger, syringe tip), and other critical sites. Solutions from ampuls should be properly filtered to remove particles. Solutions of reconstituted powders should be mixed carefully, ensuring complete dissolution of the drug with the appropriate diluent. Needle entry into vials should be performed in such a manner as to avoid coring of the vial closure. Some patients may require a latex-free admixture to avoid severe allergic reactions.[68] Latex-related policies and procedures should be developed by each institution, given the paucity of evidence that latex closures and syringe plungers are implicated in patient reactions to latex.[69,70] Before, during, and after the preparation of sterile products, the pharmacist should carefully check the identity and verify the amounts and sequence of the additives in sterile preparations against the original prescription, medication order, or other appropriate documentation (e.g., computerized patient profile, label generated from a pharmacist-verified order) before the product is released or dispensed.

RL 1.7: Process Validation[71]

Validation of aseptic processing procedures provides a mechanism for ensuring that processes consistently result in sterile products of acceptable quality.[10] In risk level 1, process validation (or process simulation) of compounding procedures is actually a method of assessing the adequacy of an operator's aseptic technique. Each individual involved in the preparation of sterile products should successfully complete a validation process on technique before being allowed to prepare sterile products. The validation process should follow written procedures.[42,43,45] Commercial kits are available for process validation; however, their ability to support microbial growth should be tested by challenging the intended kit with an indicator organism (e.g., *Bacillus stearothermophilus*) that can be purchased in known concentrations, is known not to be pathogenic, and grows only at relatively high temperatures.

Process simulation allows for the evaluation of opportunities for microbial contamination during all steps of sterile product preparation. The sterility of the final product is a cumulative function of all processes involved in its preparation and is ultimately determined by the processing step providing the lowest probability of sterility.[31] Process simulation testing is carried out in the same manner as normal production, except that an appropriate microbiological growth medium is used in place of the actual product used during sterile preparation. The same personnel, procedures, equipment, and materials are involved. Completed medium samples are incubated. If no microbial growth is detected, this provides evidence that adequate aseptic technique was used. If growth is detected, the entire sterile preparation process must be evaluated, corrective action taken, and the process simulation test performed again. No products intended for patient use should be prepared by an individual until the process simulation test indicates that the individual can competently perform aseptic procedures. It is recommended that personnel competency be revalidated at least annually, whenever the quality assurance program yields an unacceptable result, and whenever unacceptable techniques are observed; this revalidation should be documented.

RL 1.8: Expiration Dating[72]

All pharmacy-prepared sterile products should bear an appropriate expiration date. The expiration date assigned should be based on currently available drug stability information and sterility considerations. Sources of drug stability information include references (e.g.,

AHFS Drug Information,[73] *Extended Stability for Parenteral Drugs*,[74] *Handbook on Injectable Drugs*,[75] *King Guide to Parenteral Admixtures*[76]), manufacturer recommendations, and reliable, published research. When interpreting published drug stability information, the pharmacist should consider all aspects of the final sterile product being prepared (e.g., drug reservoir, drug concentration, storage conditions). Methods used for establishing expiration dates should be documented. Appropriate inhouse (or contract service) stability testing may be used to determine expiration dates when drug stability data are not readily available. Home care pharmacies are often required to assign extended beyond-use dates to sterile products, so ASHP has published guidelines for home care pharmacies that address beyond-use dating.[74,77]

RL 1.9: Labeling[78]

Sterile products should be labeled with at least the following information:

1. For patient-specific products: the patient's name and any other appropriate patient identification (e.g., location, identification number); for batch-prepared products: control or lot number,

2. All solution and ingredient names, amounts, strengths, and concentrations (when applicable),

3. Expiration date and time, when applicable,

4. Prescribed administration regimen, when appropriate (including rate and route of administration),

5. Appropriate auxiliary labeling (including precautions),

6. Storage requirements,

7. Identification (e.g., initials) of the responsible pharmacist (and technician),

8. Device-specific instructions (when appropriate), and

9. Any additional information, in accordance with state or federal requirements; for example, a prescription number for products dispensed to ambulatory care, long-term-care, and home care patients.

The label should be legible and affixed to the final container in a manner enabling it to be read while the sterile product is being administered (when possible). Written policies and procedures should address proper placement of labels on containers.[79]

RL 1.10: End-Product Evaluation[80]

The final product should be inspected when preparation is completed and again when the product is dispensed. This inspection includes an evaluation for container leaks, container integrity, solution cloudiness or phase separation, particulates in the solution, appropriate solution color, and solution volume. The responsible pharmacist should verify that the product was compounded accurately with the correct ingredients, quantities of each ingredient, containers, and reservoirs; different methods may be used for end-product verification (e.g., observation, calculation checks, documented records). Refractive index measurement may also be used to verify the addition of dextrose, for example in parenteral nutrient solutions.[81]

RL 1.11: Handling of Sterile Products Outside the Pharmacy[82]

Pharmacists should participate in developing procedures for the safe use (e.g., stability, sterility) of sterile products once they are distributed outside the pharmacy. How the product is transported from the pharmacy, how it is stored outside the pharmacy, and methods for return, recycling, and disposal should be addressed in written policies and procedures.[15,83] Sterile products should be transported so as to be protected from extremes of temperature outside their range of stability and from light if they are photosensitive. Storage containers and packaging verified as suitable for protection during transport should be specified. Transit time and conditions should also be specified and controlled. Delivery personnel should be instructed on special handling procedures. Once delivered to the end user, sterile products should be appropriately stored before use. Pharmacists should ascertain that the user has appropriate locations and equipment for storage (e.g., a refrigerator with a suitable thermometer). Special instructions for storage should be a part of the label or a separate information sheet (e.g., instructions for cleanliness, proper storage, interpretation of the expiration date and how to look for signs of product deterioration). The pharmacist should be notified if storage conditions do not remain suitable so that the pharmacist can give advice as to the disposition of the sterile products and remedies for storage problems. Pharmacists should participate in training end users on the proper care and storage of sterile products, either directly or through written instructional materials.

RL 1.12: Documentation[84]

The following should be documented and maintained on file for an adequate period of time, according to organizational policies and state regulatory requirements: (1) the training and competency evaluation of employees in sterile product procedures, (2) refrigerator and freezer temperatures, (3) certification of laminar-airflow workbenches, and (4) other facility quality control logs specific to the pharmacy's policies and procedures (e.g., cleaning logs for facilities and equipment). Pharmacists should also maintain appropriate dispensing records for sterile products, in accordance with state regulatory requirements.

Quality Assurance for Risk Level 2

Because the risks of inaccurate products are associated with more complex procedures and because instability and contamination are more likely with long-term storage and administration, more stringent requirements are appropriate for risk level 2 preparations. These requirements may be viewed as more important in circumstances where the medical need is *routine*. In circumstances where the medical need for a product is immediate (and there is not a suitable alternative) or when the preparation of such a product is rare, professional judgment should be applied to the extent to which some guidelines (e.g., cleanroom design and final product testing before product dispensing) must be applied.

RL 2.1: Policies and Procedures

In addition to all guidelines for risk level 1, a written quality assurance program should define and identify necessary environmental monitoring devices and techniques to be used to ensure an adequate environment for risk level 2 sterile product preparation. Examples include the use of airborne particle counters, air velocity and temperature meters, viable particle samplers (e.g., slit samplers), agar plates, and swab sampling of surfaces and potential contamination sites. All aspects of risk level 2 sterile product preparation, storage, and distribution, including such details as the choice of cleaning materials and disinfectants and the monitoring of equipment accuracy, should be addressed in written policies and procedures. Limits of acceptability (threshold or action levels) for environmental monitoring and process validation and actions to be implemented when thresholds are exceeded should be defined in written policies. For sterile batch compounding, written policies and procedures should be established for the use of master formulas and work sheets and for appropriate documentation. Policies and procedures should also address personnel attire in the controlled area, lot number determination and documentation, and any other quality assurance procedures unique to compounding risk level 2 sterile products.

RL 2.2: Personnel Education, Training, and Evaluation

All guidelines for risk level 1 should be met. In addition to guidelines for risk level 1, assessment of the competency of personnel preparing risk level 2 sterile products should include appropriate process validation (as described in RL 1.7: Process validation). However, process simulation procedures for assessing the preparation of risk level 2 sterile products should be representative of all types of manipulations, products, and batch sizes personnel preparing risk level 2 products are likely to encounter.[15] Personnel should also be taught which products are to undergo end-product quantitative analysis (see RL 2.10).

RL 2.3: Storage and Handling

All storage and handling guidelines for risk level 1 should be met.

RL 2.4: Facilities and Equipment

In addition to all guidelines for risk level 1, the following guidelines should be followed for risk level 2 sterile product preparation:

1. The controlled area should meet the standards of a class 10,000 cleanroom,[e] as defined by Federal Standard 209E.[85,f] A positive air pressure relative to adjacent pharmacy areas is required, as are an appropriate number of air exchanges per hour and appropriate humidity and temperature levels.[86] For open-architecture cleanrooms, it is appropriate to measure the volume of air entering the cleanroom versus the volume of air entering adjacent rooms, so as to ensure a positive pressure gradient for the cleanroom. To allow proper cleaning and disinfection, walls, floors, and ceilings in the controlled area should be nonporous. To help reduce the number of particles in the controlled area, an adjacent support area (e.g., anteroom) should be provided. A properly maintained barrier isolator also provides an acceptable environment.[57] A barrier isolator provides a class 100 environment for product preparation; therefore, the isolator itself can be in a separate area of the pharmacy but need not actually be in a cleanroom.

2. Cleaning materials (e.g., mops, sponges, and germicidal disinfectants) for use in the cleanroom should be carefully selected. They should be made of materials that generate a low amount of particles. If reused, cleaning materials should be cleaned and disinfected between uses.

3. The critical-area work surfaces (e.g., interior of the laminar-airflow workbench) should be disinfected frequently and before and after each batch-preparation process with an appropriate agent, according to written policies and procedures. Floors should be disinfected at least daily. Carpet or porous floors, porous walls, and porous ceiling tiles are not suitable in the controlled area because these surfaces cannot be properly cleaned and disinfected. Exterior workbench surfaces and other hard surfaces in the controlled area, such as shelves, carts, tables, and stools, should be disinfected weekly and after any unanticipated event that could increase the risk of contamination. Walls should be cleaned at least monthly.

4. To ensure that an appropriate environment is maintained for risk level 2 sterile product preparation, an effective written environmental monitoring program is recommended.[87] Sampling of air and surfaces according to a written plan and schedule is recommended.[31] The plan and frequency should be adequate to document that the controlled area is suitable and that the laminar-airflow workbench or biological safety cabinet meets class 100 requirements. Limits of acceptabil-

ity (thresholds or action levels) and appropriate actions to be taken in the event thresholds are exceeded should be specified. *USP* presents examples of environmental monitoring.[15] Settle plates or wipe samples can provide a simple but effective means of routinely monitoring airborne microbial contamination in controlled and critical areas.[45,88,89]

5. To help reduce the number of particles in the controlled area, an adjacent support area (e.g., anteroom) of high cleanliness, separated from the controlled area by a barrier (e.g., plastic curtain, partition, wall), is recommended. Appropriate activities for the support area include, but are not limited to, hand washing, gowning and gloving, removal of packaging and cardboard items, and cleaning and disinfecting hard-surface containers and supplies before placing these items into the controlled area.

6. Methods should be established for calibrating and verifying the accuracy and sterility of automated compounding methods used in aseptic processing.[90-96]

RL 2.5: Garb

All guidelines for risk level 1 should be met. Gloves, gowns, and masks are required for the preparation of all risk level 2 sterile products. Even when sterile gloves are used, they do not remain sterile during aseptic compounding; however, they do assist in containing bacteria, skin, and other particles that may be shed even from scrubbed hands. Clean gowns, coveralls, or closed jackets with sleeves having elastic binding at the cuff are recommended; these garments should be made of low-shedding materials. Shoe covers may be helpful in maintaining the cleanliness of the controlled area. Barrier isolators do not require the same level of gowning as laminar-airflow workstations as long as they operate as closed systems with HEPA filtration of air entering and leaving the barrier isolator and a separate area for entrance, such as an air lock for product transfers.

During sterile product preparation, gloves should be rinsed frequently with a suitable agent (e.g., 70% isopropyl alcohol) and changed when their integrity is compromised (i.e., when they are punctured or torn). Personnel should discard gloves upon leaving the cleanroom and don new gloves upon reentering the cleanroom.

RL 2.6: Aseptic Technique and Product Preparation[97-99]

All guidelines for risk level 1 sterile product preparation should be met. Relative to batch-prepared products, a master work sheet should be developed for a batch of each discrete identity and concentration of sterile product to be prepared. The master work sheet should consist of the formula, components, compounding directions or procedures, a sample label, and evaluation and testing requirements. Once the original master work sheet is approved by the designated pharmacist, a verified duplicate (e.g., a photocopy) of the master work sheet should be used as the preparation work sheet from which each batch is prepared and on which all documentation for each batch occurs. (For small-formula, frequently prepared batches, it may be more efficient to have multiple lines on the preparation work sheet for documenting more than one batch.) The preparation work sheet should be used to document the following:

1. Identity of all solutions and ingredients and their corresponding amounts, concentrations, or volumes,

2. Manufacturer lot number and expiration date for each component,

3. Component manufacturer or suitable manufacturer identification number,

4. Container specifications (e.g., syringe, pump cassette),

5. Lot or control number assigned to batch,

6. Expiration date of batch-prepared products,

7. Date of preparation,

8. Identity (e.g., initials, codes, signatures) of personnel involved in preparation,

9. End-product evaluation and testing specifications and results,

10. Storage requirements,

11. Specific equipment used during aseptic preparation (e.g., a specific automated compounding device), and

12. Comparison of actual yield with anticipated yield, when appropriate.

However documentation is done, a procedure should exist for easy retrieval of all records pertaining to a particular batch. Each batch of sterile products should bear a unique lot number. Identical lot numbers must never be assigned to different products or different batches of the same product. Lot numbers may be alphabetic, numeric, or alphanumeric.

The process of combining multiple sterile ingredients into a single sterile reservoir for subdivision into multiple units for dispensing may necessitate additional quality control procedures. A second pharmacist should verify calculations associated with this process, when possible; this verification should be documented. Because this process often involves making multiple entries into the intermediate sterile reservoir, the likelihood of contamination may be greater than that associated with the preparation of other risk level 2 sterile products.

For preparation involving automated compounding devices, a pharmacist should verify data entered into the compounding device before compounding begins. End-product checks should be performed to verify accuracy of ingredient delivery. These checks may include weighing and visually verifying the final product. For example, the expected weight (in grams) of the final product, based on the specific gravities of the ingredients and their respective volumes, can be documented on the compounding formula sheet, dated, and initialed by the responsible pharmacist. Once compounding is completed, each final product can be weighed and its weight compared with the expected weight. The product's actual weight should fall within a preestablished threshold for variance. Visual verification may be aided by marking the beginning level of each bulk container before starting the automated mixing process and checking each container after completing the mixing process to determine whether the final levels appear reasonable in comparison with expected volumes. The operator should also periodically observe the device during the mixing process to ensure that the device is operating properly (e.g., check to see that all stations are operating). If there are doubts whether a product or component has been properly prepared or stored, the product should not be used.

RL 2.7: Process Validation

Each individual involved in the preparation of risk level 2 sterile products should successfully complete a validation process, as recommended for risk level 1. Process simulation for compounding risk level 2 sterile products should be representative of all types of manipulations, products, and batch sizes that personnel preparing risk level 2 sterile products are likely to encounter.

RL 2.8: Expiration Dating

All guidelines for risk level 1 should be met.

RL 2.9: Labeling

All guidelines for risk level 1 should be met.

RL 2.10: End-Product Evaluation

All guidelines for risk level 1 should be met. For complex or toxic products, it is appropriate, when possible, to obtain quantitative testing of the accuracy of sterile additives, for example, the dextrose concentration in pediatric parenteral nutrient solutions or the potassium concentration in cardioplegia solutions.[g]

RL 2.11: Handling of Sterile Products Outside the Pharmacy

All guidelines for risk level 1 should be met.

RL 2.12: Documentation

All guidelines for risk level 1 should be met. Additionally, documentation of end-product sampling and batch-preparation records should be maintained for an adequate period, in accordance with organizational policies and procedures and state regulatory requirements.[100] Documentation for sterile batch-prepared products should include the

1. Master work sheet,
2. Preparation work sheet, and
3. End-product evaluation and testing results.

Quality Assurance for Risk Level 3

Risk level 3 addresses the preparation of products that pose the greatest potential risk to patients. The quality assurance activities described in this section are clearly more demanding—in terms of processes, facilities, and final product assessment—than for risk levels 1 and 2. Ideally, the activities described for risk level 3 would be used for all high-risk products. However, the activities may be viewed as most important in circumstances where the medical need for such high-risk products is *routine*. In circumstances where the medical need for such a product is immediate (and there is not a suitable alternative) or when the preparation of such a product is rare, professional judgment must be applied as to the extent to which some activities (e.g., strict facility design, quarantine, and final product testing before product dispensing) should be applied.

RL 3.1: Policies and Procedures

There should be written policies and procedures related to every aspect of preparation of risk level 3 sterile products. These policies and procedures should be detailed enough to ensure that all products have the identity, strength, quality, and purity purported for the product.[14,101] All policies and procedures should be reviewed and approved by the designated pharmacist. There should be a mechanism designed to ensure that policies and procedures are communicated, understood, and adhered to by personnel cleaning or working in the controlled area or support area. Written policies and procedures should define and identify the environmental monitoring activities necessary to ensure an adequate environment for risk level 3 sterile product preparation.

In addition to the policies and procedures required for risk levels 1 and 2, there should be written policies and procedures for the following:

1. Component selection, handling, and storage,

2. Any additional personnel qualifications commensurate with the preparation of risk level 3 sterile products,

3. Personnel responsibilities in the controlled area (e.g., sterilization, cleaning, maintenance, access to controlled area),

4. Equipment use, maintenance, calibration, and testing,

5. Sterilization and expiration dating,

6. Master formula and master work sheet development and use,

7. End-product evaluation and testing,

8. Appropriate documentation for preparation of risk level 3 sterile products,

9. Use, control, and monitoring of environ-

mentally controlled areas and calibration of monitoring equipment,

10. Process simulation for each risk level 3 sterile product,

11. Quarantine of products and release from quarantine, if applicable,

12. A mechanism for recalling products from patients in the event that end-product testing procedures yield unacceptable results, and

13. Any other quality control procedures unique to the preparation of risk level 3 sterile products.

RL 3.2: Personnel Education, Training, and Evaluation

Persons preparing sterile products at risk level 3 must have specific education, training, and experience to perform all functions required for the preparation of risk level 3 sterile products. However, final responsibility should lie with the pharmacist, who should be knowledgeable in pharmacy compounding practice[14] and proficient in quality assurance requirements, equipment used in the preparation of risk level 3 sterile products, and other aspects of sterile product preparation. The pharmacist should have sufficient education, training, experience, and demonstrated competency to ensure that all sterile products prepared from sterile or nonsterile components have the identity, strength, quality, and purity purported for the products.[101] In addition to the body of knowledge required for risk levels 1 and 2, the pharmacist should possess sufficient knowledge in the following areas:

1. Aseptic processing,

2. Quality control and quality assurance as related to environmental, component, and end-product testing,

3. Sterilization techniques,[98] and

4. Container, equipment, and closure system selection.

All pharmacy personnel involved in the cleaning and maintenance of the controlled area should be specially trained and thoroughly knowledgeable in the special requirements of class 100 critical-area technology and design. There should be documented, ongoing training for all employees to enable retention of expertise.

RL 3.3: Storage and Handling

In addition to guidelines for risk levels 1 and 2, risk level 3 policies and procedures for storage and handling should include procurement, identification, storage, handling, testing, and recall of nonsterile components.[14,101]

Components and finished products ready to undergo end-product testing should be stored in a manner that prevents their use before release by a pharmacist, minimizes the risk of contamination, and enables identification. There should be identified storage areas that can be used to quarantine products, if necessary, before they are released.[15]

RL 3.4: Facilities and Equipment

Preparation of risk level 3 sterile products should occur in a class 100 horizontal- or vertical-laminar-airflow workbench that is properly situated in a class 10,000 cleanroom *or* in a properly maintained and monitored class 100 cleanroom (without the workbench).[102] The cleanroom area should have a positive pressure differential relative to adjacent, less clean areas of at least 0.05 inch of water. A properly designed and maintained barrier isolator provides an aseptic environment for risk level 3 products.

To allow proper cleaning and disinfection, walls, floors, and ceilings in the controlled area should be nonporous. To help reduce the number of particles in the controlled area, an adjacent support area (e.g., anteroom) should be provided.

During the preparation of risk level 3 sterile products, access to the controlled area or cleanroom should be limited to those individuals who are required to be in the area and are properly attired. The environment of the main access areas directly adjacent to the controlled area (e.g., anteroom) should meet at least Federal Standard 209E class 100,000 requirements. To help maintain a class 100 critical-area environment during compounding, the adjacent support area (e.g., anteroom) should be separated from the controlled area by a barrier (e.g., plastic curtain, partition, wall). Written policies and procedures for monitoring the environment of the controlled area and adjacent areas should be developed.

No sterile products should be prepared in the controlled area if it fails to meet established criteria specified in the policies and procedures. A calibrated particle counter capable of measuring air particles 0.5 mm and larger should be used to monitor airborne particulate matter.[103] Before product preparation begins, the positive-pressure air status should meet or exceed the requirements. Air samples should be taken at several places in the controlled area with the appropriate environmental monitoring devices (e.g., nutrient agar plates). Surfaces on which work actually occurs, including laminar-airflow workbench surfaces and tabletops, should be monitored by using surface contact plates, the swab-rinse technique, or other appropriate methods.[104]

Test results should be reviewed and criteria should be preestablished to determine the point at which the preparation of risk level 3 sterile products will be disallowed until corrective measures are taken. When the environment does not meet the criteria specified in the policies and procedures, sterile product processing should immediately cease and corrective action should be taken. In the event that this occurs, written policies and procedures should delineate alternative methods of sterile product preparation to enable timely fulfillment of prescription orders.

Equipment should be adequate to prevent microbiological contamination. Methods should be established for the cleaning, preparation, sterilization, calibration, and documented use of all equipment.

Critical-area work surfaces should be disinfected with an appropriate agent before the preparation of each product. Floors in the controlled area should be disinfected at least daily. Exterior workbench surfaces and other hard surfaces in the controlled area, such as shelves, tables, and stools, should be disinfected weekly and after any unanticipated event that could increase the risk of contamination. Walls and ceilings in the controlled area or cleanroom should be disinfected at least weekly.

Large pieces of equipment, such as tanks, carts, and tables, used in the controlled area or cleanroom should be made of a material that can be easily cleaned and disinfected; stainless steel is recommended. Stools and chairs should be cleanroom quality. Equipment that does not come in direct contact with the finished product should be properly cleaned, rinsed, and disinfected before being placed in the controlled area. All nonsterile equipment that will come in contact with the sterilized final product should be properly sterilized before introduction into the controlled area; this precaution includes such items as tubing, filters, containers, and other processing equipment. The sterilization process should be monitored and documented.[101]

RL 3.5: Garb

All guidelines for risk levels 1 and 2 should be met. Additionally, cleanroom garb should be worn inside the controlled area at all times during the preparation of risk level 3 sterile products. Attire should consist of a low-shedding coverall, head cover, face mask, and shoe covers. These garments may be either disposable or reusable. Head and facial hair should be covered. Before donning these garments over street clothes, personnel should thoroughly wash their hands and forearms with a suitable antimicrobial skin cleanser.[25] Sterile disposable gloves should be worn and rinsed frequently with an appropriate agent (e.g., 70% isopropyl alcohol) during processing. The gloves should be changed if their integrity is compromised. If persons leave the controlled area *or* support area during processing, they should regown with clean garments before re-entering.

RL 3.6: Aseptic Technique and Product Preparation

All guidelines for risk levels 1 and 2 should be met. Methods should ensure that components and containers remain free from contamination and are easily identified as to the product, lot number, and expiration date. If components are not finished sterile pharmaceuticals obtained from licensed manufacturers, pharmacists should ensure that these components meet USP and FDA standards. Products prepared from nonsterile ingredients should be tested to ensure that they do not exceed specified endotoxin limits, unless the ingredient will denature all proteins (e.g., concentrated hydrochloric acid).[105] As each new lot of components and containers is received, the components should be quarantined until properly identified, tested, or verified by a pharmacist.[101]

The methods for preparing sterile products and using process controls should be designed to ensure that finished products have the identity, strength, quality, and purity they are intended to have. Any deviations from established methods should be documented and appropriately justified.

A master work sheet should be developed for the preparation of each risk level 3 sterile product. Once the pharmacist approves the master work sheet, a verified duplicate of the master work sheet should be used as the controlling document from which each sterile end product or batch of prepared products is compounded and on which all documentation for that product or batch occurs. The preparation work sheet should document all the requirements for risk level 2 plus the following:

1. Comparison of actual with anticipated yield,

2. Sterilization methods,[106,107]

3. Pyrogen testing,[108] and

4. Quarantine specifications.

The preparation work sheet should serve as the batch record for each time a risk level 3 sterile product is prepared. Each batch of pharmacy-prepared sterile products should bear a unique lot number, as described in risk level 2.

There should be documentation on the preparation work sheet of all additions of individual components plus the signatures or initials of those individuals involved in the measuring or weighing and addition of these components.

The selection of the final packaging system (including container and closure) for the sterile product is crucial to maintaining product integrity.[109] To the extent possible, presterilized containers obtained from licensed manufacturers should be used. If an aseptic filling operation is used, the container should be sterile at the time of the filling operation. If nonsterile containers are used, methods for sterilizing these containers should be established. Final containers selected should be capable of maintaining product integrity (i.e., identity, strength, quality, and purity) throughout the shelf life of the product.[110]

For products requiring sterilization, selection of an appropriate method of sterilization is of prime importance. Methods of product sterilization include sterile filtration, autoclaving, dry heat sterilization, chemical sterilization, and irradiation.[111,112] The pharmacist must ensure that the sterilization method used is appropriate for the product components and does not alter the pharmaceutical properties of the final product. A method of sterilization often used by pharmacists is sterile filtration.[113] In sterile filtration, the filter should be chosen to fit the chemical nature of the product, and the product should be filtered into presterilized containers under aseptic conditions. Sterilizing filters of 0.22-mm or smaller porosity should be used in this process. Colloidal or viscous products may require a 0.45-mm filter; however, extreme caution should be exercised in these circumstances, and more stringent end-product sterility testing is essential.[114]

To ensure that a bacteria-retentive filter did not rupture during filtration of a product, an integrity test should be performed on all filters immediately after filtration. This test may be accomplished by performing a bubble point test, in which pressurized gas (e.g., air in a syringe attached to the used filter) is applied to the upstream side of the filter with the downstream outlet immersed in water and the pressure at which a steady stream of bubbles begins to appear is noted.[98] The observed pressure is then compared with the manufacturer's specification for the filter. To compare the used filter with the manufacturer's specifications, which would be based on the filtration of water through the filter, it is necessary to first rinse the filter with sterile water for injection. An observed value lower than the manufacturer's specification indicates that the filter was defective or ruptured during the sterilization process. Methods should be established for handling, testing, and resterilizing any product processed with a filter that fails the integrity test.

RL 3.7: Process Validation

In addition to risk level 1 and 2 guidelines, written policies and procedures should be established to validate all processes involved in the preparation of risk level 3 sterile products (including all procedures, equipment, and techniques) from sterile or nonsterile components. In addition to evaluating personnel technique, process validation provides a mechanism for determining whether a particular process will, when performed by qualified personnel, consistently produce the intended results.[115]

RL 3.8: Expiration Dating

In addition to risk level 2 guidelines, there should be reliable methods for establishing all expiration dates, including laboratory testing of products for sterility, nonpyrogenicity, and chemical content, when necessary. These tests should be conducted in a manner based on appropriate statistical criteria, and the results documented.

RL 3.9: Labeling

All guidelines for risk levels 1 and 2 should be met.

RL 3.10: End-Product Evaluation

For each preparation of a sterile product or a batch of sterile products, there should be appropriate laboratory determination of conformity (i.e., purity, accuracy, sterility, and nonpyrogenicity) to established written specifications and policies. Any reprocessed material should undergo complete final product testing. Additionally, process validation should be supplemented with a program of end-product sterility testing, according to a formal sampling plan.[116-127] Written policies and procedures should specify measurements and methods of testing. Policies and procedures should include a statistically valid sampling plan and acceptance criteria for the sampling and testing. The criteria should be statistically adequate to reasonably ensure that the entire batch meets all specifications. Products not meeting all specifications should be rejected and discarded. There should be a mechanism for recalling all products of a specific batch if end-product-testing procedures yield unacceptable results. On completion of final testing, products should be stored in a manner that ensures their identity, strength, quality, and purity.

It is advisable to quarantine sterile products compounded from nonsterile components, pending the results of end-product testing. If products prepared from nonsterile components must be dispensed before satisfactory completion of end-product testing, there must be a procedure to allow for immediate recall of the products from patients to whom they were dispensed.

RL 3.11: Handling of Sterile Products Outside the Pharmacy

All guidelines for risk levels 1 and 2 should be met.

RL 3.12: Documentation

In addition to the guidelines for risk levels 1 and 2, documentation for risk level 3 sterile products should include

1. Preparation work sheet,
2. Sterilization records of final products (if applicable),
3. Quarantine records (if applicable), and
4. End-product evaluation and testing results.

References

1. Hughes CF, Grant AF, Lick BD et al. Cardioplegic solution: a contamination crisis. *J Thorac Cardiovasc Surg.* 1986; 91:296-302.
2. Pittsburgh woman loses eye to tainted drugs; 12 hurt. *Baltimore Sun.* 1990; Nov 9:3A.
3. ASHP gears up multistep action plan regarding sterile drug products. *Am J Hosp Pharm.* 1991; 48:386-90.
4. Dugleaux G, Coutour XL, Hecquard C et al. Septicemia caused by contaminated parenteral nutrition pouches: the refrigerator as an unusual cause. *JPEN J Parenter Enteral Nutr.* 1991; 15:474-5.
5. Solomon SL, Khabbaz RF, Parker RH et al. An outbreak of *Candida parapsilosis* bloodstream infections in patients receiving parenteral nutrition. *J Infect Dis.* 1984; 149:98-102.
6. Food and Drug Administration. Hazards of precipitation with parenteral nutrition. *Am J Hosp Pharm.* 1994; 51:427-8.
7. Pierce LR, Gaines A, Varricchio R et al. Hemolysis and renal failure associated with use of sterile water for injection to dilute 25% human albumin solution. *Am J Health-Syst Pharm.* 1998; 55:1057, 1062,1070.
8. Flynn EA, Pearson RE, Barker KN. Observational study of accuracy in compounding i.v. admixtures at five hospitals. *Am J Health-Syst Pharm.* 1997; 54:904-12.
9. Santell JP, Kamalich RF. National survey of quality assurance activities for pharmacy-prepared sterile products in hospitals and home infusion facilities—1995. *Am J Health-Syst Pharm.* 1996; 53:2591-605.
10. Kastango ES, Douglass K. Improving the management, operations and cost effectiveness of sterile-product compounding. *Int J Pharm Compd.* 1999; 3:253-8.
11. Guynn JB Jr, Poretz DM, Duma RJ. Growth of various bacteria in a variety of intravenous fluids. *Am J Hosp Pharm.* 1973; 30:321-5.
12. Hasegawa GR. Caring about stability and compatibility. *Am J Hosp Pharm.* 1994; 51:1533-4. Editorial.
13. Stability considerations in dispensing practice (general information chapter 1191). In: The United States pharmacopeia, 24th rev., and The national formulary, 19th ed. Rockville, MD: The United States Pharmacopeial Convention; 1999:2128-30.
14. Pharmacy compounding practices (general information chapter 1161). In: The United States pharmacopeia, 24th rev., and The national formulary, 19th ed. Rockville, MD: The United States Pharmacopeial Convention; 1999:2118-22.
15. Sterile drug products for home use (general information chapter 1206). In: The United States pharmacopeia, 24th rev., and The national formulary, 19th ed. Rockville, MD: The United States Pharmacopeial Convention; 1999:2130-43.
16. Good compounding practices applicable to state licensed pharmacies. *Natl Pharm Compliance News.* 1993; May:2-3, Oct:2-3.
17. Model rules for sterile pharmaceuticals. Chicago: National Association of Boards of Pharmacy; 1993:12.1-3.
18. National Advisory Group on Standards and Practice Guidelines for Parenteral Nutrition. Safe practices for parenteral nutrition formulations. *JPEN J Parenter Enteral Nutr.* 1998; 22:49-66.
19. Standard 3.3. Policies and procedures support safe medication prescription or ordering. In: 1999 Hospital accreditation standards. Chicago: Joint Commission on Accreditation of Healthcare Organizations; 1999:88.
20. Standard TX 5.1. Medications are pre-

pared safely. In: 1999-2000 Comprehensive accreditation manual for home care. Chicago: Joint Commission on Accreditation of Healthcare Organizations; 1999:182.

21. Standard TX 2.3. The pharmacy organization maintains proper conditions of sanitation, temperature, light, moisture, ventilation, segregation, safety, and security for preparing medications. 1996-1998 Standards for long term care pharmacies. Chicago: Joint Commission on Accreditation of Healthcare Organizations; 1996:70-1.

22. Standard TX 3.3. Prescribing and ordering of medications follow established procedures. 1998-99 Comprehensive accreditation manual for ambulatory care. Chicago: Joint Commission on Accreditation of Healthcare Organizations; 1998:211.

23. Food and Drug Modernization Act of 1997, Pub. L. No. 105-115, 111 Stat. 2296.

24. Centers for Disease Control. Guideline for prevention of intravascular infections. *Am J Infect Control.* 1983; 11(5):183-93.

25. Centers for Disease Control. Guideline for handwashing and hospital environmental control. *Am J Infect Control.* 1986; 4(8):110-29.

26. American Society of Hospital Pharmacists. ASHP technical assistance bulletin on handling cytotoxic and hazardous drugs. *Am J Hosp Pharm.* 1990; 47:1033-49.

27. American Society of Hospital Pharmacists. ASHP technical assistance bulletin on pharmacy-prepared ophthalmic products. *Am J Hosp Pharm.* 1993; 50:1462-3.

28. Cleanrooms and associated controlled environments—part 1: classification of air cleanliness. International standard ISO 14644-1. 1st ed. New York: American National Standards Institute; 1999.

29. Federal standard no. 209E. Airborne particulate cleanliness classes in cleanrooms and clean zones. Washington, DC: General Services Administration; 1992.

30. Microbiological evaluation of clean rooms and other controlled environments (general information chapter 1116). In: The United States Pharmacopeia, 24th rev., and The national for-

mulary, 19th ed. Rockville, MD: The United States Pharmacopeial Convention; 1999:2009-106.

31. Validation of aseptic filling for solution drug products. Technical monograph no. 22. Philadelphia: Parenteral Drug Association; 1996.

32. Formulations: *Int J Pharm Compd.* 1999; 2:297-307.

33. Buchanan EC. Policies and procedures for sterile product preparation. In: Principles of sterile product preparation. Bethesda, MD: American Society of Health-System Pharmacists; 1995:133-8.

34. Standard operating procedure of a horizontal laminar air flow hood. *Int J Pharm Compd.* 1997(Sep/Oct); 1:344-5.

35. Standard operating procedure for general aseptic procedures carried out at a laminar air flow workbench. *Int J Pharm Compd.* 1998(May/Jun); 2:242.

36. Standard operating procedure for particulate testing for sterile products. *Int J Pharm Compd.* 1997(Jan/Feb); 2:78.

37. Quality assurance of pharmacy-prepared sterile products. Bethesda, MD: American Society of Hospital Pharmacists; 1994. Videotape and workbook.

38. Safe handling of cytotoxic and hazardous drugs. Bethesda, MD: American Society of Health-System Pharmacists; 1990. Videotape and study guide.

39. Schneider PJ, Buchanan EC. Personnel education, training and evaluation. In: Principles of sterile product preparation. Bethesda, MD: American Society of Health-System Pharmacists; 1995:9-15.

40. Hunt ML. Training manual for intravenous admixture personnel. 5th ed. Chicago: Precept; 1995.

41. Gallagher M. Home care pharmacist competency assessment program. *Am J Health-Syst Pharm.* 1999; 56:1549-53.

42. Dirks I, Smith FM, Furtado D et al. Method for testing aseptic technique of intravenous admixture personnel. *Am J Hosp Pharm.* 1982; 39:457-9.

43. Brier KL. Evaluating aseptic technique of pharmacy personnel. *Am J Hosp Pharm.* 1983; 40:400-3.

44. McKinnon BT. Handling of sterile products within the pharmacy. In: Principles of sterile product preparation. Bethesda, MD: American Society of Health-System Pharmacists; 1995:111-6.

45. Morris BG, Avis KE. Quality-control plan

for intravenous admixture programs. 1: Visual inspection of solutions and environmental testing. *Am J Hosp Pharm.* 1980; 37:189-95.

46. Buchanan EC. Sterile compounding facilities. In: Principles of sterile product preparation. Bethesda, MD: American Society of Health-System Pharmacists; 1995:25-35.

47. Schneider PJ. Equipment for sterile product preparation. In: Principles of sterile product preparation. Bethesda, MD: American Society of Health-System Pharmacists; 1995:37-43.

48. Lau D, Shane R, Yen J. Quality assurance for sterile products: simple changes can help. *Am J Hosp Pharm.* 1994; 51: 1353. Letter.

49. Rahe H. Containment Technologies Group, Inc. Personal communication. 1999 Oct.

50. Hunt ML. Training manual for intravenous admixture personnel. 5th ed. Chicago: Precept; 1995:67-70.

51. Buchanan TL, Barker KN, Gibson JT et al. Illumination and errors in dispensing. *Am J Hosp Pharm.* 1991; 48:2137-45.

52. Denny VF, Kopis EM, Marsik FJ. Elements for a successful disinfection program in the pharmaceutical environment. *PDA J Pharm Sci Technol.* 1999; 53:115-24.

53. Frieben WR. Control of the aseptic processing environment. *Am J Hosp Pharm.* 1983; 40:1928-35.

54. Scheckelhoff DJ. Handling, preparation and disposal of cytotoxic and hazardous agents. In: Principles of sterile product preparation. Bethesda, MD: American Society of Health-System Pharmacists; 1995:63-9.

55. Favier M, Hansel S, Bressole F. Preparing cytotoxic agents in an isolator. *Am J Hosp Pharm.* 1993; 50: 2335-9.

56. Mosko P, Rahe H. Barrier isolation technology: a labor-efficient alternative to cleanrooms. *Hosp Pharm.* 1999; 34:834-8.

57. Pilong A, Moore M. Conversion to isolators in a sterile preparation area. *Am J Health-Syst Pharm.* 1999; 56:1978-80.

58. Tillett L. Barrier isolators as an alternative to a cleanroom. *Am J Health-Syst Pharm.* 1999; 56:1433-6.

59. Bryan D, Marback RC. Laminar air flow equipment certification: what the pharmacist needs to know. *Am J Hosp Pharm.* 1984; 41:1343-9.

60. McKinnon BT. Personnel behavior and garb use. In: Principles of sterile product preparation. Bethesda, MD: American Society of Health-System Pharmacists; 1995:57-62.

61. Coriell LL, McGarrity GJ, Horneff J. Medical applications of dust-free rooms: I. Elimination of airborne bacteria in a research laboratory. *Am J Public Health.* 1967; 57:1824-36.

62. NIOSH recommends steps for reducing work-related exposure to latex. *Am J Health-Syst Pharm.* 1997; 54:1688,1691.

63. Dasher G, Dasher T. The growing problem of latex allergies. *Infusion.* 1996; 2(Jan):23-7.

64. Hunt ML. Techniques used in preparing intravenous admixtures. In: Training manual for intravenous admixture personnel. Chicago: Precept; 1995:87-103.

65. Scheckelhoff DJ. Use of aseptic technique. In: Principles of sterile product preparation. Bethesda, MD: American Society of Health-System Pharmacists; 1995:49-56.

66. Buchanan EC. Sterile product formulation and compounding. In: Principles of sterile product preparation. Bethesda, MD: American Society of Health-System Pharmacists; 1995:17-24.

67. Kessler DA. MedWatch: The new FDA medical products reporting program. *Am J Hosp Pharm.* 1993; 50:1921-36.

68. Rice SP, Gutfeld MB. Preparation of latex-safe products. *Am J Health-Syst Pharm.* 1998; 55:1462-7.

69. Holzman RS. Latex allergy: an emerging operating room problem. *Anesth Analg.* 1993; 76:635-41.

70. McDermott JS, Gura KM. Procedures for preparing injectable medications for latex-sensitive patients. *Am J Health-Syst Pharm.* 1997; 54:2516-7.

71. Schneider PJ. Process validation. In: Principles of sterile product preparation. Bethesda, MD: American Society of Health-System Pharmacists; 1995:121-4.

72. McKinnon BT. Factors influencing expiration dates. In: Principles of sterile product preparation. Bethesda, MD: American Society of Health-System Pharmacists; 1995:95-103.

73. McEvoy GK, ed. AHFS drug information 99. Bethesda, MD: American Society of Health-System Pharmacists; 1999.

74. Bing C, ed. Extended stability for parenteral drugs. Bethesda, MD: American Society of Health-System Pharmacists; in press.

75. Trissel LA. Handbook on injectable drugs. 10th ed. Bethesda, MD: American Society of Health-System Pharmacists; 1998.

76. Catania PN, ed. King guide to parenteral admixtures. St. Louis, MO: King Guide; 1999.

77. American Society of Health-System Pharmacists. ASHP guidelines: minimum standard for home care pharmacies. *Am J Health-Syst Pharm.* 1999; 56:629-38.

78. Scheckelhoff DJ. Labeling of sterile products. In: Principles of sterile product preparation. Bethesda, MD: American Society of Health-System Pharmacists; 1995:105-9.

79. Davis NM. Optimal checking of pharmacy-prepared sterile products. *Hosp Pharm.* 1996; 31:102. Editorial.

80. Schneider PJ. End-product evaluation. In: Principles of sterile product preparation. Bethesda, MD: American Society of Health-System Pharmacists; 1995: 125-8.

81. Meyer GE, Novielli KA, Smith JE. Use of refractive index measurement for quality assurance of pediatric parenteral nutrition solutions. *Am J Hosp Pharm.* 1987; 44:1617-20.

82. Scheckelhoff DJ. Handling of sterile products outside the pharmacy. In: Principles of sterile product preparation. Bethesda, MD: American Society of Health-System Pharmacists; 1995:117-20.

83. Chamallas SN, Fishwick JJ, Riesenberg M. Special delivery, keeping the product stable during shipping. *Infusion.* 1997; 4(3):30-2.

84. McKinnon BT. Documentation of sterile product preparations. In: Principles of sterile product preparation. Bethesda, MD: American Society of Health-System Pharmacists; 1995:129-31.

85. Schumock GT, Kafka PS, Tormo VJ. Design, construction, implementation, and cost of a hospital pharmacy cleanroom. *Am J Health-Syst Pharm.* 1998; 55:458-63.

86. Gianino RR. Misconceptions about cleanrooms. *Am J Hosp Pharm.* 1994; 51:239-40. Letter.

87. Fundamentals of a microbiological environmental monitoring program. Technical report no. 13. Philadelphia: Parenteral Drug Association; 1990.

88. Whyte W. In support of settle plates. *PDA J Pharm Sci Technol.* 1996; 50:201-4.

89. Hyde HA. Origin of bacteria in the clean room and their growth requirements. *PDA J Pharm Sci Technol.* 1998; 52:154-8.

90. American Society of Health-System Pharmacists. ASHP guidelines on the safe use of automated compounding devices for the preparation of parenteral nutrition admixtures. *Am J Health-Syst Pharm.* 2000; 57:1343-8.

91. Davis NM. Unprecedented procedural safeguards needed with the use of automated iv compounders. *Hosp Pharm.* 1992; 27:488. Editorial.

92. Murphy C. Ensuring accuracy in the use of automatic compounders. *Am J Hosp Pharm.* 1993; 50:60. Letter.

93. Dickson LB, Somani SM, Herrmann G et al. Automated compounder for adding ingredients to parenteral nutrient base solutions. *Am J Hosp Pharm.* 1993; 50:678-82.

94. Fishwick JJ, Murphy CC, Riesenberg MC et al. Weight-based accuracy of parenteral nutrient solutions prepared with an automated compounder. *Am J Health-Syst Pharm.* 1997; 54:678-9.

95. Johnson R, Coles BJ, Tribble DA. Accuracy of three automated compounding systems determined by end-product laboratory testing and comparison with manual preparation. *Am J Health-Syst Pharm.* 1998; 55:1503-7.

96. Combeau D, Rey JB, Rieutord A et al. Accuracy of two filling systems for parenteral nutrient solutions. *Am J Health-Syst Pharm.* 1998; 55:1606-10.

97. Boylan JC. Essential elements of quality control. *Am J Hosp Pharm.* 1983; 40:1936-9.

98. McKinnon BT. Preparation and sterilization of batch compounds. In: Principles of sterile product preparation. Bethesda, MD: American Society of Health-System Pharmacists; 1995:71-7.

99. McKinnon BT. Batch preparation documentation. In: Principles of sterile product preparation. Bethesda, MD: American Society of Health-System Pharmacists; 1995:79-94.

100. Lima HA. Required documentation for

home infusion pharmacies—compounding records. *Int J Pharm Compd.* 1998; 2:354-9.

101. Avis KE. Assuring the quality of pharmacy-prepared sterile products. *Pharmacopeial Forum.* 1997; 23:3567-76.

102. Fontan JE, Arnaud P, Brion F. Laminar-airflow ceiling in a hospital pharmacy cleanroom. *Am J Health-Syst Pharm.* 1998; 55:182-3. Letter.

103. Chandler SW, Trissel LA, Wamsley LM et al. Evaluation of air quality in a sterile-drug preparation area with an electronic particle counter. *Am J Hosp Pharm.* 1993; 50:2330-4.

104. Schneider PJ. Environmental monitoring. In: Principles of sterile product preparation. Bethesda, MD: American Society of Health-System Pharmacists; 1995:45-8.

105. Bacterial endotoxins test (general tests and assays chapter 85). In: The United States pharmacopeia, 24th rev., and The national formulary, 19th ed. Rockville, MD: The United States Pharmacopeial Convention; 1999:1829-31.

106. Roberts JH, Wilson JD. Technical report no. 26: sterilizing filtration of liquids. *PDA J Pharm Sci Technol.* 1998; 52(suppl S1):1-31.

107. Akers MJ. Sterilization and depyrogenation: principles and methods. *Int J Pharm Compd.* 1999; 3:263-9.

108. Pyrogen test (general tests and assays chapter 151). In: The United States pharmacopeia, 24th rev., and The national formulary, 19th ed. Rockville, MD: The United States Pharmacopeial Convention; 1999:1850-1.

109. Aspects of container/closure integrity. Technical information bulletin no. 4. Philadelphia: Parenteral Drug Association; 1983.

110. Neidich RL. Selection of containers and closure systems for injectable products. *Am J Hosp Pharm.* 1983; 40:1924-7.

111. Validation of steam sterilization cycles. Technical information bulletin no. 1. Philadelphia: Parenteral Drug Association; 1978.

112. Turco S, ed. Sterile dosage forms: their preparation and clinical application. Philadelphia: Lea & Febiger; 1994:57-78.

113. McKinnon BT, Avis KE. Membrane filtration of pharmaceutical solutions. *Am J Hosp Pharm.* 1993; 50: 1921-36.

114. Eudailey WA. Membrane filters and membrane filtration processes for health care. *Am J Hosp Pharm.* 1983; 40:1921-3.

115. Wilson JD. Aseptic process monitoring—a better strategy. *PDA J Pharm Sci Technol.* 1999; 53:111-4.

116. Sterility tests (general tests and assays chapter 71). In: The United States pharmacopeia, 24th rev., and The national formulary, 19th ed. Rockville, MD: The United States Pharmacopeial Convention; 1999:1818-23.

117. Choy FN, Lamy PP, Burkhart VD et al. Sterility-testing program for antibiotics and other intravenous admixtures. *Am J Hosp Pharm.* 1982; 39:452-6.

118. Doss HL, James JD, Killough DM et al. Microbiologic quality assurance for intravenous admixtures in a small hospital. *Am J Hosp Pharm.* 1982; 39:832-5.

119. Posey LM, Nutt RE, Thompson PD. Comparison of two methods for detecting microbial contamination in intravenous fluids. *Am J Hosp Pharm.* 1981; 38:659-62.

120. Akers MJ. Progress toward a preferred method of monitoring the sterility of intravenous admixtures. *Am J Hosp Pharm.* 1982; 39:1297. Editorial.

121. Hoffman KH, Smith FM, Godwin HN et al. Evaluation of three methods for detecting bacterial contamination in intravenous solutions. *Am J Hosp Pharm.* 1982; 39:1299-302.

122. Miller CM, Furtado D, Smith FM et al. Evaluation of three methods for detecting low-level bacterial contamination in intravenous solutions. *Am J Hosp Pharm.* 1982; 39:1302-5.

123. DeChant RL, Furtado D, Smith FH et al. Determining a time frame for sterility testing of intravenous admixtures. *Am J Hosp Pharm.* 1982; 39:1305-8.

124. Bronson MH, Stennett DJ, Egging PK. Sterility testing of home and inpatient parenteral nutrition solutions. *JPEN J Parenter Enteral Nutr.* 1988; 12:25-8.

125. Levchuk JW, Nolly RJ, Lander N. Method for testing the sterility of total nutrient admixtures. *Am J Hosp Pharm.* 1988; 45:1311-21.

126. Akers MJ, Wright GE, Carlson KA. Sterility testing of antimicrobial-containing injectable solutions prepared in the pharmacy. *Am J Hosp Pharm.* 1991; 48:2414-8.

127. Murray PR, Sandrock MJ. Sterility testing of a total nutrient admixture with a biphasic blood-culture system. *Am J Hosp Pharm.* 1991; 48:2419-21.

[a]Unless otherwise stated in this document, the term sterile products refers to sterile drugs or nutritional substances that are prepared (e.g., compounded or repackaged) by pharmacy personnel.

[b]Ampuls, swabbed and opened appropriately with contents filtered upon removal, should be considered part of a "closed" system.

[c]Isolator guidelines appear under risk level 1 sections because their greatest use is likely to be in the preparation of cytotoxic sterile products, most of which are risk level 1 processes.

[d]The need to alternate germicides is controversial. According to Akers and Moore (Microbiological monitoring of pharmaceutical cleanrooms: the need for pragmatism, *J Adv Appl Contam Control.* 1998; 1[1]:23-4,26,28,30), the data do not support alternating germicides. A literature search (Kopis EM. *Cleanrooms.* 1996; 10[10]:48-50) found little evidence for periodic alternation of disinfectants; the search did find that alternating use of acidic and alkaline phenolic disinfectants reduces resistance arising in pseudomonads adhering to hard surfaces. If ethanol 70% or isopropyl alcohol 70% is used as the primary disinfectant, it should be sterile filtered through a 0.22-mm filter before use.

[e]According to Trissel and Chandler (*Am J Hosp Pharm.* 1993; 50:1858-61), pharmacy air is nearly class 10,000 cleanroom quality already. However, true cleanrooms add HEPA air filtering and designate room air changes and room air pressure differentials to ensure cleanliness (*Am J Hosp Pharm.* 1994; 51:239-40. Letter).

[f]Note that the International Organization for Sanitation (ISO) is preparing documents that should replace Federal Standard 209E. The ISO documents (numbered 14644-1 through 14644-7 and 14698-1 through 14698-3) are being prepared by a technical committee consisting of members from six countries, including the United States. Document 14644-1 is published in final form and classifies the air cleanliness of cleanrooms and associated controlled environments. In 14644-1 ISO cleanroom class 5 is equivalent to Federal Standard 209E class 100, and ISO class 7 is equivalent to Federal Standard 209E class 10,000.

[g]As in general information chapter 1206 in *USP*, which does not require sterility testing until the third risk level, this assumes that sterile components remain sterile throughout preparation. Many sterile products are prepared in batches too small or used too quickly after preparation to make sterility testing meaningful. Also, one of the purposes of process validation is to determine that personnel and processes can produce a sterile product.

Supersedes the ASHP Technical Assistance Bulletin on Quality Assurance for Pharmacy-Prepared Sterile Products, dated September 24, 1993.

Approved by the ASHP Board of Directors, on April 27, 2000 Developed through the ASHP Council on Professional Affairs

The bibliographic citation for this document is as follows: American Society of Health-System Pharmacists. ASHP Guidelines on Quality Assurance for Pharmacy-Prepared Sterile Products. *Am J Health-Syst Pharm.* 2000; 57:1150-69.

Appendix A—Glossary

Action Level: Established particulate or microbial counts or results that require corrective action when exceeded.

Aseptic Preparation or Aseptic Processing: The technique involving procedures designed to preclude contamination (of drugs, packaging, equipment, or supplies) by microorganisms during processing.

Batch Preparation: Compounding of multiple sterile product units, in a single discrete process, by the same individuals, carried out during one limited time period.

Cleanroom: A room (1) in which the concentration of airborne particles is controlled, (2) that is constructed and used in a manner to minimize the introduction, generation, and retention of particles inside the room, and (3) in which other relevant variables (e.g., temperature, humidity, and pressure) are controlled as necessary.[28] For example, the air particle count in a class 100 cleanroom cannot exceed a total of 100 particles 0.5 mm or larger per cubic foot of air.[29]

Clean Zone: Dedicated space (1) in which the concentration of airborne particles is controlled, (2) that is constructed and used in a manner that minimizes the introduction, generation, and retention of particles inside the zone, and (3) in which other relevant variables (e.g., temperature, humidity, and pressure) are controlled as necessary. This zone may be open or enclosed and may or may not be located within a cleanroom.[28] For example, an open-architecture controlled area should be a clean zone.

Closed-System Transfer: The movement of sterile products from one container to another in which the containers–closure system and transfer devices remain intact throughout the entire transfer process, compromised only by the penetration of a sterile, pyrogen-free needle or cannula through a designated closure or port to effect transfer, withdrawal, or delivery. Withdrawal of a sterile solution from an ampul through a particulate filter in a class 100 environment would generally be considered acceptable; however, the use of a flexible closure vial, when available, would be preferable.

Compounding: For purposes of these guidelines, compounding simply means the mixing of ingredients to prepare a medication for patient use. This activity would include dilution, admixture, repackaging, reconstitution, and other manipulations of sterile products.

Controlled Area: For purposes of these guidelines, a controlled area is the area designated for preparing sterile products. This is referred to as the buffer zone (i.e., the cleanroom in which the laminar-airflow workbench is located) by USP.[15]

Corrective Action: Action to be taken when the results of monitoring indicate a loss of control or when action levels are exceeded.

Critical Area: Any area in the controlled area where products or containers are exposed to the environment.

Critical Site: An opening providing a direct pathway between a sterile product and the environment or any surface coming into contact with the product or environment.

Critical Surface: Any surface that comes into contact with previously sterilized products or containers.

Designated Pharmacist: The pharmacist chosen by experience and training to be in charge of a sterile product preparation area or unit in a licensed pharmacy.

Expiration Date: The date (and time, when applicable) beyond which a product should not be used (i.e., the product should be discarded beyond this date and time). Expiration date and time should be assigned on the basis of both stability and risk level, whichever is the shorter period. **Note:** Circumstances may occur in which the expiration date and time arrive while an infusion is in progress. When this occurs, judgment should be applied in determining whether it is appropriate to discontinue that infusion and replace the product. Organizational policies on this should be clear.[15]

High-Efficiency Particulate Air (HEPA) Filter: A filter composed of pleats of filter medium separated by rigid sheets of corrugated paper or aluminum foil that direct the flow of air forced through the filter in a uniform parallel flow. HEPA filters remove 99.97% of all air particles 0.3 mm or larger. When HEPA filters are used as a component of a horizontal- or vertical-laminar-airflow workbench, an environment can be created consistent with standards for a class 100 cleanroom.

Isolator (or Barrier Isolator): A closed system made up of four solid walls, an air-handling system, and transfer and interaction devices. The walls are constructed so as to provide surfaces that are cleanable with coving between wall junctures. The air-handling system provides HEPA filtration of both inlet and exhaust air. Transfer of materials is accomplished through air locks, glove rings, or ports. Transfers are designed to minimize the entry of contamination. Manipulations can take place through either glove ports or half-suits.

Media Fill: See process validation or simulation.

Preservatives: For purposes of these guidelines, preservatives refer to any additive intended to extend the content, stability, or sterility of active ingredients (e.g., antioxidants, emulsifiers, bacteriocides).

Process Validation or Simulation: Microbiological simulation of an aseptic process with growth medium processed in a manner similar to the processing of the product and with the same container or closure system.[30] Process simulation tests are synonymous with medium fills, simulated product fills, broth trials, and broth fills.

Quality Assurance: For purposes of these guidelines, quality assurance is the set of activities used to ensure that the processes used in the preparation of sterile drug products lead to products that meet predetermined standards of quality.

Quality Control: For purposes of these guidelines, quality control is the set of testing activities used to determine that the ingredients, components (e.g., containers), and final sterile products prepared meet predetermined requirements with respect to identity, purity, nonpyrogenicity, and sterility.

Repackaging: The subdivision or transfer of a compounded product from one container or device to a different container or device, such as a syringe or an ophthalmic container.

Sterilization: A validated process used to render a product free of viable organisms.

Sterilizing Filter: A filter that, when challenged with a solution containing the microorganism *Pseudomonas diminuta* at a minimum concentration of 10^{12} organisms per square centimeter of filter surface, will produce a sterile effluent.

Temperatures (USP): Frozen means temperatures between –20 and –10 °C (–4 and 14 °F). Refrigerated means temperatures between 2 and 8 °C (36 and 46 °F). Room temperature means temperatures between 15 and 30 °C (59 and 86 °F).

Validation: Documented evidence providing a high degree of assurance that a specific process will consistently produce a product meeting its predetermined specifications and quality attributes.

Worst Case: A set of conditions encompassing upper and lower processing limits and circumstances, including those within standard operating procedures, that pose the greatest chance of process or product failure when compared with ideal conditions. Such conditions do not necessarily induce product or process failure.[31]

Appendix B—Comparison of Risk-Level Attributes

This appendix does not show all details of the guidelines, nor does it tell whether an aspect of the sterile compounding process is "required" (must be) or "advisable" (should be). Regardless of the examples given, each compounding pharmacist must decide, according to the circumstances at the time, what conditions are appropriate for compounding a sterile product. In an emergency, it may be of more benefit to a patient to receive a sterile drug prepared under lower risk-level conditions. For the immunocompromised patient, even simple, single-patient admixtures may need to be compounded under higher risk-level conditions.

Definition of Products by Risk Level

Risk Level 1	Risk Level 2	Risk Level 3
Products that are (1) stored at room temperature and completely administered within 28 hours from preparation, (2) unpreserved and sterile and prepared for administration to one patient, or batch prepared for administration to more than one patient and contain suitable preservatives, and (3) prepared by closed-system aseptic transfer of sterile, nonpyrogenic, finished pharmaceuticals obtained from licensed manufacturers into sterile final containers obtained from licensed manufacturers.	Products that are (1) administered beyond 28 hours after preparation and storage at room temperature, (2) batch prepared without preservatives and intended for use by more than one patient, or (3) compounded by complex or numerous manipulations of sterile ingredients obtained from licensed manufacturers in a sterile container obtained from a licensed manufacturer by using closed-system, aseptic transfer.	Products that are (1) compounded from nonsterile ingredients or with nonsterile components, containers, or equipment before terminal sterilization or (2) prepared by combining multiple ingredients (sterile or nonsterile) by using an open-system transfer or open reservoir before terminal sterilization.

Examples of Sterile Products by Risk Level

Risk Level 1	Risk Level 2	Risk Level 3
Single-patient admixture	Injections for use in portable pump or reservoir over multiple days	Alum bladder irrigation
Single-patient ophthalmic, preserved	Batch-reconstituted antibiotics without preservatives	Morphine injection made from powder or tablets
Single-patient syringes without preservatives used in 28 hours	Batch-prefilled syringes without preservatives	TPN solutions made from dry amino acids
Batch-prefilled syringes with preservatives	TPN solutions mixed with an automatic compounding device	TPN solutions sterilized by final filtration
Total parenteral nutrient (TPN) solution made by gravity transfer of carbohydrate and amino acids into an empty container with the addition of sterile additives with a syringe and needle		Autoclaved i.v. solutions

Policies and Procedures

Risk Level 1	Risk Level 2	Risk Level 3
Up-to-date policies and procedures for compounding sterile products should be available to all involved personnel. When policies are changed, they should be updated. Procedures should address personnel education and training, competency evaluation, product acquisition, storage and handling of products and supplies, storage and delivery of final products, use and maintenance of facilities and equipment, appropriate garb and conduct of personnel working in the controlled area, process validation, preparation technique, labeling, documentation, quality control, and material movement.	In addition to risk level 1 guidelines, procedures describe environmental monitoring devices and techniques, cleaning materials and disinfectants, equipment accuracy monitoring, limits of acceptability and corrective actions for environmental monitoring and process validation, master formula and work sheets, personnel garb, lot numbers, and other quality control methods.	Procedures cover every aspect of preparation of level 3 sterile products, so that all products have the identity, strength, quality, and purity purported for the product. Thirteen general policies and procedures, in addition to those in levels 1 and 2, are required.

Personnel Education, Training, and Evaluation

Risk Level 1	Risk Level 2	Risk Level 3
All pharmacy personnel preparing sterile products should receive suitable didactic and experiential training and competency evaluation through demonstration or testing (written or practical). In addition to the policies and procedures listed above, education includes chemical, pharmaceutical, and clinical properties of drugs and current good compounding practices.	In addition to guidelines in risk level 1, training includes assessment of competency in all types of risk level 2 procedures via process simulation. Personnel show competency in end-product testing as well.	Operators have specific education, training, and experience to prepare risk level 3 products. Pharmacist knows principles of good compounding practice for risk level 3 products, including aseptic processing; quality assurance of environmental, component, and end-product testing; sterilization; and selection and use of containers, equipment, and closures.

Storage and Handling in the Pharmacy

Risk Level 1	Risk Level 2	Risk Level 3
Solutions, drugs, supplies, and equipment must be stored according to manufacturer or USP requirements. Refrigerator and freezer temperatures should be documented daily. Other storage areas should be inspected regularly to ensure that temperature, light, moisture, and ventilation meet requirements. Drugs and supplies should be shelved above the floor. Expired products must be removed from active product storage areas. Personnel traffic in storage areas should be minimized. Removal of products from boxes should be done outside controlled areas. Disposal of used supplies should be done at least daily. Product-recall procedures must permit retrieving affected products from specific involved patients.	All guidelines for risk level 1 apply.	In addition to risk level 1 guidelines, procedures include procurement, identification, storage, handling, testing, and recall of components and finished products. Finished but untested products must be quarantined under minimal risk for contamination or loss of identity in an identified quarantine area.

Facilities and Equipment

Risk Level 1	Risk Level 2	Risk Level 3
The controlled area should be separated from other operations to minimize unnecessary flow of materials and personnel through the area. The controlled area must be clean, well lighted, and of sufficient size for sterile compounding. A sink with hot and cold water should be near, but not in, the controlled area. The controlled area and inside equipment must be cleaned and disinfected regularly. Sterile products must be prepared in a class 100 environment (the critical area), such as within a horizontal- or vertical-laminar-airflow workbench or barrier isolator. Computer entry, order processing, label generation, and record keeping should be performed outside the critical area. The critical area must be disinfected periodically. A workbench should be recertified every six months or when it is moved; prefilters should be changed periodically. Pumps should be recalibrated according to procedure.	In addition to risk level 1 guidelines, the following are recommended for risk level 2 products: controlled area must meet class 10,000 cleanroom standards; cleaning supplies should be selected to meet cleanroom standards; critical-area work surface must be cleaned between batches; floors should be disinfected daily, equipment surfaces weekly, and walls monthly; and there should be environmental monitoring of air and surfaces. An anteroom of high cleanliness is desirable. Automated compounding devices must be calibrated and verified as to accuracy, according to procedure.	Products must be prepared in a class 100 workbench in a class 10,000 cleanroom, in a class 100 cleanroom, or in a suitable barrier isolator. Access to the cleanroom must be limited to those preparing the products who are in appropriate garb. Methods are needed for cleaning, preparing, sterilizing, calibrating, and documenting the use of all equipment. Walls and ceilings should be disinfected weekly. All nonsterile equipment that is to come in contact with the sterilized final product should be sterilized before introduction into the cleanroom. An anteroom of high cleanliness (i.e., class 100,000) should be provided. Appropriate cleaning and disinfection of the environment and equipment are required.

Garb

Risk Level 1	Risk Level 2	Risk Level 3
In the controlled area, personnel wear low-particulate, clean clothing covers such as clean gowns or coverall with sleeves having elastic cuffs. Hand, finger, and wrist jewelry is minimized or eliminated. Nails are clean and trimmed. Gloves are recommended; those allergic to latex rubber must wear gloves made of a suitable alternative. Head and facial hair is covered. Masks are recommended during aseptic preparation. Personnel preparing sterile products scrub their hands and arms with an appropriate antimicrobial skin cleanser.	In addition to risk level 1 guidelines, gloves, gowns, and masks are required. During sterile preparation, gloves should be rinsed frequently with a suitable agent (e.g., 70% isopropyl alcohol) and changed when their integrity is compromised. Shoe covers are helpful in maintaining the cleanliness of the controlled area.	In addition to risk level 1 and 2 guidelines, cleanroom garb must be worn inside the controlled area at all times during the preparation of risk level 3 sterile products. Attire consists of a low-shedding coverall, head cover, face mask, and shoe covers. Before donning this garb, personnel must thoroughly wash their hands and arms. Upon return to the controlled area or support area during processing, personnel should regown with clean garb.

Aseptic Technique and Product Preparation

Risk Level 1	Risk Level 2	Risk Level 3
Sterile products must be prepared in a class 100 environment. Personnel scrub their hands and forearms for an appropriate period at the beginning of each aseptic compounding process. Eating, drinking, and smoking are prohibited in the controlled area. Talking is minimized to reduce airborne particles. Ingredients are determined to be stable, compatible, and appropriate for the product to be prepared, according to manufacturer, USP, or scientific references.

Ingredients result in final products that meet physiological norms as to osmolality and pH for the intended route of administration. Ingredients and containers are inspected for defects, expiration, and integrity before use. Only materials essential for aseptic compounding are placed in the workbench. Surfaces of ampuls and vials are disinfected before placement in the workbench. Sterile components are arranged in the workbench to allow uninterrupted laminar airflow over critical surfaces of needles, vials, ampuls, etc. Usually only one person and one preparation are in the workbench at a time. Automated devices and equipment are cleaned, disinfected, and placed in the workbench to enable laminar airflow. Aseptic technique is used to avoid touch contamination of critical sites of containers and ingredients. Sterile powders are completely reconstituted. Particles are filtered from solutions. Needle cores are avoided. The pharmacist checks before, during, and after preparation to verify the identity and amount of ingredients before release. | In addition to risk level 1 guidelines, a master work sheet containing formula, components, procedures, sample label, final evaluation, and testing is made for each product batch. A separate work sheet and lot number are used for each batch. When combining multiple sterile ingredients, a second pharmacist should verify calculations. The pharmacist should verify data entered into an automatic compounder before processing and check the end product for accuracy. | In addition to risk level 1 and 2 guidelines, non-sterile components must meet USP standards for identity, purity, and endotoxin levels, as verified by a pharmacist. Batch master work sheets should also include comparisons of actual with anticipated yields, sterilization methods, and quarantine specifications. Presterilized containers should be used if feasible. Final containers must be sterile and capable of maintaining product integrity throughout shelf life. Sterilization method is based on properties of the product. Final filtration methods require attention to many elements of product, filter, and filter integrity. |

Process Validation

Risk Level 1	Risk Level 2	Risk Level 3
All persons who prepare sterile products should pass a process validation of their aseptic technique before they prepare sterile products for patient use. Personnel competency should be reevaluated by process validation at least annually, whenever the quality assurance program yields an unacceptable result, and whenever unacceptable techniques are observed. If microbial growth is detected, the entire sterile process must be evaluated, corrective action taken, and the process simulation test performed again.	All risk level 1 guidelines apply, and process-simulation procedures should cover all types of manipulations, products, and batch sizes that are encountered in risk level 2.	In addition to risk level 1 and 2 guidelines, written policies should be made to validate all processes (including all procedures, components, equipment, and techniques) for each risk level 3 product.

Handling Sterile Products Outside the Pharmacy

Risk Level 1	Risk Level 2	Risk Level 3
Sterile products are transported so as to be protected from excesses of temperatures and light. Transit time and condition should be specified. Delivery personnel should be trained as appropriate. Pharmacists ascertain that the end user knows how to properly store products. End users notify pharmacists when storage conditions are exceeded or when products expire so that pharmacists can arrange safe disposal or return.	All guidelines for risk level 1 should be met.	All guidelines for risk level 1 should be met.

Documentation

Risk Level 1	Risk Level 2	Risk Level 3
The following must be documented according to policy, laws, and regulations: (1) training and competency evaluation of employees, (2) refrigerator and freezer temperature logs, (3) certification of workbenches, and (4) other facility quality control logs as appropriate. Pharmacists maintain appropriate records for the compounding and dispensing of sterile products.	In addition to the guidelines in risk level 1, documentation of end-product testing and batch-preparation records must be maintained according to policies, laws, and regulations.	In addition to the guidelines in risk levels 1 and 2, documentation for risk level 3 products must include (1) preparation work sheet, (2) sterilization records if applicable, (3) quarantine records if applicable, and (4) end-product evaluation and testing records.

Expiration Dating

Risk Level 1	Risk Level 2	Risk Level 3
All sterile products must bear an appropriate expiration date. Expiration dates are assigned based on current drug stability information and sterility considerations. The pharmacist considers all aspects of the final product, including drug reservoir, drug concentration, and storage conditions.	All guidelines for risk level 1 should be met.	In addition to risk level 1 and 2 guidelines, there must be a reliable method for establishing all expiration dates, including laboratory testing of product stability, pyrogenicity, and chemical content when necessary.

Labeling

Risk Level 1	Risk Level 2	Risk Level 3
Sterile products should be labeled with at least the following information: (1) for patient-specific products, the patient's name and other appropriate patient identification; for batch-prepared products, control or lot numbers, (2) all solution and ingredient names, amounts, strengths, and concentrations, (3) expiration date (and time when applicable), (4) prescribed administration regimen, (5) appropriate auxiliary labeling, (6) storage requirements, (7) identification of the responsible pharmacist, (8) any device-specific instructions, and (9) any additional information, in accordance with state and federal regulations. A reference number for the prescription or order may also be helpful. The label should be legible and affixed to the product so that it can be read while being administered.	All guidelines for risk level 1 must be met.	All guidelines for risk levels 1 and 2 must be met.

End-Product Evaluation

Risk Level 1	Risk Level 2	Risk Level 3
The final product must be inspected for container leaks, integrity, solution cloudiness or phase separation, particulates in solution, appropriate solution color, and solution volume. The pharmacist must verify that the product was compounded accurately as to ingredients, quantities, containers, and reservoirs.	In addition to risk level 1 guidelines, toxic products, like concentrated glucose and potassium chloride, should be tested for accuracy of concentration.	In addition to risk level 1 and 2 guidelines, the medium-fill procedure should be supplemented with a program of end-product sterility testing according to a formal sampling plan. Samples should be statistically adequate to reasonably ensure that batches are sterile. A method for recalling batch products should be established if end-product testing yields unacceptable results. Each sterile preparation or batch must be laboratory tested for conformity to written specifications (e.g., concentration, pyrogenicity). It is advisable to quarantine sterile products compounded from nonsterile components pending the results of end-product testing.

Appendix B | ASHP Guidelines on Pharmacy-Prepared Ophthalmic Products

Pharmacists are frequently called on to prepare sterile products intended for ophthalmic administration when a suitable sterile ophthalmic product is not available from a licensed manufacturer. These products may be administered topically or by subconjunctival or intraocular (e.g., intravitreal and intracameral) injection and may be in the form of solutions, suspensions, or ointments.

The sterility of these products, as well as accuracy in the calculation and preparation of doses, is of great importance. Ocular infections and loss of vision caused by contamination of extemporaneously prepared ophthalmic products have been reported.[1,2] Drugs administered by subconjunctival or intraocular injection often have narrow therapeutic indices. In practice, serious errors in technique have occurred in the preparation of intravitreal solutions, which resulted in concentrations up to double the intended amounts.[3] To ensure adequate stability, uniformity, and sterility, ophthalmic products from licensed manufacturers should be used whenever possible.

The following guidelines are intended to assist pharmacists when extemporaneous preparation of ophthalmic products is necessary. These guidelines do not apply to the manufacturing of sterile pharmaceuticals as defined in state and federal laws and regulations. Other guidelines on extemporaneous compounding of ophthalmic products also have been published.[4,5]

1. Before compounding any product for ophthalmic use, the pharmacist should review documentation that substantiates the safety and benefit of the product when administered into the eye. If no such documentation is available, the pharmacist must employ professional judgment in determining suitability of the product for ophthalmic administration.

2. Important factors to be considered in preparing an ophthalmic medication include the following:[6]

    a. Sterility.

    b. Tonicity.

    c. pH, buffering.

    d. Inherent toxicity of the drug.

    e. Need for a preservative.

    f. Solubility.

    g. Stability in an appropriate vehicle.

    h. Viscosity.

    i. Packaging and storage of the finished product.

3. A written procedure for each ophthalmic product compounded should be established and kept on file and should be easily retrievable. The procedure should specify appropriate steps in compounding, including aseptic methods, and whether microbiologic filtration or terminal sterilization (e.g., autoclaving) of the finished product is appropriate.

4. Before preparation of the product is begun, mathematical calculations should be reviewed by another person or by an alternative method of calculation in order to minimize error. This approach is especially important for products, such as intraocular injections, for which extremely small doses are frequently ordered, necessitating multiple dilutions. Decimal errors in the preparation of these products may have serious consequences.

5. Accuracy in compounding ophthalmic products is further enhanced by the use of larger volumes, which tends to diminish the effect of errors in measurement caused by the inherent inaccuracy of measuring devices. Larger volumes, however, also necessitate special attention to adequate mixing procedures, especially for ointments.

6. Strict adherence to aseptic technique and proper sterilization procedures are crucial in the preparation of ophthalmic products. All extemporaneous compounding of ophthalmic products should be performed in a certified laminar airflow hood (or, for preparing cytotoxic or hazardous agents, a biological safety cabinet).[5] Only personnel trained and proficient in the techniques and procedures should prepare ophthalmic products. Quality-assurance principles for compounding sterile products should be followed, and methods should be established to validate all procedures and processes related to sterile product preparation. In addition, the following should be considered:

    a. Ingredients should be mixed in sterile empty containers. Individual ingredients often can first be drawn into separate syringes and then injected into a larger syringe by insertion of the needles into the needle-free tip of the larger syringe.

The larger syringe should be of sufficient size to allow for proper mixing of ingredients.

  b. To maximize measurement accuracy, the smallest syringe appropriate for measuring the required volume should be used. When the use of a single syringe would require estimation of the volume (e.g., measuring 4.5 ml in a 5-ml syringe with no mark at the 4.5-ml level), the use of two syringes of appropriate capacities (or two separate syringe "loads") should be considered in order to provide a more accurate measurement.

  c. A fresh disposable needle and syringe should be used at each step to avoid contamination and prevent error due to residual contents.

  d. When multiple dilutions are required, the containers of interim concentrations should be labeled to avoid confusion.

  e. In the preparation of an ophthalmic product from either (1) a sterile powder that has been reconstituted or (2) a liquid from a glass ampul, the ingredients should be filtered through a 5-mm filter to remove any particulate matter.

7. For ophthalmic preparations that must be sterilized, an appropriate and validated method of sterilization should be determined on the basis of the characteristics of the particular product and container. Filtration of thepreparation through a 0.22-μm filter into a sterile final container is a commonly used method; however, this method is not suitable for sterilizing ophthalmic suspensions and ointments.[7] When an ophthalmic preparation is compounded from a nonsterile ingredient, the final product must be sterilized before it is dispensed. Sterilization by autoclaving in the final container may be possible, provided that product stability is not adversely affected and appropriate quality control procedures are followed.[6]

8. Preservative-free ingredients should be used in the preparation of intraocular injections, since some preservatives are known to be toxic to many of the internal structures of the eye.[6]

9. In the preparation of ophthalmic products from cytotoxic or other hazardous agents, the pharmacist should adhere to established safety guidelines for handling such agents.[8,9]

10. The final container should be appropriate for the ophthalmic product and its intended use and should not interfere with the stability and efficacy of the preparation.[10] Many ophthalmic liquids can be packaged in sterile plastic bottles with self-contained dropper tips or in glass bottles with separate droppers. Ophthalmic ointments should be packaged in sterilized ophthalmic tubes. Injectables that are not for immediate use should be packaged in sterile vials rather than in syringes, and appropriate overfill should be included. All containers should be adequately sealed to prevent contamination.

11. The pharmacist should assign appropriate expiration dates to extemporaneously prepared ophthalmic products; these dates should be based on documented stability data as well as the potential for microbial contamination of the product.[11] The chemical stability of the active ingredient, the preservative, and packaging material should be considered in determining the overall stability of the final ophthalmic product.[12]

12. Ophthalmic products should be clearly and accurately labeled. In some cases, it may be appropriate to label the products with both the weight and concentration of active ingredients and preservatives. Labels should also specify storage and handling requirements and expiration dates. Extemporaneously prepared ophthalmic products dispensed for outpatient use should be labeled in accordance with applicable state regulations for prescription labeling.

References

1. Associated Press. Pittsburgh woman loses eye to tainted drugs; 12 hurt. *Baltimore Sun.* 1990; Nov 9:3A.
2. Associated Press. Eye drop injuries prompt an FDA warning. *N Y Times.* 1990; 140(Dec 9):39I.
3. Jeglum EL, Rosenberg SB, Benson WE. Preparation of intravitreal drug doses. *Ophthalmic Surg.* 1981; 12:355–9.
4. Reynolds LA. Guidelines for preparation of sterile ophthalmic products. *Am J Hosp Pharm.* 1991; 48:2438–9.
5. Reynolds LA, Closson R. Ophthalmic drug formulations. A handbook of extemporaneous products. Vancouver, WA: Applied Therapeutics; (in press).

6. The United States Pharmacopeia, 22nd rev., and The National Formulary, 17th ed. Rockville, MD: The United States Pharmacopeial Convention; 1989:1692–3.

7. Allen LV. Indomethacin 1% ophthalmic suspension. *US Pharm.* 1991;16(May): 82–3.

8. American Society of Hospital Pharmacists. ASHP technical assistance bulletin on handling cytotoxic and hazardous drugs. *Am J Hosp Pharm.* 1990; 47:1033–49.

9. OSHA work-practice guidelines for personnel dealing with cytotoxic (antineoplastic) drugs. *Am J Hosp Pharm.* 1986; 43:1193–204.

10. Ansel HC, Popovich NG. Pharmaceutical dosage forms and drug delivery systems. 5th ed. Philadelphia: Lea & Febiger; 1990:354–7.

11. Stolar MH. Expiration dates of repackaged drug products. *Am J Hosp Pharm.* 1979; 36:170. Editorial.

12. Remington's pharmaceutical sciences. 19th ed. Gennaro AR, ed. Easton, PA: Mack Publishing; 1990:1581–959.

These guidelines were reviewed in 2003 by the Council on Professional Affairs and by the Board of Directors and were found to still be appropriate.

Approved by the ASHP Board of Directors, April 21, 1993. Developed by the ASHP Council on Professional Affairs.

The bibliographic citation for this document is as follows: American Society of Hospital Pharmacists. ASHP technical assistance bulletin on pharmacy-prepared ophthalmic products. *Am J Hosp Pharm.* 1993; 50:1462–3.

Appendix C

ASHP Guidelines on the Safe Use of Automated Compounding Devices for the Preparation of Parenteral Nutrition Admixtures

Purpose

Automated compounding devices are frequently used by pharmacists for the extemporaneous preparation of parenteral nutrition admixtures. This continuing shift from manual compounding procedures comes as a result of significant advances in automated technology, as well as in response to changing health care demands to provide admixture compounding in a safer, more efficient, and more accurate manner. Approximately 65% of the hospitals in the United States currently use automated compounding devices for parenteral nutrition admixtures on a daily basis.[a] Compounders are also used for other types of intravenous admixtures and in other settings, including home care and long-term-care facilities; therefore, the overall magnitude of their use may be substantial. As with other automated systems or devices, the benefits can be realized only when the technology is used appropriately. Significant patient harm may occur when safety and quality assurance measures are overlooked or circumvented.[1]

The purpose of these guidelines is to outline the key issues that should be considered to safely and cost-effectively incorporate this technology into the pharmacy operations of health care organizations. The guidelines focus on parenteral nutrition admixtures, but the safety issues are also applicable to the use of compounders for other types of i.v. admixtures. The term "health care organization" is used throughout the guidelines as a general descriptor and is intended to be inclusive of any of the practice settings and types of facilities in which compounders are used, including, for example, home infusion companies. These guidelines should be used in conjunction with the ASHP Guidelines on Quality Assurance for Pharmacy-Prepared Sterile Products and device manufacturers' instruction manuals and training materials. Pharmacists should use professional judgment in assessing their health care organization's needs for automated compounding devices and in adapting these guidelines to meet those needs.

Background

The act of extemporaneously compounding any parenteral formulation is complex and not without inherent risks; therefore, compounding tasks are best performed by personnel most qualified to do so. An incompatible, unstable, or contaminated i.v. infusion may induce significant patient morbidity and even mortality.[1] Pharmacists are specifically educated and legally responsible for performing these tasks safely. Pharmacists are also responsible for training other personnel to perform relatively simple tasks with the least risk possible.

The extemporaneous preparation of multiadditive products, such as parenteral nutrition admixture compounding, should be performed under the direct supervision of a pharmacist and in the appropriate environment.[2] The historical method of compounding these multicomponent admixtures has been to manually use gravity-driven transfers for large-volume additives, such as amino acids, dextrose, lipids, and sterile water. Small-volume additives, such as electrolytes, trace minerals, multivitamins, and drugs, have often been added manually and separately with a syringe. Thus, this compounding method is limited by the visual inspection of volumes transferred between stock containers, as well as by the precision of the calibrations marked on the stock containers or transfer devices.

The manual method of parenteral nutrition admixture compounding is labor-intensive and requires multiple manipulations of infusion containers, sets, syringes, needles, and so forth, which can lead to the extrinsic contamination of the final admixture with sterile and nonsterile contaminants. A sterile contaminant can be particulate matter from elastomeric vial enclosures (needle cores), and nonsterile contaminants can be bacteria and other infectious materials. Minimizing the number of extemporaneous manipulations of the parenteral infusion containers and supplies improves compounding efficiency and reduces the risk of extrinsic contamination and associated sequelae.[3]

The emergence of automated technology as an alternative approach to parenteral nutrition admixture compounding has led to potentially improved compounding accuracy with the use of fluid pump technology and software that controls the compounder pump. Fluid can be delivered from the source container to the final container by using either a volumetric or a gravimetric fluid pumping system. Volumetric systems transfer a specified volume of fluid from a source container to a final container via a rotary peristaltic pump. The tubing is stretched around a rotor and, as the rotor turns, solution is pulled from the source container and pushed toward the final container. Measurements are based on the theory that each rotor movement advances a constant amount of fluid through the system. The total volume delivered is calculated by the volume pulled into the tubing by each rotor movement multiplied by the number of movements. These systems usually incorporate a final check of the *actual* total bag weight by comparing it with a calculated *expected* weight.

In gravimetric systems, measurement of fluid volume delivered from the source container to the final container is determined by weighing the fluid transferred and dividing the weight by the solution's known specific gravity, thereby converting weight to volume. Two types of gravimetric pumps are available: additive and subtractive. With an additive pump, a single load cell is positioned to measure each fluid as it is delivered to the final container. With a subtractive pump, load cells are positioned beneath the source containers to measure each fluid as it is being pumped from its source container. Weight is determined by subtracting the posttransfer weight from the pretransfer weight of the container for each source solution. When all transfers are completed, the system compares the *actual* total bag weight with a calculated *expected* weight.

In addition to the compounder, dedicated software may be used to electronically transfer information to the compounding device. Automated compounding software has additional features that can enhance the management of the parenteral nutrition program. Software issues and their integrity are additional critical components unique to compounder methods and require continuous monitoring to ensure that the operations are correct.[4]

Justification for the Use of Automated Compounding Devices

When is it appropriate to use compounders, and how will decisions affect others within and outside the pharmacy department? It is incumbent upon the pharmacist to ensure that the department is fully knowledgeable about the operation of the compounder and that a minimum acceptable standard of pharmacy practice is met. First, internal decisions need to be made to justify the expenses associated with this technology. Second, policies and procedures should be in place to assess workflow, establish training programs, and standardize compounder use in the specific pharmacy practice setting. Third, changing current compounder contracts may result in more cost than the savings that might appear in the new contracts. Specifically, the initial incorporation of an automated compounder into daily pharmacy practice is a labor-intensive effort, and such transitions can be disruptive and can even increase the risk of errors. This may be particularly true during staff orientation to new devices. Such changes must be carefully reviewed; if they are determined to be worthwhile, a well-coordinated transition plan should be devised beforehand. Whether transition costs (including the potential for unused sets and supplies) can be deferred to the new contract is another factor for consideration.

The principal emphasis associated with using automated compounding devices in health care organizations should be improving patient care and enhancing efficiency while remaining cost-effective. "Cost-effectiveness" is, therefore, a relative term with respect to personnel, as the labor saved is often redirected to other aspects of pharmaceutical care that could also improve patient safety. Time that was previously spent on operations associated with parenteral nutrition admixture compounding can now be aimed at other issues, such as optimization of drug and nutritional therapies, reorganization of product utilization, quality assurance programs, and augmentation of other core pharmaceutical services. Specific objectives related to cost justification of automated compounding devices may include the following:

1. Enhanced efficiency and worker safety during the parenteral nutrition compounding process and patient safety with parenteral use.

2. Reduction in labor associated with manually compounded parenteral nutrition admixtures. Assessment of the overall labor and material costs associated with the current manual compounding methods should include hidden costs such as pharmacists' time to perform calculations, quality assurance checks, and com-

pounder set-up, as well as staff training (initial and ongoing).

3. Reduction in waste through more efficient use of base solutions and additives. Inventory can often be reduced by consolidating source solutions to a few high-concentration, large-volume additives.

In some cases in which the cost of implementing automated compounding technology in one facility is prohibitive, health care organizations have opted to explore regional compounding centers or outsourcing to contractors.

Performance Requirements and Responsibilities

The use of automated devices for compounding parenteral nutrition admixtures should be clearly defined by the health care organization and the manufacturer. This includes the ongoing responsibilities of the pharmacy department and those of the manufacturer during and after implementation of the compounder in the pharmacy practice setting.

Three areas need to be clearly defined before choosing an automated compounding system: (1) the system's performance requirements, (2) the manufacturer's responsibilities, and (3) the pharmacy department's responsibilities. The performance requirements of the automated compounding system should ensure that

1. The compounder exceeds the level of accuracy achieved with manual compounding. The automated compounding device should be accurate to within 5% of the amount programmed, with verification of the amount pumped versus the programmed amount for each ingredient.

2. The automated compounding device has inherent safeguards, including the ability to detect inadvertent source-solution mixups; the ability to detect situations that could result in inaccurate deliveries, such as occluded transfer-set tubing and empty source containers; and the ability to keep incompatible source solutions separate.

3. The automated compounding software alerts the user when formulation issues arise.

4. The automated compounding software meets the standards of the American Society for Parenteral and Enteral Nutrition for parenteral nutrition label formats.[5]

5. The automated compounding software assists the pharmacist in producing physicochemically compatible parenteral nutrition formulations.

6. The automated compounding software provides useful clinical information.

7. The automated compounding software integrates with existing pharmacy programs wherever possible to optimize patient care and avoid therapeutic duplications.

The contractual agreement with the manufacturer should provide continuous support of the compounder and software, including information updates, problem solving, and emergency coverage. FDA considers all automated compounding devices class II devices,[6] and as such they must comply with federal regulations. The manufacturer's responsibilities are as follows:

1. The manufacturer should supply, and the pharmacist should verify, that the device is 510K cleared as evidence of compliance with regulatory requirements; that the device meets the fire and safety standards established by Underwriters Laboratories (i.e., is UL-approved); that the operator's manual and other documentation support recommendations for use; and that accuracy statements and manufacturer claims are valid.

2. The manufacturer should provide 24-hour support for the compounder and its software throughout the life of the contract.

3. The manufacturer should routinely provide the latest version of the compounder software in a timely manner.

4. The manufacturer should ensure adequate availability of compounding supplies.

5. The manufacturer should provide detailed information and instructions on the appropriate use of the compounder and its software. References should be provided when appropriate.

6. The manufacturer should comply with FDA requirements for reporting adverse events.

Within the pharmacy department, specific policies and procedures should be developed that address responsibilities for compounder operations and maintenance, staff training, and monitoring compounder performance at all times. Before selecting and implementing an automated compounder, the pharmacy department should

1. Define and agree on automated compounding system needs and performance requirements.

2. Develop an implementation team with a lead person.

3. Develop a set of policies and procedures.

Control of the Automated Compounding Device in Daily Operations

The pharmacy department is responsible for the use, maintenance, and performance of the automated compounding device, including decisions about who has access to the compounder and its operations. Specific consideration should be given to the following:

1. Only designated pharmacy department personnel should have access to the compounder and its software. The level of access should correspond to the level of authority and expertise of the personnel.

2. Before being granted access to a compounder, pharmacy personnel should pass established competency-standard testing.

3. Access to and use of the compounder by pharmacy support personnel (i.e., pharmacy technicians, students, and other designated support staff) should be directly supervised by an authorized pharmacist.

4. The additive configuration or sequence of the compounder for compounding parenteral nutrition admixtures should not be altered from the established format without the authorization of a designated pharmacist.

5. The compounder should not be used for any purpose other than parenteral nutrition admixture compounding without authorization from a designated pharmacist. If the compounder is used for other extemporaneous drug preparation, this should be done separately from the schedule for parenteral nutrition admixtures. The use of the compounder in this manner will likely require the use of new compounding sets and admixture configurations.

Safety and Efficacy Features

The complexity of automated compounding device functions makes it imperative that the pharmacy department develop a specific plan for ensuring safe and efficacious use at all times. The safety and efficacy features should outline the core principles necessary for carrying out the complex tasks of parenteral nutrition compounding. The plan should identify the minimum standards that are routinely assessed through an established monitoring and surveillance program. Automated compounding devices on the market differ in hardware design, mechanisms of fluid transfer, and software applications. Consequently, sterility and quality assurance testing procedures and measures are also different, including routine assessments of accuracy in the delivery of correct amounts of nutrients. Consideration should be given to the following in accordance with the device manufacturer's specific instructions:

1. Establishing minimum competency standards for all personnel who have access to and operate the compounder. Competency standards should ensure that the compounder user has sufficient expertise to identify errors that may inadvertently bypass quality assurance systems. The competency standards should be reviewed and validated on a routine basis for all personnel operating the compounder.

2. Establishing specific procedures for the operation of the compounder that standardize its use, irrespective of the individual operator. Changes in compounder operations should occur only when authorized and should be communicated to all staff involved in compounding.

3. Including sterility and quality assurance measures to avoid extrinsic contamination and to ensure accurate delivery of parenteral nutrition additives.

4. Ensuring that compounder tubing changes occur at appropriate specified time intervals in accordance with the

manufacturer's recommendations.

5. Devising methods for assessing and calibrating the accuracy of the compounder in delivering precise levels of substrates and additives.

6. Developing a contingency plan and a readily available backup system or method for providing uninterrupted parenteral nutrition therapy to patients in the event of compounder failure.

7. Ensuring that adequate amounts of solutions and supplies for automated compounding are on hand.

Quality Assurance Monitoring and Documentation

Automated compounding devices are intended to provide a higher margin of accuracy and to streamline the labor-intensive tasks associated with the manual extemporaneous preparation of large-volume, multiadditive parenteral nutrition admixtures and other admixtures. The compounders are not designed to replace oversight functions, which require the expertise of a pharmacist.

In theory, automated compounding devices provide compounding accuracy superior to that of traditional methods of manual compounding. However, the performance of compounders must be critically challenged by the pharmacist to ensure that their manufacturing specifications are equal to the task. In the pharmaceutical industry, that process is called validation. Ongoing quality assurance measures specified by the device manufacturer for assessing the performance of the compounder, as well as corrective actions, should be clearly delineated in policies separate from those dedicated to operational tasks. "Ongoing" means daily, and whatever measures are determined to be essential should be performed each day because random checks may not detect a more insidious, intermittent flaw that could assume major clinical significance.[7,8]

The pharmacy department may work with other departments to assess the compounder's performance if such expertise is not available within the pharmacy department. For example, portions of parenteral nutrition admixtures may be sent to the health care organization's laboratory to determine dextrose content. However, laboratory methods are usu-

ally designed for biological rather than pharmaceutical systems and should be validated to meet USP requirements for the components being tested. If outside departments participate in the quality assurance program, their methods should be appropriately validated in accordance with USP specifications and the results documented within the pharmacy department records on the compounder's performance.

The pharmacy department should develop a monitoring and surveillance plan with output reports that encompasses the principles outlined under the section on safety and efficacy features. The plan should detail specific policies and procedures that will ensure the continuing operation of the automated compounding device at optimum performance levels at all times. The data generated by the monitoring procedures should be reported to the pharmacy director and other appropriate oversight personnel and kept as a permanent record of the compounder's operations. These reports should be regularly reviewed in the assessment of trends and other long-term measures of performance. Specific consideration should be given to

1. Establishing performance standards and continuous quality assurance measures for assessing the compounder's performance and product quality during setup and in-process (during compounding) and end-process testing.

2. Establishing quality assurance testing of user-defined software variables validating that the correct responses to user commands occur.

3. Validating all quality assurance testing before implementation.

4. Establishing a minimum performance standard for each quality assurance test. For example, deviations in the accuracy of delivering a single additive cannot exceed a predetermined percent error without immediate corrective actions.

5. Documenting all quality assurance data on a daily basis. A comprehensive review of the data and documentation of performance trends should be performed at scheduled intervals as necessitated by aseptic conditions. The compounder should have scheduled, routine cleaning and maintenance according to the manufacturer's recommendations to ensure proper operation.

Storage and Inventory

The pharmacy department is responsible for housing the automated compounding device, related disposable supplies, and admixture ingredients. Other departments, such as materials management, may order and store additional supplies for the compounder yet defer to the pharmacy for the selection of the components necessary for proper compounder operation. Specific consideration should be given to

1. Maintaining an adequate inventory of supplies necessary for compounder operation and patient needs.

2. Procuring all large-volume parenteral nutrition components (amino acids, dextrose, and lipids) from one manufacturer unless such combinations have adequate physicochemical data that ensure the stability, compatibility, and safety of the final formulations commensurate with the data for single-source products.[5] Any proposed substitute products should be assessed for compatibility and approved by designated pharmacy personnel qualified to do so and possibly by the pharmacy and therapeutics committee if clinical issues are identified.

3. If a health care organization's contract requires a change in the brand of parenteral products, designated pharmacy personnel should verify that the new products are compatible. If a new product is approved, designated pharmacy personnel should verify that the new product is compatible, add it to the compounder formulary, and revise the admixture requirements and instructions relevant to the compounder's operations.

Education and Training

Pharmacists, by education and training, are competent to safely compound pharmaceuticals, including parenteral nutrition admixtures. Nevertheless, the introduction of automated compounding devices requires specific training of pharmacists as well as other pharmacy personnel in the operation, maintenance, and quality assurance of compounders. Specific consideration should be given to ensuring that

1. Pharmacy administration determines the individuals who will be responsible for education and training in the use of the compounders.

2. All education and training are documented in a permanent record maintained in the pharmacy department and in personnel files.

3. All pharmacy personnel using or supervising compounder operations are tested at regular intervals to ensure that individuals meet the department's minimum competency standards.

4. Retraining, competency assessment, and appropriate documentation accompany upgrades and new versions of the compounder to ensure the continued proficiency of personnel, safety of compounder operations, and adequacy of oversight.

Device Variability

Automated compounding devices are marketed by several manufacturers. Even though there are similarities among compounders, there may be significant differences in the design, accuracy, operation, maintenance, software, and manufacturing support, among other things. The safe operation and supervision of any given compounder depend on adherence to the manufacturer's specific instructions and continuous quality assurance monitoring of compounder performance. The safe and efficient operation of an automated compounding system depends on defined responsibilities for the pharmacy and manufacturer, as well as on strict adherence to policies, procedures, and quality assurance programs.

References

1. Food and Drug Administration. Safety alert: hazards of precipitation associated with parenteral nutrition. *Am J Hosp Pharm.* 1994; 51:1427-8.

2. American Society of Hospital Pharmacists. ASHP technical assistance bulletin on quality assurance for pharmacy-prepared sterile products. *Am J Hosp Pharm.* 1993; 50:2386-98.

3. McClendon RR. A comparative evaluation of methods used to compound parenteral nutrition solutions. *Nutr Support Serv.* 1983; 3:46-9.

4. Driscoll DF. Clinical delivery of nutri-

tional therapy: automated compounders and patient-specific feeding. *Nutrition.* 1996; 12:461-2. Editorial.

5.   American Society for Parenteral and Enteral Nutrition National Advisory Group on Standards and Practice Guidelines for Parenteral Nutrition. Safe practices for parenteral nutrition formulations. *JPEN J Parenter Enteral Nutr.* 1998; 22:49-66.

6.   Trautman KA. The FDA and worldwide quality system requirements guidebook for medical devices. Milwaukee, WI: ASQ Quality Press; 1997.

7.   Driscoll DF. Delivery of nutritional therapy: quality assurance of automated compounding devices. *Nutrition.* 1996; 12:651-2. Editorial.

8.   Fields HS. Establishing core performance requirements for automated TPN compounders. *Am J Health-Syst Pharm.* 1996; 53:1607. Letter.

[a]Mihalski T, Clintec Nutrition Division, Baxter Healthcare. Personal communication. 1999 Mar 15.

Approved by the ASHP Board of Directors on April 27, 2000. Developed through the ASHP Council on Professional Affairs.

The bibliographic citation for this document is as follows: American Society of Health-System Pharmacists. ASHP Guidelines on the Safe Use of Automated Compounding Devices for the Preparation of Parenteral Nutrition Admixtures. *Am J Health-Syst Pharm.* 2000; 57:1343-8.

Appendix D

ASHP Technical Assistance Bulletin on Handling Cytotoxic and Hazardous Drugs

In 1985, the "ASHP Technical Assistance Bulletin on Handling Cytotoxic Drugs in Hospitals"[1] summarized published information on handling hazardous drugs, referred to as cytotoxics, as of July 1984. As more information became available on the types of hazardous agents that may represent a health risk to the occupationally exposed population, and as the handling of such substances became routine in hospitals, community pharmacies, home care settings, clinics, and physicians' offices, the need to revise the Technical Assistance Bulletin became apparent.

Early concerns regarding occupational exposure to hazardous agents involved primarily drugs used in cancer therapy. Therefore, the terms "antineoplastics" (drugs used to treat neoplasms) and "chemotherapy" were used in early reports and guidelines. Although any chemical used therapeutically may be referred to as chemotherapy, this term is currently used, both in the medical and lay communities, to mean drug therapy of cancer. In an attempt to be more precise, many professionals adopted the term "cytotoxic" or "cell killer." Not all antineoplastics, however, are cytotoxic, nor are all cytotoxics used exclusively in the treatment of cancer. "Cytotoxic" is often used to refer to any agent that may be genotoxic, oncogenic, mutagenic, teratogenic, or hazardous in any way. As our knowledge of the hazardous nature of many agents grows and as new hazardous agents (e.g., genotoxic biologicals and some biotechnological agents) continue to be developed, cytotoxic is a less appropriate term. In deference to the original Technical Assistance Bulletin, cytotoxic remains in the title of this revision. The remainder of the document, however, will refer exclusively to hazardous drugs or agents, except in very specific instances.

In January 1986, the Federal Occupational Safety and Health Administration (OSHA) released recommendations on safe handling of cytotoxic drugs by health-care personnel.[2] This revised Technical Assistance Bulletin includes information from these recommendations, modified by subsequent discussions with OSHA, and from published reports by the National Institutes of Health,[3] the National Study Commission on Cytotoxic Exposure,[4] and the American Medical Association's (AMA) Council on Scientific Affairs,[5] along with other published information on this issue as of June 1988.

The safe handling of hazardous drugs is an issue that must be addressed in health-care settings and one that may even affect, in a home care environment, persons other than the patient. Inasmuch as possible, the pharmacist should take the lead in establishing policies and procedures to ensure the proper handling of all hazardous drugs in any health-care setting. The recommendations contained in this Technical Assistance Bulletin should be applied to any area where hazardous drugs are handled. Procedures specific to noninstitutional care settings have been included where available.[6-8] Because of the many questions about implementing the recommendations in the original Technical Assistance Bulletin, this revision contains detailed information in those areas of greatest concern. The recommendations contained here should be supplemented with the professional judgments of qualified staff and with newer information as it develops.

Hazardous Drug Dangers

The danger to health-care personnel from handling a hazardous drug stems from a combination of its inherent toxicity and the extent to which workers are exposed to the drug in the course of carrying out their duties. This exposure may be through inadvertent ingestion of the drug on foodstuffs (e.g., workers' lunches), inhalation of drug dusts or droplets, or direct skin contact. Drugs that may represent occupational hazards include any that exhibit the following characteristics:

1. Genotoxicity [i.e., mutagenicity and clastogenicity (see Appendix A) in short-term test systems].

2. Carcinogenicity in animal models, in the patient population, or both, as reported by the International Agency for Research on Cancer (IARC).

3. Teratogenicity or fertility impairment in animal studies or treated patients.

4. Evidence of serious organ or other toxicity at low doses in animal models or treated patients.

The oncogenic and teratogenic effects of therapeutic doses of several antineoplastic agents are well established.[9-13] The mutagenic properties of some cytotoxics, immunosuppressants, antiviral agents, and biologicalresponse modifiers have also been documented.[14] The long-term effects (e.g., cancer, impaired fertility, and organ damage) of continued exposure to small amounts of one or more of such drugs remain undetermined.

For example, it is known that long-term use of potent immunosuppressive agents may result in the development of lymphoma. It is not known, however, at what drug level or over what period of time this may occur and how this correlates with possible drug levels achieved through occupational exposure during preparation and administration of hundreds or thousands of injectable and oral doses of these agents.

Studies have attempted to assess indirectly the potential exposure of hospital pharmacists and nurses to some hazardous drugs in several health-care settings including physicians' offices.[15-21] These studies examined the urine mutagenicity or evidence of chromosome damage in subjects who prepared or administered primarily antineoplastic injections. The mutagenicity and chromosome damage that were found were thought to document exposure to and absorption of the drugs that had been handled. An association may exist between carcinogenicity and chromosome breakage or mutagenicity. Therefore, one might conclude that handling hazardous drugs entails some danger to health-care personnel. These studies, although not conclusive, support the postulated occupational risks.

However, several reports make the situation slightly more ominous. Palmer and coworkers[22] measured chromosome damage in 10 patients receiving chlorambucil. They found that the damage was cumulative and was related to both the daily dose and the duration of therapy. Another report[23] described permanent liver damage in three nurses who had worked 6, 8, and 16 years, respectively, on an oncology ward. On the basis of histories, the investigators suggested that the liver injuries may have been related to the intensity and duration of exposure to certain toxic agents. The chlorambucil study involved therapeutic doses of drug, and three cases of liver damage is a small base for drawing any final conclusions. Nevertheless, this information is disturbing in view of the fact that many health-care workers prepare or administer hundreds or even thousands of doses of hazardous drugs during their careers. If low-dose

exposure to these agents is cumulative, this exposure should be minimized by strict compliance with safe handling procedures.

The value of chromosome and mutagenicity studies as indicators of the occupational risks of exposure to hazardous drugs has been questioned.[24-28] However, several researchers have employed more direct methods of determining whether or not workers have been exposed to and absorbed hazardous drugs handled in the customary manner. Demonstration that absorption has occurred would be strong support for the imposition of safety measures. (The absorption of hazardous drug is presumed to be a health risk.)

A letter[29] described a study that used the presence of thioethers in the urine as an indicator of exposure to alkylating agents (i.e., certain antineoplastic drugs). The mean urinary thioether concentration (UTC) was higher in a group of 15 oncology nurses after a 5-day rotation than it was when they returned to work after a 3-day leave ($p < 0.01$). There was no difference between the mean pre-exposure UTC and that of a group of 20 nurses who never handled antineoplastic drugs. Twelve of the 15 nurses wore gloves when handling the drugs; none wore any other form of protective apparel. Drug preparation procedures were not reported.

Using gas chromatography, Hirst's group[30] found cyclophosphamide in the urine of two nurses working in a cancer clinic who took no special precautions when handling the drug. They also demonstrated that cyclophosphamide can be absorbed through intact skin. On the other hand, another group of researchers[31] looked for (but could not detect) platinum in the urine of 10 pharmacists and nurses who frequently prepared or administered cisplatin and other platinum-containing antineoplastic agents. However, these subjects employed several protective measures when working with the drugs; this may have influenced the results (and demonstrated the effectiveness of the safety precautions employed). Also, the assay method may not have been sensitive enough.

With a different type of approach, Neal et al.[32] detected fluorouracil in the air of a drug preparation room and nearby office (where the drug was not prepared). A similar study[33] showed that routine drug manipulations in a horizontal laminar airflow hood contaminated the air in an intravenous admixture preparation room. Fluorouracil and cefazolin sodium were the test drugs employed.

Certain antineoplastic drugs have also been implicated in reproductive risks in humans. There have been reports of fetal loss or malformation occurring in pregnancies of women receiving drug therapy for cancer during the first trimester.[34] Two controlled, retrospective Finnish studies[35,36] attempted to examine the relationship between occupational exposure to antineoplastics and reproductive risks in nurses. One study of nurses reported a statistically significant correlation between the birth of children with malformations and the nurses' preparation and administration of antineoplastics more than once a week during the first trimester of pregnancy. At the time of these nurses' exposure, few protective mechanisms were used.

The second study was done in cooperation with the U.S. National Institute for Occupational Safety and Health (NIOSH); it examined only the incidence of fetal loss and did not investigate the condition of live births. The study showed a significant association between fetal loss and occupational exposure to antineoplastic drugs during the first trimester. Both studies are subject to criticism regarding recall bias and determination of exposure data. Concern about exposure of pregnant workers to hazardous drugs, at least in the first trimester, is, however, valid in light of the reproductive risk reported with therapeutic exposure to certain antineoplastics. At therapeutic doses, these drugs have also been shown to suppress testicular function and spermatogenesis.[37-39] While the relationship between occupational exposure to hazardous drugs and testicular dysfunction has not been assessed, this potential complication should be considered in light of the effects on treated patients.

To date, these reports provide the primary evidence that health-care workers exposed to hazardous drugs during the course of their work may be absorbing these drugs and may be at risk for adverse outcomes.

Additional research in this area is needed, but awareness of the problem has led to overall reduction of exposures, either by improved drug handling techniques or through the implementation of safety programs,[40,41] and thus fewer exposed health-care workers are available for study. Definitive knowledge of the occupational dangers of handling hazardous drugs may someday be available through epidemiologic studies of health-care workers.

In theory, correct and perfect preparation and handling techniques will prevent drug particles or droplets from escaping from their containers while they are being manipulated. Our opinion is that near-perfect technique is uncommon; therefore, contamination of the workplace is likely and worker exposure may increase without protective equipment and other safety measures. This is particularly true, we think, in the absence of any structured training and quality-assurance programs covering the proper handling of hazardous drugs. (Such programs are most likely to be found in health-care settings where the preparation of hazardous drugs is centralized.) Beyond problems in technique, however, contamination also will occur from inevitable spills and from the breakage of hazardous drug containers. ASHP believes that the occupational dangers of exposure to hazardous drugs can be summarized as follows:

1. If hazardous drugs are handled in the same way as other less hazardous substances (e.g., potassium chloride solutions and multivitamin tablets), contamination of the work environment is almost certain to occur.

2. The limited data available suggest that this contamination may result in exposure to and absorption of the drugs by health-care personnel and others. The amount of drug absorbed by any one individual on any given day probably is very small, except for instances of excessive exposure.

3. However, if experience with the therapeutic use of hazardous drugs indicates that the damage is cumulative, individuals whose job responsibilities require them to prepare or administer large numbers of hazardous drug doses for long periods of time (e.g., oncology or transplant nurses and pharmacy intravenous service staff) are at greater risk.

4. Considering the above, the use of procedures, equipment, and materials that demonstrably or theoretically reduce exposure to hazardous drugs in the health-care workplace is necessary.

The question remains: What safety precautions should be employed?

Safety Precautions

Ideally, the safety precautions employed to protect health-care workers handling hazardous drugs would be those whose efficacy and cost-effectiveness have been documented. Since these drugs have many different physical and chemical properties, research studies into environmental contamination and safety-garment penetration for all questionable drugs are problematic. However, several studies have attempted to demonstrate the effectiveness of certain recommended interventions. Hoy and Stump[42] concluded that a commercial air-venting device, when used with appropriate technique, effectively reduced the release of drug aerosols during reconstitution of drugs packaged in vials. A study by Anderson et al.[16] provides support for preparing hazardous drugs in a vertical laminar airflow biological safety cabinet (BSC) (NSF Class II[43]; see Appendix B) rather than a horizontal airflow clean air work station.

A more recent air-sampling study,[44] carried out in a hospital pharmacy work area where a Class II BSC was used to prepare cytotoxic drugs, detected no fluorouracil during the study period. The study was limited to one drug and two short study periods; the results indicate that a Class II BSC, in conjunction with stringent aseptic technique and recommended procedures for handling hazardous drugs, may reduce environmental contamination by these drugs.

While common sense suggests that the airflow characteristics of containment cabinets would provide greater worker protection than open airflow workstations, it should also suggest that the front opening of the Class II BSC might present potential for environmental contamination and increased worker exposure to hazardous agents. Indeed, as demonstrated by an industrial hygiene experiment,[45] a Class II BSC may cause occasional leakage toward the operator and into the environment if it is placed in an area of strong air drafts or frequent personnel traffic. The containment characteristics of the Class II BSC are compromised whenever the intake or exhaust grilles are blocked (e.g., by placing equipment or supplies on the front grille or too near the back exhaust) or by too much movement on the part of the operator.

Gloves are a major source of protection, whether the work is performed with or without a Class II BSC. The permeability of various glove materials to selected drugs has been examined.[46-49] By using various methods to determine and quantitate penetration, researchers found that permeability of the glove material varied with the drug, contact time, and glove thickness. None of the glove materials tested was impervious to all drugs, and no material was statistically superior except as related to thickness. A thicker glove material is optimal. In addition, several glove materials showed variation in permeability within a manufacturer's lot. These studies do establish that gloves can provide protection against skin contact with the tested drugs, although the degree of protection has not been substantiated. Protection from skin contact is important since many of the problem drugs are skin irritants or even vesicants and, as Hirst et al.[30] showed, at least one (cyclophosphamide) is absorbed through the skin.

Only one study[50] looked at the permeability of gown materials to drugs. Lab coats and disposable isolation gowns were penetrated immediately and were therefore inappropriate for study. Of the four other gown materials studied, Kaycel and nonporous Tyvek had greater permeability than the coated fabrics (Saranex-laminated Tyvek and polyethylene-coated Tyvek). As with gloves, permeability was drug specific. The investigators concluded that users of garments made of Kaycel and nonporous Tyvek should be aware of the potential of these materials for permeability to certain drugs. An earlier report[51] supports the wearing of gloves and gowns. Additional research is needed in the area of protective garments and equipment. Since substantive data are still lacking, health-care professionals should choose protective measures on the basis of expert recommendations, professional judgment, and common sense as well as scientifically established facts.

Recommended Safe Handling Methods

The balance of this article presents our recommendations for policies, procedures, and safety materials for controlling, preparing, administering, containing, and disposing of hazardous drugs. The recommendations are given in a format that can be used either as a base for establishing safe handling methods or for evaluating existing procedures as part of a quality-assurance program. ASHP believes these recommendations represent a conservative but reasonable approach to the precautions that should be taken.

The recommendations are in the format of evaluation criteria organized into four groups. This format should be useful in establishing a quality-assurance system for all nontherapeutic aspects of hazardous drug use. Each group begins with a broad goal, followed by a set of specific criteria and recommendations for achieving the goal. The four goals reflect the following axioms for handling hazardous drugs:

1. Protect and secure packages of hazardous drugs.

2. Inform and educate all involved personnel about hazardous drugs and train them in the safe handling procedures relevant to their responsibilities.

3. Do not let the drugs escape from containers when they are manipulated (i.e., dissolved, transferred, administered, or discarded).

4. Eliminate the possibility of inadvertent ingestion or inhalation and direct skin or eye contact with the drugs.

The handling of hazardous drugs is a complex issue, and the advice of medical experts, occupational physicians, industrial hygienists, legal counsel, and others should be obtained when organizational policy is being established.

Goal I. Accidental contamination of the health-care environment, resulting in exposure of personnel, patients, visitors, and family members to hazardous substances, is prevented by maintaining the physical integrity and security of packages of hazardous drugs.

1. *Access to all areas where hazardous drugs are stored is limited to specified authorized staff.*

2. *A method should be present for identifying to personnel those drugs that require special precautions (e.g., cytotoxics).*[52] One way to accomplish this is to apply appropriate warning labels (see Figure 1) to all hazardous drug containers, shelves, and bins where the drug products are stored.

3. *A method of identifying, for patients and family members, those drugs that require special precautions in the home should be in place.* This may be accomplished in the health-care setting by providing specific labeling for discharge medications, along with counseling and written instructions. Providers of home care and supplies should develop similar labeling and instructional material for the protection of patients and their families.

4. *Methods for identifying shipping cartons of hazardous drugs should be required from manufacturers and distributors of these drugs.*

5. *Written procedures for handling damaged packages of hazardous drugs should be maintained.* Personnel involved in shipping and receiving hazardous drugs should be trained in these procedures, including the proper use of protective garments and equipment. Damaged shipping cartons of hazardous drugs should be received and opened in an isolated area (e.g., in a laboratory fume hood, if available, not in a BSC used for preparing sterile products). Protective apparel—disposable closed-front gown or coveralls, disposable utility gloves over disposable latex gloves, NIOSH-approved[53] air-purifying half-mask respirator (may be disposable) equipped with a high-efficiency filter, and eye protection—should be worn. Broken containers and contaminated packaging materials should be placed in the designated receptacles as described in this article.

6. *Facilities (e.g., shelves, carts, counters, and trays) for storing hazardous drugs are designed to prevent breakage and to limit contamination in the event of leakage.* Bins, shelves with barriers at the front, or other design features that reduce the chance of drug containers falling to the floor should be used. Hazardous drugs requiring refrigeration should be stored separately from nonhazardous drugs in individual bins designed to prevent breakage and contain leakage.

7. *Methods for transporting hazardous drugs to the health-care setting should be consistent with environmental protection and national or local regulations for transporting hazardous substances.* When hazardous drugs are being transported to the home care setting, appropriate containers (e.g., lined cardboard boxes) and pro-

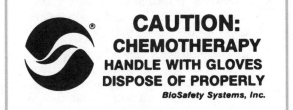

Figure 1. One example of a suitable warning label for cytotoxic and hazardous drugs. Other labels may be used.

cedures should be used to prevent breakage and contain leakage. Hazardous drug containers should be secured to prevent handling by unauthorized persons. Transportation vehicles should be kept locked at all times.

For transporting hazardous drugs within the health-care setting, methods that do not cause breakage of or leakage from drug containers should be used. Conveyances that produce severe mechanical stress on their contents (e.g., pneumatic tubes) must not be used to transport hazardous drugs. The drugs must be securely capped or sealed and properly packaged and protected during transport to reduce further the chance of breakage and spillage in a public area such as a corridor or elevator. Adequate instruction and appropriate containers should be provided to patients for transporting discharge and home care medications that require special precautions.

Goal II. The preparation of hazardous drugs does not result in contamination of the health-care work environment or excessive exposure of personnel, patients, or family members to hazardous drug powders, dusts, liquids, or mists.

1. *Written policies and standard procedures for preparing hazardous drugs are maintained.*

   a. They should include a method for identifying for health-care personnel the particular drugs covered by these policies.

   b. Policies and procedures should be consistent with applicable government regulations, professional practice standards, and the recommendations of pharmaceutical manufacturers, hospital safety

officers, and other knowledgeable parties.

c. Since several departments, such as pharmacy, nursing, transportation, maintenance, housekeeping, and medical staff, will be involved with some aspect of the hazardous drug handling issue, preparation of safe handling policies and procedures must be a collaborative effort. Pharmacy should take the lead in this effort.

d. All personnel who handle cytotoxic and other hazardous agents should have access to the procedures pertaining to their responsibilities. Deviations from the standard procedures must not be permitted except under defined circumstances.

2. *A method for orienting all involved personnel to the special nature of the hazardous drugs in question and the policies and procedures that govern their handling is present.*

   a. The orientation should include, as appropriate, a discussion of the known and potential hazards of the drugs and explanation of all relevant policies. Training done in association with the orientation should cover all relevant techniques and procedures and the proper use of protective equipment and materials. The contents of the orientation program and attendance should be well documented and sufficient to meet "worker right to know" statutes and regulations.

   b. While implementation of a safety program should reduce the risk of personnel exposure to hazardous drugs, the efficacy of such a program in protecting personnel during preparation or administration of these drugs has yet to be demonstrated. The limitations of such a program should be made known to hazardous drug handlers.

   c. Until the reproductive risks (or lack thereof) associated with handling hazardous drugs within a safety program have been substantiated, staff who are pregnant or breast-feeding should be allowed to avoid contact with these drugs. Policies should be in effect that provide these individuals with alternative tasks or responsibilities if they so desire. In general, these policies should encourage personnel to solicit recommendations from their personal physicians regarding the need for restricted duties. In the case of personnel actively trying to conceive or father a child, a similar policy should be considered, and a specific time period (e.g., 3 months) should be agreed on. Legal counsel should be sought when establishing policies.

d. Prospective temporary and permanent employees who may be required to work with hazardous drugs should be so notified and should receive adequate information about the policies and procedures pertaining to their use. This notification should be documented during the interview proc-ess and retained as part of the employment record for all employees.

e. All individuals handling hazardous drugs who do not have employee status (e.g., contract workers, students, residents, medical staff, and volunteers) should be informed through proper channels of the special nature of the drugs. If they choose to handle the hazardous drugs, then they will be expected to comply with established policies and procedures for preparing, administering, and containing hazardous drugs and their associated waste.

3. *A system for verifying and documenting acceptable staff performance of and conformance with established procedures is maintained.*

a. Methods of determining adherence to departmental safety program policies and procedures should be in place. Proper technique is essential to maintain the sterility of the product being manipulated and to reduce the generation of hazardous drug contaminants. Therefore, after initial training and at regular intervals, the knowledge and competence of personnel preparing and administering these drugs should be evaluated and documented. This evaluation should include written examinations and an observed demonstration of competence in the preparation and simulated administration of practice solutions. The monitoring of staff performance and the control of hazardous drugs usually are best achieved if the storage and preparation of the drugs are centralized within one area or department.

b. All personnel involved with the transportation, preparation, administration, and disposal of cytotoxic and hazardous substances should continually be updated on new or revised information on safe handling of cytotoxic and hazardous substances. Policies and procedures should be updated accordingly.

4. *Sufficient information is maintained on safe use of the hazardous drugs in the work area.*

a. The pharmacy should provide access to information on toxicity, treatment of acute exposure (if available), chemical inactivators, solubility, and stability of hazardous drugs (including investigational agents) used in the workplace. This information should be in addition to information required to ensure patient safety during therapy with these drugs and to be in compliance with all applicable laws and regulations. The information must be easily and readily accessible to all employees where these drugs are routinely handled.

b. Currently, a large number of investigational agents that are potentially hazardous are under clinical study. Staff members should not prepare or administer any investigational agent unless they have received adequate information and instruction about the safe and correct use of the drug. The clinical protocol should include appropriate handling and disposal techniques, if available. When information is limited, pre-clinical data should be used to assess the health risk of the agent.

5. *Appropriate engineering controls should be in place to protect the drug product from microbial contamination and to protect personnel and the environment from the potential hazards of the product.* These engineering controls should be maintained according to applicable regulations and standards.

a. Class 100 clean air work stations,[54] both horizontal and vertical airflow (with no containment characteristics), are inappropriate engineering controls for handling hazardous drugs because they provide no personnel protection and permit environmental contamination. Although there are no engineering controls designed specifically for the safe handling of hazardous chemicals as sterile products, Class II[43] contained vertical flow BSCs (biohazard cabinets) have been adopted for this use. Biohazard cabinetry is, however, designed for the handling of infectious agents, not hazardous chemicals. Therefore, the limitations of such cabinetry must be understood by purchaser and operator. Manufacturers, vendors, the National Sanitation Foundation (NSF), and some certifying agencies are appropriate sources of information regarding BSCs.

b. BSCs are available in three classes (Appendix B). Based on design, ease of use, and cost considerations, Class II contained vertical flow biohazard cabinetry is currently recommended for use in preparing sterile doses of hazardous drugs. Class II cabinetry design and performance specifications are defined in NSF Standard 49.[43] BSCs selected for use with hazardous drugs should meet NSF Standard 49 specifications to ensure the maximum protection from these engineering controls. NSF Standard 49 defines four types of Class II cabinetry, depending on the amount of contaminated air that is recirculated through high-efficiency particulate air (HEPA) filters within the cabinet (see Appendix B).

Selection criteria for Class II cabinetry should include the types and amounts of hazardous drugs prepared, the available location and amount of space, NSF Standard 49, any local requirements for handling hazardous materials and ducting contaminated air, and the cost of the cabinet and related ventilation. Minimum recommendations are a Class II, Type A cabinet (recirculating a major portion of contaminated air through a HEPA filter and back into the cabinet and exhausting a minor portion, through a HEPA filter, to the workroom). In light of the continued development of hazardous drugs having differing physical properties, selection of a Type A cabinet that can be converted to a Type B3 (greater inflow velocity, contaminated ducts and plenums under negative pressure and vented to the outside) may be a prudent investment. There are currently no data to indicate that the use of an auxiliary charcoal filter is more effective in retaining hazardous drugs than the mandatory exhaust HEPA filter of the Type A cabinet.

Type B BSCs are designed to provide more personnel protection than Type A through their greater inflow velocities and required external exhaust of contaminated air. Types B1 (exhausting approximately 70% of the contaminated air to the outside through a HEPA filter) and B2 (exhausting 100% of the contaminated air to the outside through a HEPA filter) require outside exhaust ducts with auxiliary blowers. The Type B2 cabinet is preferred, but unavailability of adequate "makeup" air may eliminate it in favor of the Type B1. All exhaust ducting of any type of BSC must meet applicable codes and ordinances. Ducting into the "dead space" in the ceiling is inappropriate and may be illegal, because it may contaminate ventilation systems and promote contamination of the environment and personnel not directly involved in hazardous drug handling.

In the selection of any BSC, ceiling height should also be considered. Several manufacturers' models have top-load HEPA filters. In workrooms with standard-height ceilings, the filters are difficult to access for certification, which may require that the entire BSC be moved when the filter must be replaced. Because of restrictions of space and cost, the 2-foot wide, Class II, Type A BSC may seem to be the only choice for smaller institutions, outpatient centers, and physician offices. There are, however, many limitations to the smaller cabinet. Because NSF testing facilities are not currently adaptable to 2-foot BSC models, no 2-foot BSC is NSF approved. Selection of a 2-foot cabinet should, therefore, include thorough investigation of cabinet design and knowledge of the reliability of the manufacturer. In all cases, the manufacturer's 2-foot cabinet should not differ extensively from designs used for its NSF-approved larger models.

c. All Class II BSCs have an open front with inward airflow forming a "curtain" or barrier to protect the operator and the environment from contaminants released in the BSC work area. Because BSCs are subject to breaks in their containment properties if there is interference with the inward airflow through the work area access opening, placement of the BSC and operator training are critical. The placement of a BSC in an area with drafts or in close proximity to other airflow devices (e.g., horizontal flow hoods, air conditioners, air vents, fans, and doors) may interfere with the inward airflow through the opening and may release contaminants into the workroom.

The horizontal motion of an operator's arms in the opening may also result in similar workroom contamination. Because smaller BSCs are more sensitive to disruption of the inward airflow barrier, the use of a 2- to 3-foot BSC is associated with a greater risk of releasing contaminants than are larger cabinets and requires that the operator be more carefully trained and monitored. It is critical that all operators know the proper method for preparing hazardous drugs in a BSC and that they understand the limitations of BSCs.

d. Class II BSCs should be certified according to specifications of NSF Standard 49 and Class 100 specifications of Federal Standard 209C.[54] Certification should take place on initial installation, whenever the cabinet is moved or repaired, and every 6 months thereafter. At present, there are no licensing requirements for individuals who certify Class II BSCs. It is, therefore, imperative that the pharmacist responsible for the intravenous preparation area be familiar with the certification requirements for Class II BSCs and the test procedures that should be performed.[55]

All BSCs should be tested for the integrity of the HEPA filter, velocity of the work access airflow and supply airflow, airflow smoke patterns, and integrity of external surfaces of the cabinet and filter housings. Testing of the integrity of the HEPA filter generally ensures that the particulate count in the work area is less than that required to meet Class 100 conditions of Federal Standard 209C.[54] Class II, Type B1 BSCs may be prone to exceed Class 100 particle counts and should have routine particulate testing as part of the certification process. Individuals certifying the BSC should be informed of the hazardous nature of the drugs being prepared in the BSC and should wear appropriate protective apparel (see section 5g).

e. BSCs should be cleaned and disinfected regularly to ensure a proper environment for preparation of sterile products. For routine cleanups of surfaces between decontaminations, water should be used (for injection or irrigation) with or without a small amount of cleaner. If the contamination is soluble only in alcohol, then 70% isopropyl or ethyl alcohol may be used in addition to the cleaner. In general, alcohol is not a good cleaner, only a disinfectant, and its use in a BSC should be limited. The BSC should be disinfected with 70% alcohol before any aseptic manipulation is begun. The excessive use of alcohol should be avoided in BSCs where air is recirculated (i.e., Class II, Type A, B3, and, to a lesser extent, B1) because alcohol vapors may build up in the cabinet.

A lint-free, plastic-backed disposable liner may be used in the BSC to facilitate spill cleanup. Problems with the use of such a liner include introduction of particulates into the work area, "lumping" of a wet liner that causes unsteady placement of drug containers, poor vis-

ibility of spills, and creation of additional contaminated disposables. If used, the liner should be changed frequently and whenever it is overtly contaminated.

f. The BSC should be operated with the blower turned on continuously, 24 hours a day, 7 days a week. Hazardous drug aerosols and spills generated in the work area of the BSC routinely accumulate in the deposits of room dust and particles under the work tray. These contaminants are too heavy to be transported to the HEPA filter located at the top of the cabinet. In addition, the plenums in all of the BSCs currently available in the United States become contaminated during use; these plenums cannot be accessed for washing. Turning off the blower may allow contaminated dust to recirculate back into the workroom, especially if other sources of air turbulence, such as horizontal hoods, air intakes, air conditioners, and fans, are located near the BSC. Whether or not the BSC is vented to the outside, the downward airflow velocity is insufficient to move and "trap" room dust, spill debris, and other contaminants on the HEPA filter. If it is necessary to turn off a BSC, first the entire cabinet, including all parts that can be reached, should be thoroughly cleaned with a detergent that will remove surface contamination and then rinsed (see section 5g). Once the BSC is clean, the blower may be turned off and the work access opening of the BSC and the HEPA exhaust area may be covered with impermeable plastic and sealed with tape to prevent any contamination from inadvertently escaping from the BSC. The BSC must be sealed with plastic whenever it is moved or left inoperative for any period of time.

g. The BSC should be decontaminated on a regular basis (ideally at least weekly) and whenever there is a spill or the BSC is moved or serviced, including for certification. While NSF Standard 49 recommends decontamination with formaldehyde to remove biohazard contamination, chemical (drug) contamination is not removed by such treatment. Currently, no single reagent will deactivate all known hazardous drugs; therefore, decontamination of a BSC used for such drugs is limited to removal of contamination from a nondisposable surface (the cabinet) to a disposable surface (e.g., gauze or towels) by use of a good cleaning agent that removes chemicals from stainless steel.

The cleaning agent selected should have a pH approximating that of soap and be appropriate for stainless steel. Cleaners containing chemicals such as quaternary ammonium compounds should be used with caution, because they may be hazardous to humans and their vapors may build up in any BSC where air is recirculated (see section 5e). Similar caution should be used with any pressurized aerosol cleaner; spraying a pressurized aerosol into a BSC may disrupt the protective containment airflow, damage the HEPA filter, and cause an accumulation of the propellant within a BSC where air is recirculated, resulting in a fire and explosion hazard.

During decontamination, the operator should wear a disposable closed-front gown, disposable latex gloves covered by disposable utility gloves, safety glasses or goggles, a hair covering, and a disposable respirator, because the glass shield of the BSC occasionally must be lifted (see 5j). The blower must be left on, and only heavy toweling or gauze should be used in the BSC to prevent it from being "sucked" up the plenum and into the HEPA filter.

Decontamination should be done from top to bottom (areas of lesser contamination to greater) by applying the cleaner, scrubbing, and rinsing thoroughly with distilled or deionized water. All contaminated disposables should be contained in sealable bags for transfer to larger waste containers. The HEPA filter must not become wet during cleaning of the protective covering (e.g., grille front). This covering, therefore, should not be cleaned with spray cleaners while it is in place. Removable parts of the BSC should be cleaned within the containment area of the BSC and should not be removed from the cabinet. The work tray usually can be lifted and placed against the back wall for cleaning of the undersurface of the tray and exposure of the very bottom (or sump) of the BSC.

The drain spillage trough area collects room dust and all spills, so it is the most heavily contaminated area and must be thoroughly cleaned (at least twice with the cleaning agent). The trough provides limited access to the side and back plenums; surfaces should be cleaned as high as possible. BSCs have sharp metal edges, so disposable utility gloves are more durable and appropriate than surgical latex gloves for decontamination. Gloves should be changed immediately if torn. All plenum surfaces must be rinsed well, with frequent changes of water and gauze. If the BSC is equipped with a drainpipe and valve, it may be used to collect rinse water. The collection vessel used must fit well around the drain valve and not allow splashing. Gauze may be used around the connection to prevent aerosol from escaping. The collection vessel must have a tight-fitting cover, and all rinse water (and gauze, if used) must be disposed of as contaminated waste. The outside of the BSC should be wiped down with cleaner to remove any drip or touch contamination.

Cleaner and rinse containers are generally contaminated during the procedure and should remain in the BSC during cleaning or be placed on a plastic-backed, absorbent liner outside the BSC. All bottles must be discarded as contaminated waste after decontamination of the BSC. All protective apparel (e.g., gown, gloves, goggles, and respirator) should be discarded as contaminated waste. Work area surfaces should be disinfected with 70% alcohol before any aseptic operation is begun. With good planning, decontamination of a 4-foot BSC should take about 1 hour.

h. Because of its design and decontamination limitations, the BSC should be considered a contaminated environment and treated as such. The use of the BSC should be restricted to the preparation of sterile dosage forms of hazardous drugs. Access to the BSC should be limited to authorized personnel wearing appropriate protective clothing.

i. If a BSC previously used for biologicals will be adopted for use with hazardous drugs, the BSC should be completely decontaminated of biohazardous agents by use of NSF Standard 49 decontamination techniques. Both HEPA filters should be replaced and the cabinet tested against the *complete* requirements of NSF Standard 49 Appendix B and the particulate limitations of Class 100 conditions of Federal Standard 209C. A BSC used for hazardous drugs that will be recycled for use with hazardous drugs in another section of the institution or in another institution must be surface decontaminated (as described in section 5g), sealed (as in section 5f), and carefully transported to its new location before the filters are replaced (as in section 5j). Once in its new location, the BSC must be recertified.

j. The HEPA filters of the BSC must be replaced whenever they restrict required airflow velocity or if they are overtly contaminated (e.g., by a breach in technique that causes hazardous drug to be introduced onto the clean side of the supply HEPA filter). Personnel and environmental protection must be maintained during replacement of a contaminated HEPA filter. Because replacement of a HEPA filter generally requires breaking the integrity of the containment aspect of the cabinet, this procedure may release contamination from the filter into the pharmacy or intravenous preparation area if carried out in an inappropriate manner.

Before replacement of a HEPA filter contaminated with hazardous drugs, the BSC service agent should be consulted for a mutually acceptable procedure for replacing and subsequently disposing of a contaminated HEPA filter. One procedure would include moving the BSC to a secluded area or using plastic barriers to segregate the contaminated area. Protective clothing and equipment must be used by the servicer. The BSC should be decontaminated before filter replacement (see section 5g). The contaminated filters must be removed, bagged in thick plastic, and prepared for disposal in a hazardous waste dump site or incinerator licensed by the Environmental Protection Agency (EPA).

When arranging for disposal, precise terms should be used to describe the hazard (e.g., "toxic chemicals" or "chemical carcinogens," not "cytotoxic" or "chemotherapy") to ensure that contractors are not inadvertently misled in the classification of the hazard. Disposal of an entire contaminated BSC should be approached in the same manner. The filters should be removed, bagged, and disposed of separately from the BSC. If no available service company will arrange for removal of the filter (or entire BSC) and its ultimate disposal, a licensed hazardous waste contractor should be used. The use of triple layers of thick plastic (e.g., 2-mil low-linear or 4-mil plastic) for initial covering of the filter or cabinet and then the construction of a plywood crate for transport to an EPA-licensed hazardous waste dump site or incinerator is suggested.

6. *Engineering controls should be supplemented with personal protective apparel and other safety materials.* Policies and procedures should be in place to ensure that these materials are used properly and consistently.

a. Workers should wear powder-free, disposable surgical latex gloves of good quality when preparing hazardous drugs. Selection criteria for gloves should include thickness (especially at the fingertips where stress is the greatest), fit, length, and tactile sensation. While no glove material has been shown to be impervious to all hazardous drugs or to be statistically superior in limiting drug penetration, thickness and time in contact with drug are crucial factors affecting permeability.[47-49]

The practice of double gloving is supported by research that indicates that many glove materials vary in drug permeability even within lots[48,49]; therefore, double gloving is recommended. This recommendation is based on currently available research findings. Evidence to show that single gloves are sufficiently protective might make this recommendation unnecessary. In general, surgical latex gloves fit better, have appropriate elasticity for double gloving and maintaining the integrity of the glove-gown interface, and have sufficient tactile sensation (even during double gloving) for stringent aseptic procedures.

b. Powdered gloves increase the particulate level in the filtered air environment of the BSC and leave a powder residue on the surfaces of supplies, final product, and the hands that may absorb contamination generated in the BSC; therefore, powdered gloves should be avoided. The use of sterile gloves is unnecessary during operations involving nonsterile surfaces. Hands must be thoroughly washed and dried before gloves are donned and when a task or batch is completed. If only powdered gloves are available, all powder must be washed off the outside of the outer glove before any operation is begun, and hands should be washed once gloves have been removed.

c. Two pairs of fresh gloves should be put on when beginning any task or batch. The outer glove should be changed immediately if contaminated. Both gloves should be changed if the outer glove is torn, punctured, or overtly contaminated with drug (as in a spill) and every hour during batch operations. During removal of gloves, care should be taken to avoid touching the inside of the glove or the skin with the contaminated glove fingers. To limit transfer of contamination from the BSC into the work area, outer gloves should be removed after each batch and should be placed in "zipper"-closure plastic bags or other sealable containers for disposal.

d. The worker should wear a protective disposable gown made of lint-free, low-permeability fabric with a solid front, long sleeves, and tight-fitting elastic or knit cuffs when preparing hazardous drugs. Washable garments are immediately penetrated by liquids and therefore provide little, if any, protection. In addition, washable garments require laundering and thus potentially expose other personnel to contamination.

e. When double gloving, one glove should be placed under the gown cuff and one over. The glove-gown interface should be such that no skin on the arm or wrist is exposed. Gloves and gowns should not be worn outside the immediate preparation area. On completion of each task or batch, the worker should, while wearing outer gloves, wipe all final products with gauze. The outer gloves should then be removed and placed, along with the gauze, in a sealable container (e.g., a zipper-closure plastic bag) within the BSC. All waste bags in the BSC should be sealed and removed for disposal. The gown should be removed and placed in a sealable container before removal of the inner gloves. The inner gloves should be removed last and placed in the container with the gown.

f. Workers who are not protected by the containment environment of a BSC should use respiratory protection when handling hazardous drugs. Respiratory protection should be an adjunct to and not a substitute for engineering controls.

g. Surgical masks of all types provide no respiratory protection against powdered or liquid aerosols of hazardous drugs.

h. In situations where workers may be exposed to potential eye contact with hazardous drugs, an appropriate plastic face shield or splash goggles should be worn. Eyewash fountains should be available in areas where hazardous drugs are routinely handled. Inexpensive alternatives include an intravenous bag of 0.9% sodium chloride solution (normal saline) or irrigation bottle of water or saline with appropriate tubing.

7. *Proper manipulative technique to maintain the sterility of injectable drugs and to prevent generation of hazardous drug contaminants is used consistently.*

a. Proper manipulative technique must be taught to all workers who will be required to prepare hazardous drugs.[56] Preparers should demonstrate competence in these techniques once training has been completed and at least annually thereafter.

b. Systems to ensure that these techniques are adhered to should exist, along with systems to ensure patient safety by providing that drugs are properly selected, calculated, measured, and delivered.

c. The work area should be designed to provide easy access to those items necessary to prepare, label, and transport final products; contain all related waste; and avoid inadvertent contamination of the work area.

d. Maintenance of proper technique requires an organized approach to the preparation of sterile doses of hazardous drugs in a BSC. All drug and nondrug items required for completing a dose or batch and for containing the waste should be assembled and placed in the BSC; care should be taken not to overload the BSC work area. All calculations and any label preparation should be completed at this time. Appropriate gowning, hand washing and gloving (or glove changing), and glove washing should be completed before any manipulations are begun. Unnecessary moving in and out of the BSC should be avoided during aseptic manipulations.

e. Syringes and intravenous sets with Luer-lock type fittings should be used for preparing and administering hazardous drug solutions, since they are less prone to accidental separation than friction fittings. Care must be taken to ensure that all connections are secure. Syringes should be large enough so that they are not full when containing the total drug dose. This is to ensure that the plunger does not separate from the syringe barrel. Doses should be dispensed in several syringes when this problem arises.

f. The contents of an ampul should be gently tapped down from the neck and top portion of the ampul before it is opened. The ampul should be wiped with alcohol before being opened. A sterile gauze pad should be wrapped around the neck of the ampul when it is opened.

g. Substantial positive or negative deviations from atmospheric pressure within drug vials and syringes should be avoided.

h. For additional worker protection, equipment such as venting devices with 0.2-

mm hydrophobic filters and 5-mm filter needles or "straws" may be used. It is critical that the worker be proficient with these devices before using them with hazardous drugs. Improper use of these devices may result in increased, rather than decreased, risk of exposure.

i. Final products should be dispensed in ready-to-administer form. If possible, intravenous administration sets should be attached to the bag or bottle in the BSC and primed with plain fluid before the hazardous drug is added. However, if total volume is a concern, intravenous sets may be primed with diluted drug solution, which is discarded into an appropriate container within the BSC. Potential disadvantages to this approach include difficulty in selecting the appropriate administration set when several methods of administering hazardous drugs exist, potential contamination of the outside of the intravenous set, and the risk of the intravenous set becoming dislodged from the bag or bottle during transport.

j. The outside of bags or bottles and intravenous sets (if used) should be wiped with moist gauze to remove any inadvertent contamination. Entry ports should be wiped with sterile, alcohol-dampened gauze pads and covered with appropriate seals or caps.

k. Final products should be placed in sealable containers (e.g., zipper-closure plastic bags) to reduce the risk of exposing ancillary personnel or contaminating the environment. Containers should be designed such that damage incurred during storage or transport is immediately visible and any leakage is fully contained. For offsite transport, appropriate storage conditions (e.g., refrigerated, padded, and locked carriers) should also be used.

l. Excess drug should be returned to the drug vial whenever possible or discarded into a closed container (empty sterile vial). Placing excess drug in any type of open container, even while working in the BSC, is inappropriate. Discarding excess drug into the drainage trough of the BSC is also inappropriate. These practices unnecessarily increase the risk of exposure to large amounts of hazardous drug.

m. All contaminated materials should be placed in leakproof, puncture-resistant containers within the contained environment of the BSC and then placed in larger containers outside the BSC for disposal. To minimize aerosolization, needles should be discarded in puncture-resistant containers without being clipped.

8. *Procedures for the preparation and dispensing of noninjectable dosage forms of hazardous drugs are established and followed.*

a. Although noninjectable dosage forms of hazardous drugs contain varying proportions of drug to nondrug (nonhazardous) components, there is potential for personnel exposure and environmental contamination with the hazardous components. Procedures should be developed to avoid the release of aerosolized powder or liquid into the environment during manipulation of these drugs.

b. Drugs designated as hazardous should be labeled or otherwise identified as such to prevent their improper handling.

c. Tablet and capsule forms of these drugs should not be placed in automated counting machines, which subject them to stress and may introduce powdered contaminants into the work area.

d. During *routine handling* of hazardous drugs and contaminated equipment, workers should wear one pair of gloves of good quality and thickness.

e. The counting and pouring of hazardous drugs should be done carefully, and clean equipment dedicated for use with these drugs should be used. Contaminated equipment should be cleaned initially with water-saturated gauze and then further cleaned with detergent and rinsed. The gauze and rinse should be disposed of as contaminated waste.

f. During *compounding* of hazardous drugs (e.g., crushing, dissolving, and preparing an ointment), workers should wear low-permeability gowns and double gloves. Compounding should take place in a protective area such as a disposable glove box. If compounding must be done in the open, an area away from drafts and traffic must be selected, and the worker should use appropriate respiratory protection.

g. When hazardous drug tablets in unit-of-use packaging are being crushed, the package should be placed in a small sealable plastic bag and crushed with a spoon or pestle; caution should be used not to break the plastic bag.

h. Disposal of unused or unusable oral or topical dosage forms of hazardous drugs should be performed in the same manner as for hazardous injectable dosage forms and waste.

9. *Personnel know the procedures to be followed in case of accidental skin or eye contact with hazardous drugs.*

   a. Each health-care setting should have an established first aid protocol for treating cases of direct contact with hazardous drugs, many of which are irritating or caustic and can cause tissue destruction. Medical care providers in each setting should be contacted for input into this protocol. The protocol should include immediate treatment measures and should specify the type and location of medical followup and work-injury reporting. Copies of the protocol, highlighting emergency measures, should be posted wherever hazardous drugs are routinely handled.

   b. Hazardous drug work areas should have a sink (preferably with an eyewash fountain) and appropriate first aid equipment to treat accidental skin or eye contact according to the protocol.

   c. In settings where hazardous drug handlers are offsite (e.g., home use), protocols must be part of orientation programs, and copies of the procedures should be immediately accessible to handlers, along with appropriate first aid equipment and emergency phone numbers to call for followup and reporting.

10. *All hazardous drugs are labeled with a warning label stating the need for special handling.*

    a. A distinctive warning label with an appropriate CAUTION statement should be attached to all hazardous drug materials, consistent with state laws and regulations. This would include, for example, syringes, intravenous containers, containers of unit-dose tablets and liquids, prescription vials and bottles, waste containers, and patient specimens that contain hazardous drugs.

    b. The hazardous drugs discussed in this Technical Assistance Bulletin are chemical hazards and *not* infectious hazards. Because the term "biohazard" refers to an infectious hazard, the use of this term or the biohazard symbol (in any variation) on the label of drugs that are chemical hazards is inappropriate and may be misleading to staff and contract workers who are familiar with the biohazard symbol. An example of a suitable label is shown in Figure 1.

    c. All staff and contract workers should be informed about the meaning of the label

and the special handling procedures that have been established.

    d. In settings where patients or their families will be responsible for manipulating these drugs, they should be made aware of the need for special handling and the reasons behind it.

Goal III. Procedures for administering hazardous drugs prevent the accidental exposure of patients and staff and contamination of the work environment.

1. *A method for informing and training health-care professionals in these procedures is maintained.*

   a. Only individuals trained to administer hazardous drugs should be allowed to perform this function. Training programs should contain information on the therapeutic and adverse effects of these drugs and the potential, long-term health risk to personnel handling them. Each individual's knowledge and technique should be evaluated before administration of these drugs. This should be done by written examination and direct observation of the individual's performance.

2. *Standard procedures for the safe administration of hazardous drugs are established and followed.* These procedures ensure the safety of both the patient and health-care personnel.

   a. Intravenous administration sets (e.g., vented, nonvented, and minidrip) and infusion devices appropriate for use with the final product should be selected.

   b. Syringes and intravenous sets with Luer-lock fittings should be used whenever possible.

   c. Preparation of the final product for administration should take place in a clean, uncluttered area separate from other activities and excessive traffic. A plastic-backed absorbent liner should be used to cover the work area to absorb accidental spills. A single pair of disposable latex gloves and a disposable gown should be worn. The glove and gown cuffs should be worn in a manner that produces a tight fit (e.g., loose glove tucked under gown cuff; tight glove fitted over gown cuff). Hands must be thoroughly washed before gloves are donned.

   Administration sets should be attached with care (if not attached during drug

311

preparation). Administration sets and devices should be monitored for leakage.

d. Priming of intravenous sets should not allow any drug to be released into the environment. Hazardous drug solutions may be "piggybacked" into primary intravenous solutions and primed by retrograde flow of the primary solution into the secondary tubing. All Y-site connections should be taped securely. Alternatively, the intravenous set may be primed with plain solution before the hazardous drug solution bag or bottle is connected. Some intravenous sets can be primed so that the fluid enters the medication port of the intravenous bag. The priming fluid may also be discarded into a sealable plastic bag containing absorbent material if care is taken not to contaminate the sterile needle tip. Likewise, a sterile gauze pad should be placed close to the sterile needle tip when air is expelled from a syringe. The syringe plunger should first be drawn back to withdraw liquid from the needle before air is expelled. Care should be taken not to contaminate the sterile needle with gauze fibers or microorganisms.

e. Intravenous containers designed with venting tubes should not be used. If such containers must be used, gauze should be placed over the tube when the container is inverted to catch any hazardous drug solution trapped in the tube. If containers with solid stoppers are used, any vacuum present should be eliminated before the container is attached to a primary intravenous or to a manifold. If a series of bags or bottles is used to deliver the drug, the intravenous set should be discarded with each container because removing the spike from the container is associated with a greater risk of environmental contamination than priming an intravenous set. (Use of secondary sets for administration of hazardous drugs reduces the cost of this recommendation and the risk of priming.)

f. A plastic-backed absorbent liner should be placed under the intravenous tubing during administration to absorb any leakage and prevent the solution from spilling onto the patient's skin. The use of sterile gauze around any "push" sites will reduce the likelihood of releasing drug into the environment.

g. The use of eye protection (safety glasses or goggles) during work with hazardous drugs, especially vesicants, should be considered. Work at your waist level, if possible; avoid working above the head or reaching up for connections or ports.

h. All contaminated gauze, syringes, intravenous sets, bags, bottles, etc., should be placed in sealable plastic bags and placed in a puncture-resistant container for removal from the patient-care area.

i. Gloves should be discarded after each use and immediately if contaminated. Gowns should be discarded on leaving the patient-care area and immediately if contaminated. Hands must be washed thoroughly after hazardous drugs are handled.

j. Gloves should be worn when urine and other excreta from patients receiving hazardous drugs are being handled. Skin contact and splattering should be avoided during disposal. While it may be useful to post a list of drugs that are excreted in urine and feces and the length of time after drug administration during which precautions are necessary, an alternative is to select a standard duration (e.g., 48 hours) that covers most of the drugs and is more easily remembered.

k. Disposable linen or protective pads should be used for incontinent or vomiting patients. Nondisposable linen contaminated with hazardous drug should be handled with gloves and treated similarly to that for linen contaminated with infectious material. One procedure is to place the linen in specially marked water-soluble laundry bags. These bags (with the contents) should be prewashed; then the linens should be added to other laundry for an additional wash. Items contaminated with hazardous drugs should not be autoclaved unless they are also contaminated with infectious material.

3. *Appropriate apparel and materials needed to protect staff and patients from exposure and to protect the work environment from contamination are readily available.* Supplies of disposable gloves and gowns, safety glasses, disposable plastic-backed absorbent liners, gauze pads, hazardous waste disposal bags, hazardous drug warning labels, and puncture-resistant containers for disposal of needles and ampuls should be conveniently located for all areas where hazardous drugs are handled. Assembling a "hazardous drug preparation and administration kit" is one way to furnish nursing and medical personnel with the materials needed to reduce the risk of preparing and administering a hazardous drug.

4. *Personnel know the procedures to be followed in case of accidental skin or eye contact with hazardous drugs. (See Goal II9.)*

Goal IV. The health-care setting, its staff, patients, contract workers, visitors, and the outside environment are not exposed to or contaminated with hazardous drug waste materials produced in the course of using these drugs. (See Figure 2 for proposed flow chart for handling contaminated items.)

1. *Written policies and procedures governing the identification, containment, collection, segregation, and disposal of hazardous drug waste materials are established and maintained.* All health-care workers who handle hazardous drugs or waste must be oriented to and must follow these procedures.

2. *Throughout institutional health-care facilities and in alternative health-care settings, hazardous drug waste materials are identified, contained, and segregated from all other trash.*

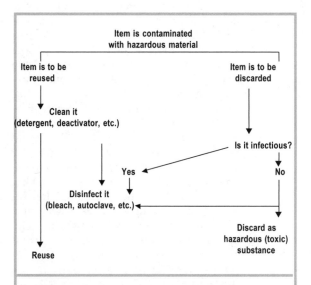

Figure 2. Proposed flow chart for handling chemical hazards versus biohazards. Disinfection of a disposable item contaminated with both infectious and hazardous material may not be necessary, depending on the degree of infectious hazard (e.g., human immunodeficiency virus versus *Escherichia coli*) and depending on the method of disposal (e.g., burial versus incineration).

a. Hazardous drug waste should be placed in specially marked (specifically labeled CAUTION: HAZARDOUS CHEMICAL WASTE) thick plastic bags or leakproof containers. These receptacles should be kept in all areas where the drugs are commonly used. All and only hazardous drug waste should be placed in them. Receptacles used for glass fragments, needles, and syringes should be puncture resistant. Hazardous drug waste should not be mixed with any other waste. Waste containers should be handled with uncontaminated gloves.

b. Health-care personnel providing care in a patient's home should have with them all the equipment and supplies necessary to contain properly any hazardous drug waste that is generated during the visit. Contaminated needles and syringes, intravenous containers, intravenous sets, and any broken ampuls should be placed in leakproof, puncture-resistant containers. Gloves, gowns, drug vials, etc., should be sealed in specially labeled (CAUTION: HAZARDOUS CHEMICAL WASTE) thick plastic bags or leakproof containers. All waste should be removed from the patient's home and transported to a designated area. Additional precautions should be taken during transport, including temporary storage in a spill-resistant container and ensuring that the vehicle is locked at all times. Hazardous waste should be securely stored at a designated area until it is picked up for appropriate disposal. Patients or their caregivers should be instructed on methods for the proper handling of excreta from patients receiving hazardous drugs.

c. Unless restricted by state or local regulations, hazardous drug waste may be further divided into trace and bulk-contaminated waste, if desired, to reduce costs of disposal. As defined by the EPA, bulk-contaminated materials are solutions or containers whose contents weigh more than 3% of the capacity of the container.[57,58] For example, empty intravenous containers and intravenous administration sets usually are considered trace waste; half-empty vials of hazardous drugs and unused final doses in syringes or intravenous containers are considered bulk-contaminated waste. If trace and bulk-contaminated waste are handled separately, bulk-contaminated waste should be segregated into more secure receptacles for containment and disposal as toxic waste. While this may allow for less expensive overall disposal of hazardous waste, it also requires close monitoring of the containment and segregation process to prevent the accidental discarding of a bulk-contaminated container into a trace-waste receptacle.

d. All hazardous waste collected from drug preparation and patient-care areas should be held in a secure place in labeled, leak-proof drums or cartons (as required by state or local regulation or disposal contractor) until disposal. This waste should be disposed of as hazardous or toxic waste in an EPA-permitted, state-licensed hazardous waste incinerator. Transport to an offsite incinerator should be done by a contractor licensed to handle and transport hazardous waste. (While licenses are generally required to transport infectious waste as well as hazardous waste, these are different classes of contractors and may not be interchanged. Verification of possession and type of license should be documented before a contractor is engaged.)

e. If access to an appropriately licensed incinerator is not available, transport to and burial in an EPA-licensed hazardous waste dump site is an acceptable alternative. While there are concerns that destruction of carcinogens by incineration may be incomplete, newer technologies and stringent licensing criteria have improved this disposal method. (Again, the existence and type of license should be verified before use of a contract incinerator.)

f. Chemical deactivation of hazardous drugs should be undertaken only by individuals who are thoroughly familiar with the chemicals and the procedures required to complete such a task. The IARC recently published a monograph describing methods for chemical destruction of some cytotoxic (antineoplastic) drugs in the laboratory setting.[59] The chemicals and equipment described, however, are not generally found in the clinical setting, and many of the deactivating chemicals are toxic and hazardous. Most procedures require the use of a chemical fume hood. The procedures are generally difficult, and the deactivation is not always complete. Serious consideration should be given to the negative aspects of chemical deactivation before one commits to such a course of action.

3. *Materials to clean up spills of hazardous drugs are readily available and personnel are trained in their proper use.* A standard cleanup protocol is established and followed.

a. "Spill kits" containing all materials needed to clean up spills of hazardous drugs should be assembled or purchased. These kits should be readily available in all areas where hazardous drugs are routinely handled. If hazardous drugs are being prepared or administered in a nonroutine area (home setting or unusual patient-care area), a spill kit should be obtained by the drug handler. The kit should include two pairs of disposable gloves (one outer pair of utility gloves and one inner latex pair); low permeability, disposable protective garments (coveralls or gown and shoe covers); safety glasses or splash goggles; respirator; absorbent, plastic-backed sheets or spill pads; disposable toweling; at least two sealable thick plastic hazardous waste disposal bags (prelabeled with an appropriate warning label); a disposable scoop for collecting glass fragments; and a puncture-resistant container for glass fragments.

b. All individuals who routinely handle hazardous drugs must be trained in proper spill management and cleanup procedures. Spills and breakages must be cleaned up immediately according to the following procedures. If the spill is not located in a confined space, the spill area should be identified and other people should be prevented from approaching and spreading the contamination. Wearing protective apparel from the spill kit, workers should remove any broken glass fragments and place them in the puncture-resistant container. Liquids should be absorbed with a spill pad; powder should be removed with damp disposable gauze pads or soft toweling. The hazardous material should be completely removed and the area rinsed with water and then cleaned with detergent. The spill cleanup should proceed progressively from areas of lesser to greater contamination. The detergent should be thoroughly rinsed and removed. All contaminated materials should be placed in the disposal bags provided and sealed and transported to a designated containment receptacle.

c. Spills occurring in the BSC should be cleaned up immediately; a spill kit should be used if the volume exceeds 150 ml or the contents of one drug vial or ampul. If there is broken glass, utility gloves should be worn to remove it and place it in the puncture-resistant container located in the BSC. The BSC, including the drain spillage trough, should be thoroughly cleaned. If the spill is not easily and thoroughly contained, the BSC should be decontaminated after cleanup. If the spill contaminates the HEPA filter, use of the BSC should be suspended until the cabinet has been decontaminated and the HEPA filter replaced. (See Goal II 5j.)

d. If hazardous drugs are routinely prepared or administered in carpeted areas, special equipment is necessary to remove the spill. Absorbent powder should be substituted for pads or sheets and left in place on the spill for the time recommended by the manufacturer. The powder should then be picked up with a small vacuum unit reserved for hazardous drug cleanup. The carpet should then be cleaned according to usual procedures. The vacuum bag should be removed and discarded or cleaned, and the exterior of the vacuum cleaner should be washed with detergent and rinsed before being covered and stored. The contaminated powder should be discarded into a sealable plastic bag and segregated with other contaminated waste materials. Alternatively, inexpensive wet or dry vacuum units may be purchased for this express use and used with appropriate cleaners. All such units are contaminated, once used, and must be cleaned, stored, and ultimately discarded appropriately (i.e., like BSCs).

e. The circumstances and handling of spills should be documented. Health-care personnel exposed during spill management should also complete an incident report or exposure form.

4. *Hazardous drug waste is disposed of in accordance with all applicable state, federal, and local regulations for the handling of hazardous and toxic waste.*

a. Regulatory agencies such as the EPA and state solid and hazardous waste agencies and local air and water quality control boards must be consulted regarding the classification and appropriate disposal of drugs that are defined as hazardous or toxic chemicals. EPA categorizes several of the antineoplastic agents (including cyclophosphamide and daunorubicin) as toxic wastes, while many states are more stringent and include as carcinogens certain cytotoxic drugs (azathioprine) and hormonal preparations (diethylstilbestrol and conjugated estrogens). EPA also allows exemptions from toxic waste regulations for "small quantity generators,"[57] whereas certain states do not. It is critical to research these regulations when disposal procedures are being established.

Other Hazardous Drug Issues

The handling of hazardous drugs, some of which are defined by the EPA as toxic chemicals, has implications that go beyond the health-care setting. Disposal of hazardous materials and toxic chemicals continues to be a controversial issue of which the disposal of hazardous drugs is but a small part. The EPA currently issues permits for both burial and incineration of hazardous waste. Some such facilities may purport to possess permits to handle these types of hazardous agents when, in fact, they do not meet the requirements or are only in the initial stages of obtaining permits. It is imperative that health-care facilities verify the license or permit status of any contractor used to remove or dispose of infectious or hazardous waste. In addition, many hazardous drugs are excreted unchanged or as equally toxic metabolites. The amount of hazardous drug transferred to the environment (primarily through the water supply) from this source may exceed that resulting from the hospital trash pathway. No good methods for reducing this source of contamination are currently known.

Definitive risks of handling these drugs may never be fully determined without epidemiologic data from a national registry of handlers of hazardous drugs (and chemicals). There is no method available for routine monitoring of personnel for evidence of hazardous drug exposure. Tests for the presence of mutagens or chromosomal damage are not drug specific and are of value only in controlled studies. Chemical analysis of urine for the presence of hazardous drugs at the sensitivity level needed to detect occupational exposure is limited to a few drugs and is not yet commercially available.

This document is designed to identify areas of risk in the handling of hazardous drugs and to provide recommendations for reducing that risk. A safety program should be coupled with a strong quality-assurance program that periodically evaluates and verifies staff adherence to and performance of the established safe handling policies and procedures. Until some type of external monitoring of exposure levels from handling hazardous drugs is commercially available, development of and compliance with a safety program remain the most logical means for minimizing occupational risk.

References

1. American Society of Hospital Pharmacists. ASHP technical assistance bulletin on handling cytotoxic drugs in hospitals. *Am J Hosp Pharm.* 1985; 42:131–7.
2. Yodaiken R. Safe handling of cytotoxic drugs by health care personnel. Washington, DC: Occupational Safety and Health Administration; 1986 Jan 29. (Instructional publication 8-1.1).
3. U.S. Public Health Service, National Institutes of Health. Recommendations for the safe handling of parenteral antineoplastic drugs. Washington, DC: U.S. Department of Health and Human Services; 1983. (NIH publication 83-2621).
4. Recommendations for handling cytotoxic agents. Providence, RI: National Study Commission on Cytotoxic Exposure; 1987 Sep.
5. AMA Council on Scientific Affairs. Guidelines for handling parenteral antineoplastics. *JAMA.* 1985; 253:1590–2.
6. Scott SA. Antineoplastic drug information and handling guidelines for office-based physicians. *Am J Hosp Pharm.* 1984; 41:2402–3.
7. Barstow J. Safe handling of cytotoxic agents in the home. *Home Healthc Nurse.* 1986; 3:46–7.
8. Barry LK, Booher RB. Promoting the responsible handling of antineoplastic agents in the community. *Oncol Nurs Forum.* 1985; 12:40–6.
9. Berk PD, Goldberg JD, Silverstein MN, et al. Increased incidence of leukemia in polycythemia vera associated with chlorambucil therapy. *N Engl J Med.* 1981; 304:441–7.
10. Penn I. Occurrence of cancer in immune deficiencies. *Cancer.* 1974; 34:858–66.
11. Schafer AI. Teratogenic effects of antileukemic therapy. *Arch Intern Med.* 1981; 141:514–5.
12. Stephens JD, Golbus MS, Miller TR, et al. Multiple congenital abnormalities in a fetus exposed to 5-fluorouracil during the first trimester. *Am J Obstet Gynecol.* 1980; 137:747–9.
13. IARC monographs on the evaluation of the carcinogenic risk of chemicals to humans. Geneva, Switzerland: World Health Organization; 1981.
14. Benedict WF, Baker MS, Haroun L, et al. Mutagenicity of cancer chemotherapeutic agents in the *Salmonella*/microsome test. *Cancer Res.* 1977; 37:2209–13.
15. Falck K, Grohn P, Sorsa M, et al. Mutagenicity in urine of nurses handling cytostatic drugs. *Lancet.* 1979; 1:1250–1.
16. Anderson RW, Puckett WH, Dana WJ, et al. Risk of handling injectable antineoplastic agents. *Am J Hosp Pharm.* 1982; 39:1881–7.
17. Norppa H, Sorsa M, Vainio H, et al. Increased sister chromatid exchange frequencies in lymphocytes of nurses handling cytostatic drugs. *Scand J Work Environ Health.* 1980; 6:299–301.
18. Waksvik H, Klepp O, Brogger A. Chromosome analyses of nurses handling cytostatic agents. *Cancer Treat Rep.* 1981; 65:607–10.
19. Nikula E, Kiviniitty K, Leisti J, et al. Chromosome aberrations in lymphocytes of nurses handling cytostatic agents. *Scand J Work Environ Health.* 1984; 10:71–4.
20. Chrysostomou A, Morley AA, Sehadri R. Mutation frequency in nurses and pharmacists working with cytotoxic drugs. *Aust N Z J Med.* 1984; 14:831–4.
21. Rogers B, Emmett EA. Handling antineoplastic agents: urine mutagenicity in nurses. *Image J Nurs Sch.* 1987; 19:108–13.
22. Palmer RG, Dore CJ, Denman AM. Chlorambucil-induced chromosome damage to human lymphocytes is dose-dependent and cumulative. *Lancet.* 1984; 1:246–9.
23. Sotaniemi EA, Sutinen S, Arranto AJ, et al. Liver damage in nurses handling cytostatic agents. *Acta Med Scand.* 1983; 214:181–9.
24. How real is the hazard? *Lancet.* 1984; 1:203.
25. Tuffnell PG, Gannon MT, Dong A, et al. Limitations of urinary mutagen assays for monitoring occupational exposure to antineoplastic drugs. *Am J Hosp Pharm.* 1986; 43:344–8.
26. Cloak MM, Connor TH, Stevens KR, et al. Occupational exposure of nursing per-

sonnel to antineoplastic agents. *Oncol Nurs Forum.* 1985; 12:33–9.

27. Connor TH, Anderson RW. Demonstrating mutagenicity testing using the Ames test. *Am J Hosp Pharm.* 1985; 42:783–4.

28. Connor TH, Theiss JC, Anderson RW, et al. Re-evaluation of urine mutagenicity of pharmacy personnel exposed to antineoplastic agents. *Am J Hosp Pharm.* 1986; 43:1236–9.

29. Jagun O, Ryan M, Waldrom HA. Urinary thioether excretion in nurses handling cytotoxic drugs. *Lancet.* 1982; 2:443–4.

30. Hirst M, Tse S, Mills DG, et al. Occupational exposure to cyclophosphamide. *Lancet.* 1984; 1:186–8.

31. Venitt S, Crofton-Sleigh C, Hunt J, et al. Monitoring exposure of nursing and pharmacy personnel to cytotoxic drugs: urinary mutation assays and urinary platinum as markers of absorption. *Lancet.* 1984; 1:74–6.

32. Neal A deW, Wadden RA, Chiou WL. Exposure of hospital workers to airborne antineoplastic agents. *Am J Hosp Pharm.* 1983; 40:597–601.

33. Kleinberg ML, Quinn MJ. Airborne drug levels in a laminar flow hood. *Am J Hosp Pharm.* 1981; 38:1301–3.

34. Gililland J, Weinstein L. The effects of chemotherapeutic agents on the developing fetus. *Obstet Gynecol Surv.* 1983; 38:6–13.

35. Hemminki K, Kyyronen P, Lindbohm ML. Spontaneous abortions and malformations in the offspring of nurses exposed to anesthetic gases, cytostatic drugs and other potential hazards in hospitals, based on registered information of outcome. *J Epidemiol Community Health.* 1985; 39:141–7.

36. Selevan SH, Lindbohm ML, Hornung RW, et al. A study of occupational exposure to antineoplastic drugs and fetal loss in nurses. *N Engl J Med.* 1985; 333:1173–8.

37. Richter P, Calamera JC, Morgenfeld MC, et al. Effect of chlorambucil on spermatogenesis in the human with malignant lymphoma. *Cancer.* 1970; 25:1026–30.

38. Maguire LC. Fertility and cancer therapy. *Postgrad Med.* 1979; 65:293–5.

39. Sherins JJ, DeVita VT Jr. Effect of drug treatment for lymphoma on male reproductive capacity. *Ann Intern Med.* 1973; 79:216–20.

40. Gregoire RE, Segal R, Hale KM. Handling antineoplastic-drug admixtures at cancer centers: practices and pharmacist attitudes. *Am J Hosp Pharm.* 1987; 44:1090–5.

41. Cohen IA, Newland SJ, Kirking DM. Injectable-antineoplastic-drug practices in Michigan hospitals. *Am J Hosp Pharm.* 1987; 44:1096–105.

42. Hoy RH, Stump LM. Effect of an air-venting filter device on aerosol production from vials. *Am J Hosp Pharm.* 1984; 41:324–6.

43. National Sanitation Foundation Standard: Class II (laminar flow) Biohazard Cabinetry. Standard 49. Ann Arbor, MI: National Sanitation Foundation; 1987 Jun.

44. McDiarmid MA, Egan T, Furio M, et al. Sampling for airborne fluorouracil in a hospital drug preparation area. *Am J Hosp Pharm.* 1986; 43:1942–5.

45. Clark RP, Goff MR. The potassium iodide method for determining protection factors in open-fronted microbiological safety cabinets. *J Appl Biol.* 1981; 51:461–73.

46. Connor TH, Laidlaw JL, Theiss JC, et al. Permeability of latex and polyvinyl chloride gloves to carmustine. *Am J Hosp Pharm.* 1984; 41:676–9.

47. Laidlaw JL, Connor TH, Theiss JC, et al. Permeability of latex and polyvinyl chloride gloves to 20 antineoplastic drugs. *Am J Hosp Pharm.* 1984; 41:2618–23.

48. Slevin ML, Ang LM, Johnston A, et al. The efficiency of protective gloves used in the handling of cytotoxic drugs. *Cancer Chemother Pharmacol.* 1984; 12:151–3.

49. Stoikes ME, Carlson JD, Farris FF, et al. Permeability of latex and polyvinyl chloride gloves to fluorouracil and methotrexate. *Am J Hosp Pharm.* 1987; 44:1341–6.

50. Laidlaw JL, Connor TH, Theiss JC, et al. Permeability of four disposable protective-clothing materials to seven antineoplastic drugs. *Am J Hosp Pharm.* 1985; 42:2449–54.

51. Falck K, Sorsa M, Vainio H. Use of the bacterial fluctuation test to detect mutagenicity in urine of nurses handling cytostatic drugs. *Mutat Res.* 1981; 85:236–7.

52. Myers CE. Preparing a list of cytotoxic agents. *Am J Hosp Pharm.* 1987; 44:1296, 1298. Questions and Answers.

53. National Institute of Occupational Safety and Health. Respirator decision logic. Washington, DC: U.S. Department of Health and Human Services; 1987. (DHHS, NIOSH publication 87-108).

54. Commissioner, Federal Supply Service, General Serv-ices Administration. Federal Standard 209C. Clean room and work station requirements, controlled environments. Washington, DC: U.S. Government Printing Office; 1988.

55. Bryan D, Marback MA. Laminar-airflow equipment certification: what the pharmacist needs to know. *Am J Hosp Pharm.* 1984; 41:1343–9.

56. Wilson JP, Solimando DA. Aseptic technique as a safety precaution in the preparation of antineoplastic agents. *Hosp Pharm.* 1981; 15:575–81.

57. F40 CFR 261.5.

58. Vaccari PL, Tonat K, DeChristoforo R, et al. Disposal of antineoplastic wastes at the National Institutes of Health. *Am J Hosp Pharm.* 1984; 41:87–93.

59. Castegnaro M, Adams J, Armour MA, et al., eds. Laboratory decontamination and destruction of carcinogens in laboratory wastes: some antineoplastic agents. International Agency for Research on Cancer Scientific Publication 73. Fair Lawn, NJ: Oxford University Press; 1985.

Appendix A—Glossary

Biohazard: An infectious agent presenting a real or potential risk to humans and the environment.

Carcinogen: Any cancer-producing substance.

Chemotherapy: The treatment of disease by chemical means; first applied to use of chemicals that affect the causative organism unfavorably but do not harm the patient; currently used to describe drug (chemical) therapy of neoplastic diseases (cancer).

Clastogenic: Giving rise to or inducing disruption or breakage, as of chromosomes.

Contamination: The deposition of potentially dangerous material where it is not desired, particularly where its presence may be harmful or constitute a hazard.

Cytotoxic: Possessing a specific destructive action on certain cells; used commonly in referring to antineoplastic drugs that selectively kill dividing cells.

Decontamination: Removal, neutralization, or destruction of a toxic (harmful) agent.

Exposure: The condition of being subjected to something, as to chemicals, that may have a harmful effect. Acute exposure is exposure of short duration, usually exposure of heavy intensity; chronic exposure is long-term exposure, either continuous or intermittent, usually referring to exposure of low intensity.

Genotoxic: Damaging to DNA; pertaining to agents (radiation or chemical substances) known to damage DNA, thereby causing mutations or cancer.

Hazardous: Dangerous; risky; representing a health risk.

Mutagen: Chemical or physical agent that induces or increases genetic mutations by causing changes in DNA.

Plenum: Space within a biohazard cabinet where air flows; plenums may either be under positive (greater than atmospheric pressure) or negative pressure, depending on whether the air is "blown" or "sucked" through the space.

Respirator: A National Institute of Occupational Safety and Health (NIOSH) approved, air-purifying half-mask respirator equipped with a high-efficiency filter; may be disposable (discarded after the end of its recommended period of use).

Trough: Drain spillage trough; an area below the biological safety cabinet's work surface, provided to retain spillage from the work area.

Utility Gloves: Heavy, disposable gloves, similar to household latex gloves.

Appendix B—Classification of Biohazard Cabinetry

(Biological Safety Cabinets)[43]

Class I: A ventilated cabinet for personnel and environmental protection, with an unrecirculated inward airflow away from the operator.

Note: The cabinet exhaust air is treated to protect the environment before it is discharged to the outside atmosphere. This cabinet is suitable for work with low- and moderate-risk bio-

logical agents when no product protection is required.

Class II: A ventilated cabinet for personnel, product, and environmental protection, having an open front with inward airflow for personnel protection, high-efficiency particulate air (HEPA) filtered laminar airflow for product protection, and HEPA-filtered exhausted air for environmental protection.

Note: When toxic chemicals or radionuclides are used as adjuncts to biological studies or pharmaceutical work, Class II cabinets designed and constructed for this purpose should be used.

- *Type A (formerly designated Type 1):* Cabinets that (1) maintain minimum calculated average inflow velocity of 75 feet per minute (fpm) through the work area access opening; (2) have HEPA-filtered downflow air from a common plenum (i.e., plenum from which a portion of the air is exhausted from the cabinet and the remainder is supplied to the work area); (3) may exhaust HEPA-filtered air back into the laboratory; and (4) may have positive-pressure-contaminated ducts and plenums. Type A cabinets are suitable for work with low- to moderate-risk biological agents in the absence of volatile toxic chemicals and volatile radionuclides.

- *Type B1 (formerly designated Type 2):* Cabinets that (1) maintain a minimum (calculated or measured) average inflow velocity of 100 fpm through the work area access opening; (2) have HEPA-filtered downflow air composed largely of uncontaminated recirculated inflow air; (3) exhaust most of the contaminated downflow air through a dedicated duct exhausted to the atmosphere after it passes through a HEPA filter; and (4) have all biologically contaminated ducts and plenums under negative pressure or surrounded by negative-pressure ducts and plenums. Type B1 cabinets are suitable for work with low- to moderate-risk biological agents. They may also be used with biological agents treated with minute quantities of toxic chemicals and trace amounts of radionuclides required as an adjunct to microbiological studies if work is done in the directly exhausted portion of the cabinet or if the chemicals or radionuclides will not interfere with the work when recirculated in the downflow air.

- *Type B2 (sometimes referred to as "total exhaust"):* Cabinets that (1) maintain a minimum (calculated or measured) average inflow velocity of 100 fpm through the work area access opening; (2) have HEPA-filtered downflow air drawn from the laboratory or the outside air (i.e., downflow air is not recirculated from the cabinet exhaust air); (3) exhaust all inflow and down-flow air to the atmosphere after filtration through a HEPA filter without recirculation in the cabinet or return to the laboratory room air; and (4) have all contaminated ducts and plenums under negative pressure or surrounded by directly exhausted (nonrecirculated through the work area) negative-pressure ducts and plenums. Type B2 cabinets are suitable for work with low- to moderate-risk biological agents. They may also be used with biological agents treated with toxic chemicals and radionuclides required as an adjunct to microbiological studies.

- *Type B3 (sometimes referred to as "convertible cabinets"):* Cabinets that (1) maintain a minimum (calculated or measured) average inflow velocity of 100 fpm through the work access opening; (2) have HEPA-filtered downflow air that is a portion of the mixed downflow and inflow air from a common exhaust plenum; (3) discharge all exhaust air to the outdoor atmosphere after HEPA filtration; and (4) have all biologically contaminated ducts and plenums under negative pressure or surrounded by negative-pressure ducts and plenums. Type B3 cabinets are suitable for work with low- to moderate-risk biological agents treated with minute quantities of toxic chemicals and trace quantities of radionuclides that will not interfere with the work if recirculated in the downflow air.

- *Other Types:* Other cabinets may be considered Class II if they meet these requirements for performance, durability, reliability, safety, operational integrity, and cleanability.

Class III: A totally enclosed, ventilated cabinet of gas-tight construction. Operations in the cabinet are conducted through attached rubber gloves. The cabinet is maintained under negative air pressure of at least 0.5 inch (12.7 mm) water gauge (wg). Supply air is drawn into the cabinet through HEPA filters. The exhaust air is treated by double HEPA filtration or by HEPA filtration and incineration.

This Technical Assistance Bulletin was reviewed in 1996 by the Council on Professional Affairs and by the ASHP Board of Directors and was found to still be appropriate.

Revised by ASHP's Clinical Affairs Department in collaboration with Luci A. Power, M.S., Senior Consultant, Power Enterprises, San Francisco, CA. Reviewed by the officers of the ASHP Special Interest Group (SIG) on Oncology Pharmacy Practice and approved by the ASHP Council on Professional Affairs, September 20, 1989. Approved by the ASHP Board of Directors, November 15–16, 1989. Supersedes a previous version approved by the Board of Directors on November 14, 1984.

The bibliographic citation for this document is as follows: American Society of Hospital Pharmacists. ASHP technical assistance bulletin on handling cytotoxic and hazardous drugs. *Am J Hosp Pharm.* 1990; 47:1033–49.

Appendix E

Sec. 460.100 Hospital Pharmacies—Status as Drug Manufacturer (CPG 7132.06)

Policy

1. Compounding in hospitals—registration
2. Application of the "current good manufacturing practices" regulations to hospital pharmacies
3. Labeling of "prepackaged drugs"
4. Investigational drugs
5. New drug applications
6. Prepacking
7. Antibiotic certification

Policy

1. Compounding in hospitals— registration

We interpret Section 510 of the Federal Food, Drug, and Cosmetic Act as not requiring registration by the hospital pharmacy that compounds medication for inpatient dispensing, outpatient dispensing (sale or free), mailing to a patient within the State or out of the State, or for transferral to another unit of the same hospital (within the State or in another State) for dispensing by that unit of the hospital. However, if the hospital pharmacy compounds medication which it sells to another hospital or a drugstore, such sale is not at "retail" and registration is required.

2. Application of the "current good manufacturing practices" regulations to hospital pharmacies

Section 501(a)(2)(B) of the Act provides that a drug shall be deemed to be adulterated if "the methods used in, or the facilities or controls used for its manufacture, processing, packing, or holding do not conform to current good manufacturing practice..." This section, through the operation of Section 301(k) is applicable to hospital pharmacies, as well as to manufacturers, whether or not the establishments are required to register with FDA under Section 510. However, the CGMP regulations set forth in 21 CFR 211 apply to those establishments which are both required to register under Section 510 and which prepare dosage forms. Therefore, if the hospital pharmacy is not required to register as described in paragraph one above, 21 CFR 211 does not apply. It is the policy of FDA not to routinely inspect such pharmacies for compliance with Section 501(a)(2)(B) if they operate within state or local laws governing the practice of pharmacy. However, when a hospital pharmacy is engaged in repacking or relabeling operations that are beyond the usual conduct of dispensing or selling drugs at retail, the exemptions in the Act cease to apply; the establishment is required to register and is subject to regular inspections under Section 704 of the Act.

3. Labeling of "prepackaged drugs"

We believe that drugs packaged for use as ward stock should be labeled with the information required by regulation 201.100(b).

4. Investigational drugs

We do not believe that preparation of investigational drugs by a hospital pharmacy for use by an investigator in the hospital or in another hospital, requires registration under Section 510 of the Act. However, if the new drug has been or is to be shipped in interstate commerce for clinical trials, the "sponsor" of the investigation should file a "Notice of Claimed Investigational Exemption for a New Drug" before the shipment is made or the trials started. This "Notice" would necessarily include the name and address of the pharmacy and provide information regarding manufacture of the new drug by the pharmacy.

Submission of Forms FD-1571, 1572, and 1573 is only required when the finished new drug or the "new drug substance" used in its manufacture, is in interstate commerce.

When interstate commerce is involved and the various forms must be submitted, the hospital or some other responsible person may act as the "sponsor" and file the Form FD-1571. Such "sponsor" should obtain completed Form FD-1572 or 1573 as appropriate from the actual investigators.

The physician-investigator may delegate to a hospital pharmacist responsible to him, or any other person responsible to him, the maintenance of the required records concerning the use of the investigational drug.

5. New drug applications

We recognize that a physician may prescribe an unusual preparation that requires compounding by the pharmacy from drugs readily available for other uses and which is not generally regarded as safe and effective for the intended use. If the pharmacy merely acts to fill each individual prescription as received, it is our opinion that clearance under the "new drug" provisions of the Act is not required.

If the hospital prepares a bulk quantity of an unusual drug in anticipation of prescriptions from the physician who developed the formula, or from other physicians who have been induced to use the unusual medication, we believe the situation would then differ from the one described in the preceding paragraph. If such drug is shipped interstate or a major ingredient used in manufacturing the drug is received from an out-of-state supplier, we would regard the article as a "new drug" in interstate commerce and therefore subject to the investigational new drug regulations.

6. Prepacking

We do not believe that "prepackaging" by the hospital pharmacy for dispensing within the hospital, or for outpatient dispensing, or for transferral to another unit of the hospital, would require registration under Section 510 of the Act. However, repacking of a drug which is sold to another hospital, whether or not such other hospital is under the control of the same corporation, would require registration under Section 510.

7. Antibiotic certification

Hospital pharmacies are not exempt from the antibiotic certification regulations. Antibiotic preparations compounded by the hospital pharmacy are subject to the applicable regulations, regardless of whether the item that is compounded by the hospital pharmacy is available in the usual commercial channels. However, we point out that the pharmacist may, without further certification, compound an antibiotic preparation on the basis of a prescription issued by a licensed practitioner, if the antibiotic ingredient used for compounding the prescription is taken from a certified container packaged for dispensing. The compounded prescription is exempt from certification "for a reasonable time to permit the delivery of the drug compounded on such prescription."

Issued: 10/1/80

Appendix F

Compliance Policy Guide— Compliance Policy Guidance for FDA Staff and Industry[1]

Chapter—4
Sub Chapter—460
Sec. 460.200 Pharmacy Compounding

Guidance for FDA Staff and Industry Compliance Policy Guides Manual Sec. 460.200 Pharmacy Compounding

Submit written comments regarding this guidance document to the Dockets Management Branch (HFA-305), 5630 Fishers Lane, rm.1061, Rockville, MD 20852. Additional copies of this document may be obtained by sending a request to the Division of Compliance Policy (HFC-230), Food and Drug Administration, 5600 Fishers Lane, Rockville, MD 20857, or from the Internet at: http://www.fda.gov/ora/compliance_ref/cpg/default.htm U.S. Department of Health and Human Services Food and Drug Administration Office of Regulatory Affairs Center for Drug Evaluation and Research May 2002

This guidance represents the Food and Drug Administration's (FDA's) current thinking on this topic. It does not create or confer any rights for or on any person and does not operate to bind FDA or the public. An alternative approach may be used if such approach satisfies the requirements of the applicable statutes and regulations.

Introduction

This document provides guidance to drug compounders and the staff of the Food and Drug Administration (FDA) on how the Agency intends to address pharmacy compounding of human drugs in the immediate future as a result of the decision of the Supreme Court in Thompson v. Western States Medical Center, No. 01-344, April 29, 2002. FDA is considering the implications of that decision and determining how it intends to regulate pharmacy compounding in the long term. However, FDA recognizes the need for immediate guidance on what types of compounding might be subject to enforcement action under current law. This guidance describes FDA's current thinking on this issue.

Background

On March 16, 1992, FDA issued a compliance policy guide (CPG), section 7132.16 (later renumbered as 460.200) to delineate FDA's enforcement policy on pharmacy compounding. That CPG remained in effect until 1997 when Congress enacted the Food and Drug Administration Modernization Act of 1997.

On November 21, 1997, the President signed the Food and Drug Administration Modernization Act of 1997 (Pub. L. 105-115) (the Modernization Act). Section 127 of the Modernization Act added section 503A to the Federal Food, Drug, and Cosmetic Act (the Act), to clarify the status of pharmacy compounding under Federal law. Under section 503A, drug products that were compounded by a pharmacist or physician on a customized basis for an individual patient were entitled to exemptions from three key provisions of the Act: (1) the adulteration provision of section 501(a)(2)(B) (concerning the good manufacturing practice requirements); (2) the misbranding provision of section 502(f)(1) (concerning the labeling of drugs with adequate directions for use); and (3) the new drug provision of section 505 (concerning the approval of drugs under new drug or abbreviated new drug applications). To qualify for these statutory exemptions, a compounded drug product was required to satisfy several requirements, some of which were to be the subject of FDA rulemaking or other actions.

Section 503A of the Act took effect on November 21, 1998, one year after the date of the enactment of the Modernization Act. In November, 1998, the solicitation and advertising provisions of section 503A were challenged by seven compounding pharmacies as an impermissible regulation of commercial speech. The U.S. District Court for the District of Nevada ruled in the plaintiffs' favor. FDA appealed to the U.S. Court of Appeals for the Ninth Circuit. On February 6, 2001, the Court of Appeals declared section 503A invalid in its entirety (Western States Medical Center v. Shalala, 238 F.3rd 1090 (9th Cir. 2001)). The government petitioned for a writ of certiorari to the U.S. Supreme Court for review of the circuit court opinion. The Supreme Court granted the writ and issued its decision in the case on April 29, 2002.

The Supreme Court affirmed the 9th Circuit Court of Appeals decision that found section 503A of the Act invalid in its entirety because it contained unconstitutional restrictions on commercial speech (i.e., prohibitions on soliciting prescriptions for and advertising specific compounded drugs). The Court did not rule on, and therefore left in place, the 9th Circuit's holding that the unconstitutional restrictions on commercial speech could not be severed from the rest of section 503A. Accordingly, all of section 503A is now invalid. FDA has therefore determined that it needs to issue guidance to the compounding industry on what factors the Agency will consider in exercising its enforcement discretion regarding pharmacy compounding.

Discussion

FDA recognizes that pharmacists traditionally have extemporaneously compounded and manipulated reasonable quantities of human drugs upon receipt of a valid prescription for an individually identified patient from a licensed practitioner. This traditional activity is not the subject of this guidance.

FDA believes that an increasing number of establishments with retail pharmacy licenses are engaged in manufacturing and distributing unapproved new drugs for human use in a manner that is clearly outside the bounds of traditional pharmacy practice and that violates the Act. Such establishments and their activities are the focus of this guidance. Some "pharmacies" that have sought to find shelter under and expand the scope of the exemptions applicable to traditional retail pharmacies have claimed that their manufacturing and distribution practices are only the regular course of the practice of pharmacy. Yet, the practices of many of these entities seem far more consistent with those of drug manufacturers and wholesalers than with those of retail pharmacies. For example, some firms receive and use large quantities of bulk drug substances to manufacture large quantities of unapproved drug products in advance of receiving a valid prescription for them. Moreover, some firms sell to physicians and patients with whom they have only a remote professional relationship. Pharmacies engaged in activities analogous to manufacturing and distributing drugs for human use may be held to the same provisions of the Act as manufacturers.

Policy

Generally, FDA will continue to defer to state authorities regarding less significant violations of the Act related to pharmacy compounding of human drugs. FDA anticipates that, in such cases, cooperative efforts between the states and the Agency will result in coordinated investigations, referrals, and follow-up actions by the states.

However, when the scope and nature of a pharmacy's activities raise the kinds of concerns normally associated with a drug manufacturer and result in significant violations of the new drug, adulteration, or misbranding provisions of the Act, FDA has determined that it should seriously consider enforcement action. In determining whether to initiate such an action, the Agency will consider whether the pharmacy engages in any of the following acts:

1. Compounding of drugs in anticipation of receiving prescriptions, except in very limited quantities in relation to the amounts of drugs compounded after receiving valid prescriptions.

2. Compounding drugs that were withdrawn or removed from the market for safety reasons. Appendix A provides a list of such drugs that will be updated in the future, as appropriate.

3. Compounding finished drugs from bulk active ingredients that are not components of FDA approved drugs without an FDA sanctioned investigational new drug application (IND) in accordance with 21 U.S.C. § 355(i) and 21 CFR 312.

4. Receiving, storing, or using drug substances without first obtaining written assurance from the supplier that each lot of the drug substance has been made in an FDA-registered facility.

5. Receiving, storing, or using drug components not guaranteed or otherwise determined to meet official compendia requirements.

6. Using commercial scale manufacturing or testing equipment for compounding drug products.

7. Compounding drugs for third parties who resell to individual patients or offering compounded drug products at wholesale to other state licensed persons or commercial entities for resale.

8. Compounding drug products that are commercially available in the marketplace or that are essentially copies of commercially available FDA-approved drug products. In certain circumstances, it may be

appropriate for a pharmacist to compound a small quantity of a drug that is only slightly different than an FDA-approved drug that is commercially available. In these circumstances, FDA will consider whether there is documentation of the medical need for the particular variation of the compound for the particular patient.

9. Failing to operate in conformance with applicable state law regulating the practice of pharmacy. The foregoing list of factors is not intended to be exhaustive. Other factors may be appropriate for consideration in a particular case.

Other FDA guidance interprets or clarifies Agency positions concerning nuclear pharmacy, hospital pharmacy, shared service operations, mail order pharmacy, and the manipulation of approved drug products.

Regulatory Action Guidance

District offices are encouraged to consult with state regulatory authorities to assure coherent application of this guidance to establishments that are operating outside of the traditional practice of pharmacy.

FDA-initiated regulatory action may include issuing a warning letter, seizure, injunction, and/or prosecution. Charges may include, but need not be limited to, violations of 21 U.S.C. §§ 351(a)(2)(B), 352(a), 352(f)(1), 352(o), and 355(a) of the Act.

Issued: 3/16/1992
Reissued: 5/29/2002

Appendix A—List of Compounding Drugs That Were Withdrawn or Removed from the Market for Safety Reasons

Adenosine phosphate: All drug products containing adenosine phosphate.

Adrenal cortex: All drug products containing adrenal cortex.

Aminopyrine: All drug products containing aminopyrine.

Astemizole: All drug products containing astemizole.

Azaribine: All drug products containing azaribine.

Benoxaprofen: All drug products containing benoxaprofen.

Bithionol: All drug products containing bithionol.

Bromfenac sodium: All drug products containing bromfenac sodium.

Butamben: All parenteral drug products containing butamben.

Camphorated oil: All drug products containing camphorated oil.

Carbetapentane citrate: All oral gel drug products containing carbetapentane citrate.

Casein, iodinated: All drug products containing iodinated casein.

Chlorhexidine gluconate: All tinctures of chlorhexidine gluconate formulated for use as a patient preoperative skin preparation.

Chlormadinone acetate: All drug products containing chlormadinone acetate.

Chloroform: All drug products containing chloroform.

Cisapride: All drug products containing cisapride.

Cobalt: All drug products containing cobalt salts (except radioactive forms cobalt and its salts and cobalamin and its derivatives).

Dexfenfluramine hydrochloride: All drug products containing dexfenfluramine hydrochloride.

Diamthazole dihydrochloride: All drug products containing diamthazole dihydrochloride.

Dibromsalan: All drug products containing dibromsalan.

Diethylstilbestrol: All oral and parenteral drug products containing 25 milligrams or more of diethylstilbestrol per unit dose.

Dihydrostreptomycin sulfate: All drug products containing dihydrostreptomycin sulfate.

Dipyrone: All drug products containing dipyrone.

Encainide hydrochloride: All drug products containing encainide hydrochloride.

Fenfluramine hydrochloride: All drug products containing fenfluramine hydrochloride.

Flosequinan: All drug products containing flosequinan.

Gelatin: All intravenous drug products containing gelatin.

Glycerol, iodinated: All drug products containing iodinated glycerol.

Gonadotropin, chorionic: All drug products containing chorionic gonadotropins of animal origin.

Grepafloxacin: All drug products containing grepafloxacin.

Mepazine: All drug products containing mepazine hydrochloride or mepazine acetate.

Metabromsalan: All drug products containing metabromsalan.

Methamphetamine hydrochloride: All parenteral drug products containing methamphetamine hydrochloride.

Methapyrilene: All drug products containing methapyrilene.

Methopholine: All drug products containing methopholine.

Mibefradil dihydrochloride: All drug products containing mibefradil dihydrochloride.

Nitrofurazone: All drug products containing nitrofurazone (except topical drug products formulated for dermatalogic application).

Nomifensine maleate: All drug products containing nomifensine maleate.

Oxyphenisatin: All drug products containing oxyphenisatin.

Oxyphenisatin acetate: All drug products containing oxyphenisatin acetate.

Phenacetin: All drug products containing phenacetin.

Phenformin hydrochloride: All drug products containing phenformin hydrochloride.

Pipamazine: All drug products containing pipamazine.

Potassium arsenite: All drug products containing potassium arsenite.

Potassium chloride: All solid oral dosage form drug products containing potassium chloride that supply 100 milligrams or more of potassium per dosage unit (except for controlled-release dosage forms and those products formulated for preparation of solution prior to ingestion).

Povidone: All intravenous drug products containing povidone.

Reserpine: All oral dosage form drug products containing more than 1 milligram of reserpine.

Sparteine sulfate: All drug products containing sparteine sulfate.

Sulfadimethoxine: All drug products containing sulfadimethoxine.

Sulfathiazole: All drug products containing sulfathiazole (except those formulated for vaginal use).

Suprofen: All drug products containing suprofen (except ophthalmic solutions).

Sweet spirits of nitre: All drug products containing sweet spirits of nitre.

Temafloxacin hydrochloride: All drug products containing temafloxacin.

Terfenadine: All drug products containing terfenadine.

3,3',4',5-tetrachlorosalicylanilide: All drug products containing 3,3',4',5-tetrachlorosalicylanilide.

Tetracycline: All liquid oral drug products formulated for pediatric use containing tetracycline in a concentration greater than 25 milligrams/milliliter.

Ticrynafen: All drug products containing ticrynafen.

Tribromsalan: All drug products containing tribromsalan.

Trichloroethane: All aerosol drug products intended for inhalation containing trichloroethane.

Troglitazone: All drug products containing troglitazone.

Urethane: All drug products containing urethane.

Vinyl chloride: All aerosol drug products containing vinyl chloride.

Zirconium: All aerosol drug products containing zirconium.

Zomepirac sodium: All drug products containing zomepirac sodium.

---

[1] This guidance has been prepared by the Office of Regulatory Policy and the Office of Compliance in the Center for Drug Evaluation and Research (CDER) at the Food and Drug Administration.

[2] With respect to such activities, 21 U.S.C. 360(g)(1) exempts retail pharmacies from the registration requirements of the Act. The exemption applies to "Pharmacies" that operate in accordance with state law and dispense drugs "upon prescriptions of practitioners licensed to administer such drugs to patients under the care of such practitioners in the course of their professional practice,

and which do not manufacture, prepare, propagate, compound, or process drugs or devices for sale other than in the regular course of their business of dispensing or selling drugs or devices at retail" (emphasis added). See also 21 U.S.C. §§ 374(a)(2) (exempting pharmacies that meet the foregoing criteria from certain inspection provisions) and 353(b)(2) (exempting drugs dispensed by filling a valid prescription from certain misbranding provisions).[7]

Hypertext created: June 3, 2002 (tc)

Appendix G | Model Rules for Sterile Pharmaceuticals*

*National Association of Boards of Pharmacy. Model state pharmacy act and model rules of the National Association of Boards of Pharmacy. June 2003. www.nabp.net. Accessed 09/02/04.

Section 1. Purpose and Scope

The purpose of this section is to assure positive patient outcomes through the provision of standards for 1) pharmaceutical care; 2) the preparation, labeling, and distribution of sterile pharmaceuticals by pharmacies, pursuant to or in anticipation of a prescription drug order; and 3) product quality and characteristics. These standards are intended to apply to all sterile pharmaceuticals, notwithstanding the location of the patient (e.g., home, hospital, nursing home, hospice, doctor's office).

Section 2. Definitions

(a) "Biological safety cabinet" means a containment unit suitable for the preparation of low to moderate risk agents where there is a need for protection of the product, personnel, and environment, according to National Sanitation Foundation (NSF) Standard 49.

(b) "Class 100 environment" means an atmospheric environment which contains fewer than 100 particles 0.5 microns in diameter per cubic foot of air, according to Federal Standard 209E.

(c) "Cytotoxic" means a pharmaceutical that has the capability of killing living cells.

(d) "Enteral" means within or by way of the intestine.

(e) "Parenteral" means a sterile preparation of drugs for injection through one or more layers of the skin.

(f) "Positive patient outcomes" include the cure or prevention of disease, elimination or reduction of a patient's symptoms, or arresting or slowing of a disease process so as to improve the patient's quality of life.

(g) "Product quality and characteristics" include: sterility, potency associated with environmental quality, preparation activities, and checks and tests.

(h) "Sterile pharmaceutical" means any dosage form devoid of viable microorganisms, including, but not limited to, parenterals, injectables, and ophthalmics.

Section 3. Policy and Procedure Manual

A policy and procedure manual shall be prepared and maintained for the compounding, dispensing, delivery, administration, storage, and use of sterile pharmaceutical prescription drug orders.

(a) The policy and procedure manual shall include a quality assurance program for the purpose of monitoring patient care and pharmaceutical care outcomes, adverse drug reactions, personnel qualifications, training and performance, product integrity, equipment, facilities, infection control, and guidelines regarding patient education.

(b) The policy and procedure manual shall be current and available for inspection by a board of pharmacy-designated agent.

Section 4. Physical Requirements

(a) The pharmacy shall have a designated area with entry restricted to designated personnel for preparing parenteral products. This area shall be structurally isolated from other areas with restricted entry or access, and must be designed to avoid unnecessary traffic and airflow disturbances from activity within the controlled facility. It shall be used only for the preparation of these specialty products. It shall be of sufficient size to accommodate a laminar airflow hood and to provide for the proper storage of drugs and supplies under appropriate conditions of temperature, light, moisture, sanitation, ventilation, and security.

(b) The pharmacy preparing parenteral products shall have:

(1) appropriate environmental control devices capable of maintaining at least Class 100 conditions in the workplace where critical objects are exposed and critical activities are performed; furthermore, these devices are capable of maintaining Class 100 conditions during normal activity. Examples of appropriate devices include laminar airflow hoods and zonal laminar flow of high efficiency particulate air (HEPA) filtered air;

(2) appropriate disposal containers for used needles, syringes, etc., and, if applicable,

for cytotoxic waste from the preparation of chemotherapy agents and infectious wastes from patients' homes;

(3) when cytotoxic drug products are prepared, appropriate environmental control also includes appropriate biohazard cabinetry;

(4) temperature-controlled delivery container;

(5) infusion devices, if appropriate.

(c) The pharmacy shall maintain supplies adequate to maintain an environment suitable for the aseptic preparation of sterile products.

(d) The pharmacy shall have sufficient current reference materials related to sterile products to meet the needs of pharmacy staff.

Section 5. Records and Reports

In addition to standard record and reporting requirements, the following records and reports must be maintained for sterile pharmaceuticals:

(a) A policy and procedure manual, including policies and procedures for cytotoxic and/or infectious waste, if applicable; and

(b) Lot numbers of the components used in compounding sterile prescriptions.

Section 6. Delivery Service

The pharmacist-in-charge shall assure the environmental control of all products shipped. Therefore, any compounded, sterile pharmaceutical must be shipped or delivered to a patient in appropriate temperature-controlled (as defined by USP Standards) delivery containers and stored appropriately in the patient's home.

Section 7. Disposal of Cytotoxic and/or Hazardous Wastes

The pharmacist-in-charge is responsible for assuring that there is a system for the disposal of cytotoxic and/or infectious waste in a manner so as not to endanger the public health.

Section 8. Emergency Kit

When sterile pharmaceuticals are provided to home care patients, the dispensing pharmacy may supply the nurse or patient with emergency drugs, if the physician has authorized the use of these drugs by a protocol, in an emergency situation (e.g., anaphylactic shock).

Section 9. Cytotoxic Drugs

In addition to the minimum requirements for a pharmacy established by rules of the board, the following requirements are necessary for those pharmacies that prepare cytotoxic drugs to ensure the protection of the personnel involved.

(a) All cytotoxic drugs should be compounded in a vertical flow, Class II, biological safety cabinet. Other products should not be compounded in this cabinet.

(b) Protective apparel shall be worn by personnel compounding cytotoxic drugs. This shall include disposable masks, gloves, and gowns with tight cuffs.

(c) Appropriate safety and containment techniques for compounding cytotoxic drugs shall be used in conjunction with the aseptic techniques required for preparing sterile products.

(d) Disposal of cytotoxic waste shall comply with all applicable local, state, and federal requirements.

(e) Written procedures for handling both major and minor spills of cytotoxic agents must be developed and must be included in the policy and procedure manual.

(f) Prepared doses of cytotoxic drugs must be dispensed, labeled with proper precautions inside and outside, and shipped in a manner to minimize the risk of accidental rupture of the primary container.

Section 10. Patient Education and Training

If appropriate, the pharmacist must demonstrate or document the patient's training and competency in managing this type of therapy provided by the pharmacist to the patient in the home environment. A pharmacist must be involved in the patient training process in any area that relates to drug compounding, labeling, administration, storage, stability, compatibility, or disposal. The pharmacist must be responsible for seeing that the patient's competency in the above areas is reassessed on an ongoing basis.

Section 11. Quality Assurance/ Compounding and Preparation of Sterile Pharmaceuticals

There shall be a documented, ongoing quality assurance control program that monitors personnel performance, equipment, and facilities. Appropriate samples of finished products shall be examined to assure that the pharmacy is capable of consistently preparing sterile pharmaceuticals meeting specifications.

(a) All cleanrooms and laminar flow hoods shall be certified by an independent contractor according to Federal Standard 209E, or National Sanitation Foundation Standard 49, for operational efficiency at least every 6 months. Appropriate records shall be maintained.

(b) There shall be written procedures developed requiring sampling if microbial contamination is suspected.

(c) If bulk compounding of parenteral solutions is performed using nonsterile chemicals, extensive end-product testing must be documented prior to the release of the product from quarantine. This process must include appropriate tests for particulate matter and testing for pyrogens.

(d) There shall be written justification of the chosen beyond-use dates for compounded products.

(e) There shall be documentation of quality assurance audits at regular, planned intervals, including infection control and sterile technique audits.

Section 12. Pharmaceutical Care Outcomes

There shall be a documented, ongoing quality assurance control program that monitors patient care and pharmaceutical care outcomes, including but not limited to the following:

(a) routine performance of prospective drug regimen review and patient monitoring functions by a pharmacist, as defined in the rules of the board;

(b) patient monitoring plans that include written outcome measures and systems for routine patient assessment (examples include infection rates, rehospitalization rates, and the incidence of adverse drug reactions);

(c) documentation of patient training as specified in Section 10; and

(d) appropriate collaboration with other health care professionals.

Appendix H

Preventing Occupational Exposures to Antineoplastic and Other Hazardous Drugs in Healthcare Settings*

*www.cdc.gov/niosh/docs/2004-HazDrugAlert/pdfs/2004-HazDrugAlert.pdf. Accessed 08/16/04.

Warning!

Healthcare workers who prepare or administer hazardous drugs or who work in areas where these drugs are used may be exposed to these agents in air or on work surfaces, contaminated clothing, medical equipment, patient excreta, or other sources. Studies have associated workplace exposures to hazardous drugs with health effects such as skin rashes and adverse reproductive events (including infertility, spontaneous abortions or congenital malformations) and possibly leukemia and other cancers. The health risk is influenced by the extent of the exposure and the potency and toxicity of the hazardous drug. Potential health effects can be minimized through sound procedures for handling hazardous drugs, engineering controls and proper use of protective equipment to protect workers to the greatest degree possible.

SCOPE

The purpose of this Alert is to warn healthcare workers of the potential hazards associated with working with *hazardous drugs*, and to alert them and their employers of appropriate measures for protecting their health. The term *hazardous drug*, as used throughout this Alert, refers to particular drugs that have been associated with or suspected of causing adverse health effects from workplace exposures. Appendix A includes examples of drugs that are considered hazardous by several sources. This Alert addresses workers in the healthcare setting who handle hazardous drugs, but not those in the drug manufacturing sector.

Employers of healthcare workers should:

- Ensure that written policies address medical surveillance of healthcare workers and all phases of hazardous drug handling including receipt and storage, preparation, administration, housekeeping, deactivation and cleanup and disposal of unused drugs and contaminated spills and patient wastes.

- Formally seek input from employees who handle drugs in developing a program for preventing exposure.

- Prepare a written inventory identifying all hazardous drugs used in the workplace and establish a procedure for regular review and update of the inventory.

- Make guidance documents, Material Safety Data Sheets (MSDSs) and other information available to those who handle hazardous drugs or work in an area where hazardous drugs are handled.

- Provide training to employees on the recognition, evaluation and control of hazardous drugs.

- Ensure that horizontal laminar flow workstations that move the air from the drug towards the worker are never used for the preparation of hazardous drugs.

- For hazardous drug preparation, provide and maintain ventilated cabinets designed for worker protection. Examples of these include biological safety cabinets (BSCs) and containment isolators that are designed to prevent hazardous drugs inside the cabinet from escaping into the surrounding environment. The exhaust from these cabinets should be HEPA-filtered and whenever feasible exhausted to the outdoors (away from air intake locations). Additional equipment, such as closed-system drug-transfer devices, glove bags and needleless systems will further protect workers from exposures when used properly.

- Establish and oversee the implementation of appropriate work practices when hazardous drugs, patient wastes and contaminated materials are handled.

- Ensure training in and the availability and use of proper personal protective equipment (PPE) to reduce exposure via inhalation, ingestion, skin absorption, and injection of hazardous drugs as required based on the results of a risk assessment and the OSHA PPE Standard. PPE includes chemotherapy gloves, low-lint, low-permeability disposable gowns and sleeve covers, and eye and face protection. NIOSH-certified respiratory protection is needed when equipment such as biological safety cabinets are not adequate to protect against inhalation exposure. Surgical masks do not provide adequate respiratory protection.

- Provide syringes and intravenous (IV) sets with Luer-lock fittings for preparing and administering hazardous drugs, as well as containers for their disposal. Closed-system, drug-transfer devices and needleless systems should be considered to protect nursing personnel during drug administration.

- Complete a periodic evaluation of workplace hazardous drugs, equipment, training effectiveness, policies and procedures to reduce exposures to the greatest degree possible.

- Comply with all relevant U.S. Environmental Protection Agency/Resource Conservation and Recovery Act (USEPA/RCRA) regulations related to the handling, storage and transportation of hazardous waste.

Healthcare workers should:

- Participate in standardized training on the hazards of the drugs handled and equipment and procedures used to prevent exposure.

- Review guidance documents, MSDSs and other information resources for hazardous drugs handled.

- Be familiar with and be able to recognize sources of exposure to hazardous drugs.

- Prepare these agents in a dedicated area where access is restricted to authorized personnel only.

- Prepare these agents within a ventilated cabinet designed to protect workers and adjacent personnel from exposure and to provide product protection for all drugs that require aseptic handling.

- Use two pairs of powder-free, disposable chemotherapy gloves with the outer one covering the gown cuff whenever there is risk of exposure to hazardous drugs.

- Avoid skin contact by using a disposable gown made of a low-lint and low permeability fabric. The gown should have a closed front, long sleeves and elastic or knit closed cuffs and should not be re-used.

- Wear a face shield to avoid splash incidents involving eyes, nose, or mouth when adequate engineering controls are not available.

- Wash hands with soap and water immediately before using and after removing personal protective clothing, such as disposable gloves and gowns.

- Use syringes and IV sets with Luer-lock fittings for preparing and administering these agents and place drug-contaminated syringes and needles in chemotherapy sharps containers for disposal.

- When additional protection is necessary, use closed-system, drug-transfer devices, glove bags and needle-less systems within the ventilated cabinet.

- Handle hazardous wastes and contaminated materials separately from other trash.

- Decontaminate work areas before and after each activity with hazardous drugs and at the end of each shift.

- Clean up spills immediately while using appropriate safety precautions and personal protective equipment (PPE) unless the spill is large enough to require an environmental services specialist.

Please tear out and post. Distribute copies to workers. See back of sheet to order complete Alert.

For additional information, see NIOSH Alert: Preventing Occupational Exposures to Antineoplastic and other Hazardous Drugs in Healthcare Settings. Single copies of the Alert are available from the following:

NIOSH–Publications Dissemination
4676 Columbia Pkwy.
Cincinnati, OH 45226-1998
Telephone: 1-800-35-NIOSH
 (1-800-356-4674)
Fax: 1-513-533-8573
E-mail: pubstaft@cdc.gov

Or visit the NIOSH Web site: www.cdc.gov/NIOSH

Department of Health and Human Services
Centers for Disease Control and Prevention
National Institute for Occupational Safety and Health

Glossary

Active ingredient—The chemical, substance or other component of articles intended for use in the diagnosis, cure, mitigation, treatment, or prevention of diseases in humans or other animals or for use as nutritional supplements.

Added substances—Ingredients that are necessary to prepare the preparation but are not intended or expected to cause a human pharmacologic response if administered alone in the amount or concentration contained in a single dose of the compounded preparations. Synonymous terms are *inactive ingredients*, *excipients*, and *pharmaceutic ingredients*.

Air lock—An enclosed transition area with two or more doors that control access to the controlled and outside environments of the isolator. The purpose of the air lock is to control airflow between the environments while transferring materials between the two environments.

Ampul—A single-use container composed entirely of glass.

Anteroom—Any area adjacent to buffer or cleanroom where unsterilized products, in-process components, materials, and containers are handled (see also Controlled area).

Antibody—a specific substance (immunoglobulin) produced by specialized blood cells (plasma cells) as a reaction to an antigen for the purpose of host defense. Antibodies are blood proteins that are produced in response to a foreign substance or antigen.

Antigen—A macromolecule that elicits an immune response in the body. The most common antigens are proteins (e.g., natural rubber latex) and polysaccharides (e.g., starch). Antigens may be either exogenous or endogenous to the body.

Aseptic technique—The methods used to manipulate sterile products so that they remain sterile.

Batch compounding—Compounding of multiple sterile preparation units, in a single discrete process, by the same individuals, carried out during one limited time period.

Beyond-use dating—The maximum time period in which 90% or greater of a labeled active ingredient is measurable in the solu-tion and container specified, under the stated storage or administration conditions.

Buffer zone—The space is designated for compounding sterile preparations (see also Cleanroom).

Certification—The process by which a nongovernmental agency or organization grants recognition to an individual who has met certain predetermined qualifications specified by that agency or organization. Certification is usually voluntary and involves passing a validated, standardized examination.

Chemotherapy drug—A chemical agent used to treat diseases. The term usually refers to a drug used to treat cancer.

Cleanroom—A room in which the concentration of airborne particles is controlled, and which is constructed and used in a manner to minimize the introduction, generation, and retention of particles inside the room, and in which other relevant parameters e.g., temperature, humidity, and pressure are controlled as necessary.

Clean zone—Dedicated space in which the concentration of airborne particles is controlled, and which is constructed and used in a manner to minimize the introduction, generation, and retention of particles inside the zone, and in which other relevant parameters, e.g., temperature, humidity, and pressure, are controlled as necessary. This zone may be open or enclosed and may or may not be located within a cleanroom.

Closed system transfer—The movement of sterile products from one container to another in which the container-closure system and transfer devices remain intact throughout the entire transfer process, compromised only by the penetration of a sterile, pyrogen-free needle or cannula through a designated stopper or port to effect transfer, withdrawal, or delivery. Withdrawal of a sterile solution from an ampul in an ISO Class 5 environment would generally be considered a closed system transfer.

Cold temperatures—Temperature not exceeding 8° C (46° F).

Color-coding—systematic, standard application of color to aid in classification and identification.

Compounding—The preparation, mixing, assembling, packaging, and labeling of a drug or device in accordance with a licensed practitioner's prescription under an initiative based on the practitioner/patient/pharmacist/compounder relationship in the course of professional practice.

Container—That which holds the preparations and is or may be in direct contact with the preparation. The closure is part of the container.

Continuing education—Teaching and learning usually approved by an accrediting organization. Continuing education is designed to update the knowledge of a competent practitioner.

Controlled area—The space designated for compounding sterile preparations. This is referred to as the buffer zone (i.e., the cleanroom in which the laminar-airflow workbench is located) in USP <797>.

Cool temperatures—Temperature between 8° C and 15° C (46° F and 59° F).

Critical area—Any part of the controlled area where preparations or containers are exposed to the environment.

Documentation—A record of how a drug was processed and what quality attributes it possesses.

Expiration date—The longest time period during which 90% or more of the labeled active ingredient is available for delivery (see also Shelf life).

Extemporaneous compounding—The preparation of drugs or solutions that have no commercially available equivalents.

Freezer—A cold place in which the temperature is maintained thermostatically between -20° C and -10° C (-4° F and 14° F).

Hazard analysis, critical control points (HACCP)—Analyzing the compounding process and flow charting it to ensure that it reflects the actual procedure that is performed. Once the procedure has been clearly identified, the hazards within the procedures are identified.

Hazardous drug—Any drug that is identified by at least one of the six criteria. These include: carcinogenicity; teratogenicity or developmental toxicity; reproductive toxicity in humans; organ toxicity at low doses in humans or animals; genotoxicity; or new drugs that mimic existing hazardous drugs in structure or toxicity.

High-efficiency particulate air (HEPA) filter—A filter that retains airborne particles and microorganisms, and its use decreases the chance of contamination of compounded preparations.

Hydrolysis—The attack of labile bonds in dissolved drug molecules by water with resultant molecular changes.

Incompatibility—A physical or chemical phenomenon that reduces the concentration of the active ingredient(s) (see also Physical and visual incompatibility).

In-process testing—A method to verify that the compounding environment and the actual preparation meet established criteria.

Isolator—An isolator is a controlled environment that is defined by fixed walls, floor, and ceiling. Transfers of materials into and out of the environment as well as the interaction technologies are separated by barriers such as gloves, sleeves, and airlocks.

Laminar airflow workbenches (LAFWs)—A controlled environment created by a high-efficiency particulate air (HEPA) filter to retain airborne particles and microorganisms. Its use decreases the chance of contamination of compounded preparations.

Licensure—The process by which a government agency or board grants permission to an individual to engage in a given occupation or professional practice. Licensure is contingent upon an applicant's successful completion of certain specified minimal levels of competency necessary to ensure the public's health, safety, and welfare.

Manufacturing—The production, propagation, conversion, or processing of a drug or device, either directly or indirectly, by extraction of the drug from substances of natural origin or by means of chemical or biological synthesis.

Mass reconstitution—Reconstitution of parenteral drugs in bulk and then refrigerating or freezing them for later use.

Media fills—A test that mimics an actual and entire compounding procedure, using a suitable growth medium such as tryptic soy broth (TSB) instead of using ingredients to prepare a finished compounded preparation (see also Process validation).

Microbial bioburden—The amount of viable microoganisms on an item or within an area.

Open reservoir mixing— Combining either sterile or nonsterile ingredients using an open-system transfer or an open reservoir before terminal sterilization or subdivision into units.

Orientation—On-the-job training necessary for an individual to understand the policies and procedures used at a specific practice site.

Particulates—Airborne particle found in the environment are pollen, dust, bacteria, miscellaneous living and dead organisms, skin flakes, hair, clothing lint, cosmetics, respiratory gases, and bacteria from perspiration.

Percentage of fresh air—The amount of air not recirculated from within enclosed spaces.

PhaSeal—An ancillary device manufactured by Carmel Pharma ab, Goteborg, Sweden, and distributed by BAXA, Denver. PhaSeal is a proprietary, closed-system hazardous drug handling device comprising a number of interlocking parts for reconstituting, injecting, and administering doses of hazardous drugs.

Photodegradation—The catalysis of degradation reactions by light (see also Photolysis).

Photolysis—The catalysis of degradation reactions by light (see also Photodegradation).

Physical incompatibility—Visible changes in a preparation, such as precipitation, cloudiness or haziness, color change, viscosity change, cracking, and effervescence (see also Visual incompatibility).

Policy—A general statement that provides a basis for decision-making. It addresses what must be done and, occasionally, why and when it must be done.

Pooling—Preparations are made by combining sterile ingredients in a sterile closed system, by aseptic transfer, before subdivision into patient units.

Pressure differential—The measurement of air pressures between two adjoining areas where the air pressure in the more stringently classified area is higher than the pressure of the next classified area.

Procedure—A how-to document that provides methods for carrying out a policy. Procedures outline the complete cycle of a task, step by step, and assign responsibility to specific personnel.

Process validation—A test that mimics an actual and entire compounding procedure using a suitable growth medium such as TSB instead of using ingredients to prepare a finished compounded preparation (see also Media fills).

Quality assurance—A set of activities used to ensure that the processes used in the compounding of sterile preparations lead to preparations that meet predetermined standards of quality.

Refrigerator—A cold place in which the temperature is maintained thermostatically between 2° C and 8° C (36° F to 46° F).

Registration—The process of including a person's name on a registry with a state agency or regulatory board. Registration is the lowest form of "regulating" a group of individuals, and it enables the agency or board to track where those individuals are registered to practice.

Regulations—Rules promulgated by a state or federal agency as needed to apply the concepts encompased in a law or statute.

Relative humidity (RH)—The ratio of the amount of water vapor present in the air relative to the greatest amount possible of water vapor at the same temperature.

Shelf life—The longest time period during which 90% or more of the labeled active ingredient is available for delivery (see also Expiration date).

Sorption—Drug is lost (from the solution to be administered) by adsorption to the surface or absorption into the matrix of the container material, administration set, or filter.

Stability—The extent to which a preparation retains, within specified limits, and throughout its period of storage and use, the same properties and characteristics that it possessed at the time of compounding.

Sterility assurance level (SAL)—The probability of an item being nonsterile after it has been exposed to a validated sterilization process (steam, ionizing radiation, or ethylene oxide).

Sterilization—A vailidated process used to render a preparation free of viable organisms.

Sterilizing filter—A filter that, when challenged with a solution containing the microorganizm *Pseudo onas diminuta* at a minimum concentration of 10^{12} organisms per square centimeter of filter surface, will produce a sterile effluent.

Surface safe—A commercially available product designed to decontaminate the surface of a biological safety cabinet or isolator by deactivating various hazardous drugs. The twin-pack system provides a solution of sodium hypochlorite bleach with detergent on one towelette and thiosulfate to neutralize the bleach and deactivate several of the drugs that do not oxidize readily (platinum-containing drugs) on the second towelette.

Temperature—The degree of hotness or coldness measured on a definite scale. Units of measure are either in Fahrenheit (U.S.) or Celsius (metric).

Total nutrient admixture (TNA)—Dextrose, amino acids, and fat emulsions/lipids combined in one container.

Training—The process of becoming prepared to perform a skill or facilitating that process for others.

Validation—Documented evidence providing a high degree of assurance that a specific process will consistently produce a product meeting its predetermined specifications and quality attributes.

Ventilated control—A device, such as a biological safety cabinet or isolator, that vents exhaust away from the critical area.

Vial—A plastic or glass container with a rubber closure secured to its top by a metal ring.

Visual incompatibility—Visible changes in a preparation, such as precipitation, cloudiness or haziness, color change, viscosity change, cracking, and effervescence (see also Physical incompatibility).

Worst-case scenario—Situation in which compounding operations are at their greatest risk of introducing contamination into sterile products.

Zone of turbulence—The pattern of flow of air from the HEPA filter created behind an object placed within the LAFW pulling or allowing contaminated room air into the aseptic environment.